Surgical
Rehabilitation
of the Upper Limb
in Tetraplegia

Commissioning Editor: *Deborah Russell*
Project Development Manager: *Kim Benson*
Project Manager: *Katharine Eyston*
Illustration Manager: *Mick Ruddy*
Designer: *Jayne Jones*

Surgical Rehabilitation of the Upper Limb in Tetraplegia

Vincent R Hentz MD FACS
Professor of Surgery
Stanford University
Consultant: Spinal Cord Injury Unit
Veterans Affairs Palo Alto Health Care System
Palo Alto
California, USA

Caroline Leclercq MD
Hand Surgeon
Institut de la Main
Clinique Jouvenet
Paris, France

Illustrator: Kathy Hirsch

 W.B. SAUNDERS

LONDON EDINBURGH NEW YORK PHILADELPHIA ST LOUIS SYDNEY TORONTO 2002

WB SAUNDERS
An imprint of Elsevier Science Limited

First published 2002

ISBN 0 7020 2271 3

British Library Cataloguing in Publication Data
A catalogue record for this book is available from the British Library

Library of Congress Cataloging in Publication Data
A catalog record for this book is available from the Library of Congress

Note
Medical knowledge is constantly changing. As new information becomes available, changes in treatment, procedures, equipment and the use of drugs become necessary. The authors and the publishers have taken care to ensure that the information given in this text is accurate and up to date. However, readers are strongly advised to confirm that the information, especially with regard to drug usage, complies with the latest legislation and standards of practice.

The
publisher's
policy is to use
**paper manufactured
from sustainable forests**

Printed in China by RDC Group Limited

Contents

Preface

More than 25 years ago Erik Moberg of Goteborg, Sweden created a 100 page monograph entitled 'The Upper Limb in Tetraplegia: A New Approach to Surgical Rehabilitation.' In spite of Moberg's reputation as Sweden's foremost hand surgeon, he was unable to find a publisher interested in printing the work until he received a generous guarantee from a Stockholm medical foundation that covered the publisher's costs. The monograph was published in 1978, shortly following the first International Conference on surgical rehabilitation in tetraplegia, attended by 26 surgeons, physiatrists and therapists. At that time, most spinal cord centers had no experience in upper limb functional surgery for their patients, and only a small number of patients were undergoing surgery in just a few centers.

In the intervening years, much has changed for the patient who suffers a cervical spinal cord injury. Since 1978, six additional International Congresses have been held with attendance now measured in the hundreds. Upper limb rehabilitation surgery is being regularly performed in more and more spinal cord injury centers, a consequence of contemporary physiatrists and rehabilitation medicine specialists recognizing the role of surgery for their tetraplegic patients. For example, in the United States, in order to be designated as a 'model' spinal cord injury center, the facility must be able to provide upper limb functional surgery to appropriate patients. Questions regarding surgical rehabilitation are now commonly included in Physical Medicine and Rehabilitation in-service training and board examinations. Lectures on this topic are a regular part of the curriculum for Spinal Cord Injury Board Certification review courses.

In Europe, considerable interest was aroused by Moberg himself, who, after retirement, continuously and indefatigably visited his colleagues, convincing them to start an experience in that field. Numerous centers now perform this surgery routinely, and for example France has at least five such centers.

Through exposure to physiatrist colleagues, greater numbers of surgeons have become increasingly knowledgeable about the special conditions imposed by this devastating injury and the many reasons why the tetraplegic is so different from other patients who are candidates for upper limb functional reconstructive surgery. In addition, the surgeon's armamentarium has grown as additional procedures have been found to pass the test of time.

The rights of the disabled and their role in society have changed since 1978, through such seemingly disparate events as the 'Special Olympics' or the 'International Paraplegia Games' and the 'Americans with Disability Act' or ADA, passed by the United States Congress and signed into law by the then President Bush in 1990. In much of the industrialized world, there is the realization that even the tetraplegic patient can contribute to society, can become an asset rather than a societal liability through skillful physical and psychological rehabilitation and vocational education.

These trends strongly re-emphasize the contention expressed by Erik Moberg in his 1978 monograph, that 'the possibility of improving the function of the hands and arms (of tetraplegics) would be an important contribution, as there is much truth in the saying that "their hands are their life."' Aside from the brain, the tetraplegic patient's upper limbs represent their most important functional resource. In a survey of male patients, 75% rated restoration of normal function of arms and hands as more important than the return of normal bowel and bladder, legs and sexual function. Thus, while much has changed, the tetraplegic patient's desire for improved function has not.

It is time, perhaps past time, for updating in a monograph form the advances in surgical rehabilitation for the tetraplegic upper limb that have taken place since Moberg's 1978 monograph. Our goal is to provide information regarding the acute and long-term care of the upper limb in the tetraplegic patient, care provided by professionals with varying backgrounds and expertise, including physiatrists, physical and occupational therapists, plastic and orthopedic surgeons. Therefore, we have tried to provide both general and detailed information that would be useful to all professionals who care for these patients. The initial chapters are devoted to a discussion of the relevant anatomy, and pathology of cervical cord injuries written for the non-expert, especially therapists and surgeons. Middle chapters discuss upper limb management in the acute and early rehabilitation setting, and practical information on evaluating the neurologically stable patient who might be a surgical candidate. After introducing a specific classification scheme and general principles of surgical rehabilitation, the later chapters follow this scheme in discussing specific treatment options and our personal preferences for patients injured at various cervical cord levels. The final chapters deal with the horizons including functional neuromuscular stimulation and outcome instruments. We conclude with an appendix section that includes treatment protocols and guidelines, formats to guide patient evaluation and other information perhaps useful for someone wishing to establish their own upper limb 'team.'

Vincent R Hentz, Stanford, California, USA
Caroline Leclercq, Paris, France

Dedication

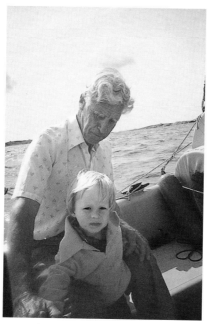

Erik Moberg MD (1905–1993)

Erik Moberg began relatively late in his professional career to study hand function in tetraplegic patients, concentrating on the high-level injured patient. He developed a very conservative surgical philosophy of doing less rather than more where any loss of function through complication or surgical misadventure was intolerable. Erik Moberg devoted the last two decades of his life to teaching other physicians and surgeons how to make the tetraplegic patient more independent through carefully conceptualized surgery.

Moberg's absolute honesty and single-mindedness of purpose served to slowly overturn the bias held by many spinal cord specialists, physiatrists and others against hand surgery for these patients. Moberg continuously stressed that 'the tetraplegic's upper limbs are, after the brain, the most important remaining functional resource.' For most surgeons currently involved in the surgical rehabilitation of the tetraplegic upper extremity, Moberg's basic philosophy, as espoused in his 1978 monograph 'The Upper Limb in Tetraplegia,' remains the foundation of surgical decision-making.

The authors feel blessed to have studied with and learned from Erik Moberg, and to be able to continue promoting his strongly held conviction that the great majority of tetraplegic patients can benefit from surgical rehabilitation. This book is a tribute to our mentor, Eric Moberg, and it is to Erik's memory that we dedicate this book.

Acknowledgments

Many individuals have contributed to this monograph, both directly and indirectly. We wish to thank the following individuals for their specific contributions:

Janet Weis OTR (Palo Alto, California, USA) for contributions to Chapter 4, The Acute and Early Rehabilitation Period.

Laurence Floris OTR (Coubert, France), **Catherine Dif OTR** (Coubert, France), and **Marie-Annie Le Mouel MD** (Coubert, France) for their contributions to Chapter 5, The Tetraplegic and the Environment.

MJ Mulcahey MS OTR (Philadelphia, USA) for her contributions regarding the pediatric population included in Chapter 16.

We are indebted to our UK colleagues at WB Saunders, Deborah Russell, Dr Kim Benson and Katharine Eyston, for their support and guidance through the lengthy process from conception to publication, and our illustrator Kathy Hirsch. We also acknowledge the critical role of our surgical mentors and colleagues, and especially our tetraplegic patients. To try to list them all from memory would only expose our cerebral frailties.

Finally, we thank our respective families, Marti, Andrew and Kirsten, and Guy, Thomas and Margaux for their forbearance and gracious acceptance of time spent away.

History of surgical rehabilitation

Changing philosophy

Prior to the 1950s, relatively few individuals who suffered transection of the cervical spinal cord survived the acute injury period. Most succumbed to the global effects of this injury, usually from respiratory or urinary failure, or they died from the complications of pressure sores.

The aggregation of various medical disciplines in specialty centers and better coordination of the multiple levels of care required for survival have resulted in greater numbers of individuals surviving their injury and leaving the hospital. These patients needed to learn how to survive outside the hospital using their remaining intellectual and physical resources, and for the tetraplegic individual their upper limbs represent the most important potential functional resource. This realization led to the development of various philosophies of upper limb acute care and rehabilitation designed to take better advantage of remaining shoulder, arm, and hand functions. For example, in the C6 tetraplegic patient, the functional goal was the development of a greater-than-normal force between the thumb and adjacent fingers when the patient actively extended the wrist. This was achieved by purposeful immobilization of the patient's hands during the early post-injury period in a posture that encouraged tightening of the finger flexor muscle groups. This encouraged the development of the presumably helpful flexion contracture of those muscles responsible for finger flexion, so that, when the wrist was extended, the patient could exert a few grams of force between the thumb and the adjacent index and middle fingers. With these few grams of force, the skillful use of balance, and the effect of gravity, the patient could be taught to obtain and manipulate light objects. Though terribly limited by normal standards,

when the functional starting point is zero, any gain can become enormous.

For patients at other neurological levels, different goals were developed, such as increasing function with the aid of a splint or orthosis.

Earliest surgery for upper limb rehabilitation

The historical record of surgery to further upper limb rehabilitation in the tetraplegic patient begins in the 1940s with the publication of occasional reports that describe the application in tetraplegics of procedures developed to restore function in the upper limb paralyzed by poliomyelitis. Standard procedures such as tenodeses (anchoring of a tendon to an adjacent firm structure), fusions (surgically uniting two bones by removing the intervening joint), and muscle-tendon transfers (by redirecting the action of a donor muscle and its tendon) were performed. The surgical literature of this period is unclear on how often tetraplegic patients were referred and evaluated for surgery. However, in the literature of this period related to the spinal cord there is little mention of the role of upper limb surgery. Upper limb surgery that was reported focused on tetraplegic patients who maintained good control of wrist motion, who but lacked finger and thumb extension or flexion. In his 1949 Instructional Course Lectures, Sterling Bunnell recognized that, for the tetraplegic patient the wrist is the key joint of the hand.[1]

Bunnell's position as the pre-eminent hand surgeon in the USA was established by the publication of his text on hand surgery in 1944,[2] and his influence as a teacher of hand reconstruction was great. Bunnell believed that the reconstruction of thumb opposition was an important goal where this function was absent, such as in the tetraplegic hand. His goal was the creation of a pinch between the tip of the thumb and the tips of the index and middle fingers. This is variously termed a three-jaw chuck pinch, akin to the three gripping surfaces in the common drill-chuck.

Since most tetraplegic patients lacked voluntary control of the muscles that position the thumb for pinch and grasp, Bunnell recommended utilizing either a tenodesis procedure or tendon transfer procedure to position the thumb in opposition to the other fingers. For tetraplegic patients functioning at the C6–C7 level, Bunnell recommended tenodesis of the flexor and extensor tendons of the fingers and thumb to the radius. A separate tendon graft attached the thumb to the ulna. Wrist extension automatically tightened the fingers into a grip and pulled the thumb into opposition. Supination of the forearm further brought the thumb into opposition. Flexing the wrist automatically opened the hand (*Fig. 1.1*).

For tetraplegic patients functioning at the C7–C8 level, Bunnell recommended multiple muscle–tendon transfers rather than tenodeses. The goal was active finger flexion and thumb opposition. Bunnell and others achieved useful results in the short term, but long-term results went unreported.

Surgical reconstruction of the tetraplegic's hand had few proponents during the 1940s and 1950s. In 1949, Hendry indicated his preference for tenodeses to achieve an automatic hand grasp.[3] He described

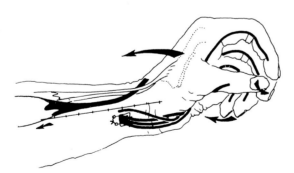

Figure 1.1 Illustrated is Bunnell's recommended procedure for the tetraplegic patient who has retained the ability to extend the wrist actively. Finger and thumb flexor tendons were tenodesed to the radius. A third tenodesis attached the thumb to the ulna so that when the wrist was voluntarily extended, the fingers automatically flexed and the thumb rotated to oppose the index and middle fingertips.

tenodesis of both flexors and extensors to the radius so that with supination the wrist extended and fingers closed and with forearm pronation, the wrist flexed and the fingers extended.

In 1956, Wilson reported his experience with four tetraplegic patients.[4] Similar to Bunnell, Wilson tenodesed the thumb and digital flexors into the radius. One patient had the profundus of the index finger powered by transfer of the pronator teres as a trigger finger. Wilson reported that useful function was obtained in all cases.

In 1958, Paul Lipscomb and colleagues from the Mayo Clinic reported a series of 12 reconstructed patients.[5] Lipscomb noted that in their experience patients injured at the C6–C7 level predominated. A two-stage approach was adopted. At the first stage, the extensor carpi radialis longus was transferred to the digital and thumb extensors. If an accessory slip of the extensor carpi radialis brevis was present, it was transferred to the abductor pollicis longus. Some time later, at a second stage, the flexor carpi radialis was lengthened with a tendon graft and transferred for thumb opposition using the flexor carpi ulnaris as a pulley. The pronator teres was similarly lengthened with a tendon graft and transferred to the digital flexors and the brachioradialis (BR) was transferred to the thumb flexor.

In 1959, Street reviewed the various methods to restore upper limb function in tetraplegic patients and his experience between 1949 and 1957 in 17 operations on 12 tetraplegic patients.[6] He championed transfer of the BR for many purposes including:

- into the thumb flexor distal to the tenodesis;
- into the extensor mechanism to assist finger opening;
- to the thumb flexor to provide voluntary lateral or key pinch; and
- to the thumb extensor to keep the thumb outside of finger grasp.

He described six different tenodesis techniques and believed that tenodesis of both profundus and superficialis tendons provided a better result. Street described using a block of bone placed under the tenodesed tendons distal to site of tenodesis to increase the moment of the tendons at the wrist and thus their 'power'.

Street reported that 10 of 12 cases achieved 'excellent' function, although two experienced flexion contractures of the proximal and/or distal inter-phalangeal joints. Street mentions the need to vary grasp size in bilateral hand surgery. He did not observe any tendency for the tendons to stretch out over time, although the average time of follow-up was 29 months and the longest follow-up was 8 years.

An early appraisal of surgery

The medical literature of that period indicates that upper limb surgery was not felt to be particularly beneficial by the physiatrists and others in whose care the tetraplegic patient remained. Various reasons have been given for this lack of enthusiasm to build on the early recommendations of Bunnell and others to apply to the tetraplegic patient the same procedures successfully used to restore hand function for patients who suffered from the effects of polio. Moberg has made the strong case that some early surgeons probably inappropriately applied procedures that succeeded in one paralyzed population (i.e., those with poliomyelitis) to tetraplegic patients, who had a similar presentation but very different etiology and functional detail.[7] Moberg makes large of the long-term consequences of the absence of sensation and the presence of spasticity, two features not present in the patient paralyzed by polio. The consequences of poor or absent sensation became visible as fusions and tenodeses gave way under the stress of years of weight bearing on insensate hands. Function, once present, was gradually lost. The consequences of spasticity became evident as once-supple hands became clawed and contracted secondary to contracture of spastic muscles, especially where no active or strong passive antagonist existed.

Some biomechanically well-designed automatic grasp-and-release procedures, such as that reported by Nickel and his colleagues from the Rancho Los Amigos Center in California,[8] were very technically demanding, requiring precise positions of the fusions to achieve function. This procedure, termed the 'flexor-hinged hand', involved fusion of the thumb metacarpal in a widely opposed position. To accomplish this, a large bone block was inserted between the base of the first and second metacarpals with the thumb in 35° of palmar flexion and rotated under the index finger, that is flexed across the palm (*Fig. 1.2*).

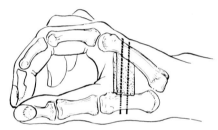

Figure 1.2 Nickel's procedure for the patient with active wrist extension is illustrated. A bone block was used to fuse the first metacarpal in full palmar opposition to the second metacarpal. When the wrist was extended, a flexor tenodesis pulled the index and middle fingers toward the rigidly positioned thumb.

A

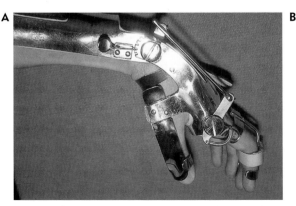

B

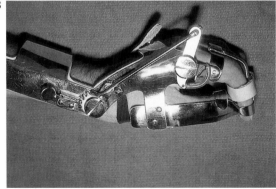

Figure 1.3 The wrist extension, finger flexion orthosis, as developed by physicians and engineers at Rancho Los Amigos Rehabilitation Facility, is shown in its (A) open and (B) closed postures. This functional orthosis is described more fully in Chapter 4.

If finger flexor or extensor power was available it was used to power the index and middle fingers. If only wrist power was available, then the superficialis flexors were anchored to the radius so that pinch was achieved at 15° of wrist extension. The common digital extensors of digits two and three were anchored to radius so that with 10° of wrist flexion, the fingers began to extend. In addition, the interphalangeal joints of the thumb, index, and middle finger were fused. The goal was to provide tip-to-tip pinch between the rigidly positioned thumb and the index and middle finger tips using the residual flexion–extension motion at the metacarpophalangeal joints of these digits, as the wrist extended.

Nickel's reported his surgical experience with 22 complete flexor hinge hands. Inability of the tips of the digits to meet was the most common cause of failure. He mentions problems of acceptance as a product of neglect and the development of negative attitudes that could be overcome in part by a graduated program of activities. In addition to the surgical procedure, Nickel and his colleagues developed an orthosis (*Fig.1.3*) that positioned the thumb and fingers similarly to the surgical procedure. Nickel's philosophy was that the brace was to be used for a particular period of time and the patient should be made aware of this. Surgery is mentioned as a means of removing the braces and as a step in progress. Nickel believed that this surgery was indicated only for the most severely paralyzed hand; when these procedures were used for less severely paralyzed hands, the results were less acceptable.

Nickel's results were difficult for others to duplicate. In addition, such procedures resulted in occasional patients who were dissatisfied with their somewhat stiff and inflexible hands. Gradually, most other surgeons abandoned this operative procedure.

For whatever reason or reasons, by the 1960s and early 1970s, various influential texts that guided the rehabilitation recommendations for tetraplegic patients exhibited strong to absolute bias against a role for surgery in upper limb rehabilitation.[9] In his comprehensive text on spinal cord injury management, Guttman advised that only a tiny minority, perhaps no more than 7%, of tetraplegic patients might benefit from upper limb surgery.[9]

This increased pessimism regarding the usefulness of surgery for the tetraplegic patient led to many surgeons abandoning surgery for tetraplegic patients, and few physiatrists referred patients for surgery. Greater emphasis was placed on the development of adaptive aids and external orthoses, many of which were designed to mimic the goals of certain surgical procedures.

The era of functional orthoses

In 1963, Nickel and his colleagues from the Rancho Los Amigos Center reviewed their philosophy regarding upper limb rehabilitation and their work in orthotics for tetraplegic patients.[10] Nickel believed that the principal goal was to stabilize the hand in one selected position and then use all residual muscle power to provide active grasp and release. Necessary activities of self-care and sedentary activities require only a light pinch between the thumb and first two fingers. Therefore, it is necessary to consider only the three radial digits. Nickel stated that lateral or key pinch requires four levels of control, while palmar pinch requires only two controls.

Nickel's goal was to place the thumb and the index and middle fingers in a stable position with motion sufficient to open and close the resultant grasp. The entire thumb should be immobilized by splint or surgery in the position of opposition, and the index and middle fingers immobilized in semiflexion at the proximal and distal interphalangeal joints. This hand resembled the terminal device developed by the Army Prosthetics Research Laboratory and is termed the APRL hand. With these joints appropriately immobilized, all that is needed for control is flexion and extension at the metacarpophalangeal joints.

Nickel utilized the biomechanical goals of certain surgical procedures and constructed an external orthotic equivalent. For example, the Rancho group designed and constructed both passive and active varieties of a dynamic orthosis that mimicked their operatively created automatic three-jaw chuck pinch grasp described above (*Fig. 1.3*). Interestingly, Street, in his 1959 publication, mentions trying but abandoning such a device.[6] The device constrained all the joints of the hand, save the metacarpophalangeal joints of the fingers, in a position that allowed wrist movement to generate finger flexion and extension. The device also stabilizes and pre-positions the thumb so that the closing index and middle finger tips contact the tip of the thumb. This design, referred to as the 'Rancho splint' or the wrist-driven, flexor-hinge splint (FHS), remains a mainstay of upper limb rehabilitation today, more than 40 years after its introduction, its basic design relatively unchanged during this period.

Nickel recommended use of the FHS at a specific time during rehabilitation. When the patient is ready for multiple functions that require too many aids to be attached to the static splint, he or she is ready to have the FHS. Nickel's policy was to use the splint before making the hand surgically like the splint. Either finger or wrist motors drive the orthosis. If finger motion is present a finger-driven FHS can be prescribed. If power exists in only one direction, a spring is added. Better function is achieved if the spring is needed for opening.

If only wrist power is available, the wrist-driven FHS can be used. With appropriate leverage, 7 cm (3 inches) of opening is possible with grasp force equivalent to 75% of wrist power.

If more distal muscles were not available, Nickel researched the use of a cable-driven FHS. This was not very successful because more proximal muscles typically were not at full power. This led to the development of the external power FHS. Nickel and his colleagues described the artificial muscle, a covered rubber bladder with active expansion and passive deflation. As the bladder expands the sleeve shortens and produces a pull, up to a point. The pull is proportional to the amount of gas put into the bladder. Typical sources of power to control this are shoulder elevation, scapular abduction, and chest expansion. Between 1958 and 1962 at Rancho, 62 hands were fitted with this artificial muscle.

Only a few patients accepted such devices as permanent. Frequently mentioned sources of discontent included mild discomfort and the inconvenience, especially when others had to put on the device.

It is of interest that Nickel's 'Rancho' surgically created flexor-hinge hand operation has passed into history while its orthotic corollary, the wrist-driven FHS remains frequently prescribed today.

Surgical islands

During the 1960s and 1970s a few surgeons continued to recommend and perform surgical reconstruction of upper limb function in this population.

Most often, surgery was carried out for patients whose injuries had spared the muscles that control wrist function. There were few surgical indications for patients who had weak or absent wrist extension, even though these patients constituted the majority of 'complete' tetraplegic patients. Only those surgeons fortunate enough to work in specialty centers or with access to these were able to generate sufficient numbers of cases for analysis, publication, and recommendations.

In 1967, Alvin Freehafer, working in Cleveland, USA,[11] reported his results using primarily tendon transfers to improve active wrist extension in six patients. Four were able to grasp effectively postoperatively. Three could use a wrist-driven FHS while the other two had improved posture. Freehafer mentioned the possibility of performing a simultaneous flexor tenodesis, but no patient had this. Freehafer was the first to advocate extensive proximal dissection of the BR muscle as part of the preparation for transfer.

In 1971, Douglas Lamb, working in Edinburgh, published his extensive experience with 113 tetraplegic patients.[12] In the 25 patients who had elected surgery, 72 muscle tendon transfers were performed during the course of 52 operations. Lamb's primary goal depended on the remaining functioning muscles. For patients who possessed strong wrist extension, he transferred the extensor carpi radialis longus to the profundus tendons and the BR to the thumb flexor. He experienced failure secondary to overstretching in all the attempts to fashion thumb opposition by opponens tenodesis. Lamb was the first surgeon to publicly advocate preferential restoration of a side or key pinch rather than opposition pinch. Lamb stated that 11 of 13 patients were improved by surgery.

For those patients who possessed strong wrist flexion, the flexor carpi radialis was used as an opponens transfer. The functionality of all five patients in this group improved. A small group of patients who lacked intrinsic function only also improved with more traditional transfers.

The French experience in that era is that of Maury and colleagues from the Fontainebleau rehabilitation center. They published their experience with tendon transfer in nine patients in 1968,[13] and then 17 patients in 1973.[14] They performed various muscle–tendon transfers for finger flexion, thumb opposition, and thumb abduction. In both series, they report roughly 50% significant improvement, 25% minor improvement, and 25% failures. All their transfers for abduction and for opposition of the thumb failed. The three cases in which they tried a simultaneous transfer of the agonist and the antagonist failed. They were more satisfied with the transfers to the flexor digitorum profundus and flexor pollicis longus, although for the latter they routinely experienced the development of a stiff, flexed interphalangeal joint. This resulted in a pinch between the dorsal aspect of the thumb terminal phalanx and the index finger. They state that fusion of the interphalangeal joint of the thumb 'is certainly not the solution to this problem', because they felt the extended phalanx would become caught under the fingers during grasp.

In 1975, Eduardo Zancolli, working in Buenos Aires, Argentina, published his analysis of 97 tetraplegic patients studied between 1947 and 1974.[15] Of these, 76 elected to undergo surgery. Almost 75% of his patients possessed wrist extension, with many also retaining active forearm pronation and/or some active wrist flexion. Zancolli opined that, in the absence of contraindications, surgery was always preferred over splinting. Surgery helps the morale of the entire center.

Surgery should be delayed until the patient can sit in bed. In bed the arms supinate; when sitting, the arms can pronate. Sitting also improves wrist flexion, which in turn improves digital extension. Wrist flexion was an important goal and could be achieved by gravity, by residual action of the flexor carpi radialis, or by transfer of the pronator teres to the flexor carpi radialis. Pronation was an equally important goal and when the patient could not pronate, Zancolli advocated re-routing the biceps to make it a pronator of the forearm rather than a supinator.[16]

Zancolli recognized that supernumerary muscles and tendons existed, especially those related to the two radial wrist extensors, and that if these extra structures were present, they could provide a valuable reconstructive resource.[17] He advocated seeking their presence during the initial stage of surgery. Two key muscles must be left undisturbed – the extensor carpi radialis brevis and the flexor carpi radialis – since wrist motion is the fundamental motion to produce finger function.

Zancolli recommended a two-stage approach for each hand.[18] The initial stage provided extension or

opening of the hand and the second closure of the hand. He advocated looking for extra muscles at the first operation so that they could be used in the second procedure. The first procedure involved fusion of the thumb carpometacarpal joint and transfer of the BR muscle to the thumb and finger extensors. The second procedure involved transfer of the extensor carpi radialis longus to the digital flexor tendons and transfer of the supernumerary muscle to the thumb flexor or tenodesis of the thumb flexor to the remaining radial wrist extensor. Zancolli provided no information regarding the functional results of his procedures.

The modern era

The role for upper limb surgery in the restoration of function for tetraplegics found a new and enthusiastic champion in the person of Erik Moberg of Gothenburg, Sweden. As he approached 65 years of age, Moberg was facing enforced retirement from his role as Head of Sweden's principal hand surgery unit. His long-term interest in sensation had led him to examine the hands of tetraplegic patients. Moberg began relatively late in his professional career to study hand function in tetraplegic patients and to consider different options for specific groups of patients whose level of injury had previously discouraged most surgeons from considering them as surgical candidates.

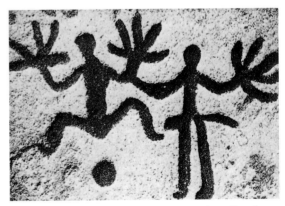

Figure 1.4 This rock carving was made in Sweden about 4000 years ago. The artist was aware of the importance of the hands in human contact. From Moberg (1978),[7] with permission of Georg Thieme Publishers.

Moberg also possessed a high reputation and a certain single-mindedness of purpose that served to slowly overturn the bias held by many spinal cord specialists, physiatrists, and others against hand surgery for these patients. Moberg continuously stressed the belief that the tetraplegic's upper limbs were, after the brain, the most important remaining functional resource (*Fig. 1.4*). He began by concentrating on those patients with high-level injuries and developed a very conservative surgical philosophy of doing less rather than more where any loss of function through complication or other surgical misadventure was felt intolerable. For many surgeons involved in the surgical rehabilitation of the tetraplegic upper extremity, Moberg's basic philosophy remains the foundation of surgical decision-making today, more than 25 years after Moberg published his espousal, first as a journal article in 1975,[19] and then expanded in his monograph published in 1978.[7]

For these patients with very few functional resources remaining to them, Moberg concentrated on restoring one prime hand function, a simply achieved key-type pinch between the pulp of the thumb and the side of the index finger, rather than the more complicated opposition pinch preferred by his surgical predecessors. He followed the suggestion of Merle D'Aubigne et al.,[20] who first proposed using part of the deltoid muscle to restore elbow extension, and demonstrated how to restore another useful function in this population, active elbow extension, by transferring the posterior half of the deltoid muscle into the triceps tendon (*Fig. 1.5*). More importantly, he traveled and spoke constantly to, essentially, anyone who would listen, promulgating his strong opinion that the majority of tetraplegic patients could benefit from carefully chosen and performed surgical procedures. Moberg stimulated the interest of surgeons from many countries and must be given credit for achieving the 'critical mass' of renewed surgical interest in this area.

Since the publication of Moberg's monograph in 1978,[7] more than 100 articles devoted to recommendations, indications, techniques, and outcomes of surgical rehabilitation of the upper limb in the tetraplegic population have been published. At the time of writing, seven international congresses on surgical rehabilitation have been held with constantly rising attendance and interest. Most physicians who care for these patients now recognize the value of surgical reconstruction of the tetraplegic's upper limb.

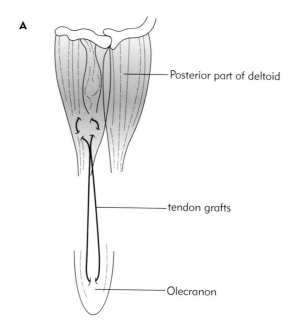

A

Posterior part of deltoid

tendon grafts

Olecranon

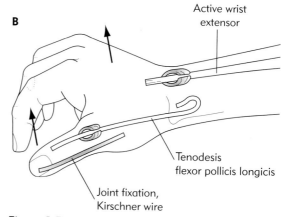

B

Active wrist extensor

Tenodesis flexor pollicis longicis

Joint fixation, Kirschner wire

Figure 1.5 Moberg's most important surgical contributions, as illustrated in his 1975 publication,[19] included restoring active elbow extension by (A) transfer of the posterior half of the deltoid and (B) a simply performed tenodesis procedure to provide a key pinch. (Reproduced with permission.)

References

1. Bunnell S. Tendon transfers in the hand and forearm. American Academy of Orthopedic Surgery – Instructional Course Lectures. St Louis: CV Mosby; 1949:102–112.
2. Bunnell S. Surgery of the Hand. Philadelphia: JB Lippincott; 1944.

3. Hendry A. The treatment of residual paralysis after brachial plexus injury. J Bone Joint Surg 1949; 31B:42–49.

4. Wilson J. Providing automatic grasp by flexor tenodesis. J Bone Joint Surg 1956; 38A:1019–1024.

5. Lipscomb P, Elkins E, Henderson E. Tendon transfers to restore function of hands in tetraplegia, especially after fracture–dislocation of the sixth cervical vertebra on the seventh. J Bone Joint Surg 1958; 40:1071–1080.

6. Street D, Stambaugh H. Finger flexor tenodesis. Clin Orthop 1959; 13:155–163.

7. Moberg E. The Upper Limb in Tetraplegia. A new approach to surgical rehabilitation. Stuttgart: George Thieme; 1978.

8. Nickel V, Perry J. The flexor hinged hand. J Bone Joint Surg 1958; 40A:971.

9. Guttman L. Spinal Cord Injuries. Oxford: Blackwell Scientific; 1973.

10. Nickel V, Perry J, Garrett A. Development of useful function in the severely paralyzed hand. J Bone Joint Surg 1963; 45A(5):933–952.

11. Freehafer A, Mast W. Transfer of the brachioradialis to improve wrist extension in high spinal cord injury. J Bone Joint Surg 1967; 49A:648.

12. Lamb DW, Landry R. The hand in quadriplegia. The Hand 1971; 3(1):31–37.

13. Masse P, Maury M, Bidart Y, et al. A propos des transplantations tendineuses pour la réanimation de la main du tétraplégique (9 cas sur 100 malades). Ann Méd Phys 1968; 11:351–369.

14. Maury M, Guillamat M, Francois N. Our experience of upper limbs transfers in cases of tetraplegia. Paraplegia 1973; 11:245–251.

15. Zancolli E. Surgery for the quadriplegic hand with active, strong wrist extension preserved. Clin Orthop Rel Res 1975; 112:101–113.

16. Zancolli EA. Paralytic supination contracture of the forearm. J Bone Joint Surg 1967; 49A:1275–1284.

17. Zancolli E, Zancolli E. Tetraplegies traumatiques. In: Tubiana R, ed. Traite' de Chirurgie de la Main. Paris: Masson; 1991.

18. Zancolli E. Structural and Dynamic Basis of Hand Surgery. 2nd edn. Philadelphia: JB Lippincott; 1979.

19. Moberg E. Surgical treatment for absent single-hand grip and elbow extension in quadriplegia. J Bone Joint Surg 1975; 57A(2):196–206.

20. Merle D'Aubigne, Seddon H, Hendry A, et al. Tendon transfers. Proc Royal Soc Med 1949; 48:831.

2

Anatomy of the cervical spine and cord

The spinal cord lies in continuity with the brain and, together, they constitute the central nervous system. Both are covered by a thin envelope, the meninges, which encloses a space filled with cerebrospinal fluid. The spinal cord is surrounded by vertebrae and lies within the vertebral canal. It is shaped as a stem (*Fig. 2.1*) with two spindle-shaped enlargements in the cervical and lumbar regions, which correspond to the emergence of the nerve roots for the upper and lower limbs. Its lower end, the conus medullaris, is prolonged by a fine thread, the filum terminale.

The spinal cord is divided in two symmetrical halves by two fissures, the anterior median fissure on its anterior aspect, and the posterior median fissure on its posterior aspect. Nerve fibers emerge dorsolaterally and ventrolaterally from each side of the spinal cord and merge into posterior and anterior roots, which eventually unite into the spinal nerves. The spinal nerves leave the spine between vertebral arches. At the level of the two spinal enlargements they first form plexuses, the brachial plexus in the cervical area and the lumbosacral plexus in the lumbar area. Of the 31 pairs of spinal nerves there are eight pairs of cervical nerves, the first pair emerging between the occipital bone and the atlas, and the final one between the seventh cervical and the first dorsal vertebra.

Gray and white matter

The spinal cord itself is not segmented. Rather, it is composed of two substances, gray and white matter.

Gray matter

The gray matter, or substantia grisea, lies in the central part and appears, in cross section, as a

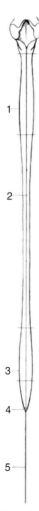

Figure 2.1 The spinal cord with (1) the cervical enlargement, (2) the dorsal area, (3) the lumbar enlargement, (4) the conus medullaris, and (5) the filum terminale.

butterfly shape. It contains the nervous medullary centers. It is composed of two large anterior horns, which contain the motor anterior horn cells from which the motor fibers emerge, and two thin posterior horns, which contain neurons of the afferent system on which sensory fibers from the dorsal root ganglion cells terminate. In the middle lies the central intermediate substance, which surrounds the central (or ependymal) canal. It contains vegetative neurons of the sympathetic system.

White matter

The white matter, or substantia alba, surrounds the gray matter. It carries nerve (dendritic) bundles, some of which are ascending, others descending, and others interconnecting (associative) bundles. It is subdivided into a posterior column from the posterior septum to the posterior horn (funiculus posterior), a lateral column from the posterior horn to the anterior horn (funiculus lateralis), and an anterior column from the anterior horn to the anterior fissure. The anterior and lateral columns combine as the anterolateral column (funiculus anterolateralis). The two halves of the white matter are joined ventrally by the commissura alba (*Fig. 2.2*).

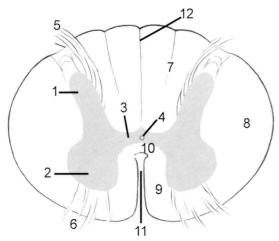

Figure 2.2 The cervical spinal cord. The gray matter: (1) posterior horn, (2) anterior horn, (3) central intermediate substance, (4) central canal, (5) fibers of the posterior roots, and (6) fibers of the anterior roots. The white matter: (7) posterior column, (8) lateral column, (9) anterior column, (10) commissura alba, (11) anterior fissure, and (12) posterior fissure. (Adapted from Kahle 1984,[1] with permission.)

The amount of white matter increases from distal to proximal, and the amount of gray matter increases at the two enlargements (cervical and lumbar). Also, the butterfly configuration of the gray matter varies in shape at different levels. In the cervical cord, the posterior horn is narrower and terminates in a cap-like 'zona spongiosa', whereas the anterior horn is widely expanded and contains several identifiable cell groups (motor nuclei) concentrated into medial and lateral groups.

Segmental topography

The medullary reflex (reflex arc)

Sensory neurons, the cell bodies of which lie in the spinal (dorsal) ganglia, reach the posterior horn. They transmit sensory impulses to the brain via the posterior horn cells. They can also run directly to the anterior horn cells and transmit impulses to them, either directly (simple reflex arc) or via interposed intermediate neurons (multisynaptic reflex arc).

Afferent (sensory) neurons

Afferent neurons may be of three different kinds, which carry different sensations and travel in different areas of the posterior horn (Fig. 2.3):

● exteroceptive fibers carry cutaneous and subcutaneous sensory impulses (primarily touch,

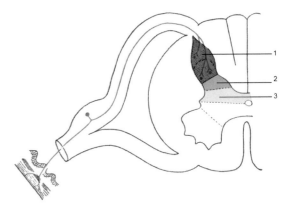

Figure 2.3 Afferent neurons enter the posterior horn and reach (1) the exteroceptive area, (2) the proprioceptive area, or (3) the interoceptive area. (Adapted from Delmas 1973,[2] with permission.)

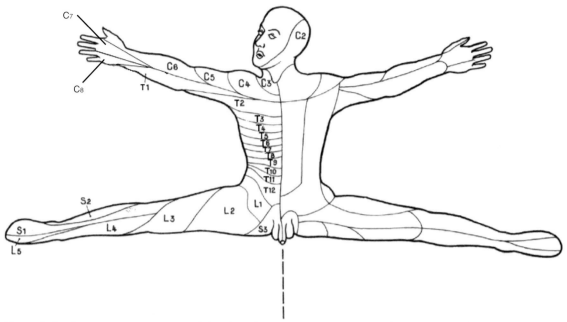

Figure 2.4   Segmentary innervation of the skin: dermatomes. (Adapted from Delmas 1973,[2] with permission.)

temperature, pain, and pressure sensations), and they reach the most posterior part of the posterior horn;

- proprioceptive fibers carry impulses from muscles, bones, and joints (primarily pain, pressure, and the status of the muscle), and they lie anterior to the exteroceptive fibers;
- interoceptive fibers carry sensation from the viscera and reach the area anterior to the proprioceptive fibers.

The sensory fibers of the spinal nerves supply segmental areas of skin, called dermatomes. Each dermatome depends on a medullary segmental center and is innervated by a segmentary nerve. Segmentary nerves in the cervical cord innervate the head (C2), the neck (C3–C4), and the upper limb (C5–C8; *Fig. 2.4*). The first cervical root does not have a representation on the body surface.

The presence or absence of sensation in specific dermatomes is a very good indicator of the extent and location of injury to the spinal cord. However, the dermatomes overlap one another somewhat, so the loss of a single posterior root cannot usually be demonstrated, because its dermatome is also partially supplied from adjacent dermatomes.

Efferent (motor) neurons

Cell bodies of the motoneurons lie in the anterior horn. The visceromotor area contains the motoneurons of the vegetative system in the posterior part of the horn, and the somatomotor area contains the motoneurons for the striated muscles in the most anterior part of the horn (*Fig. 2.5*). The anterior horn

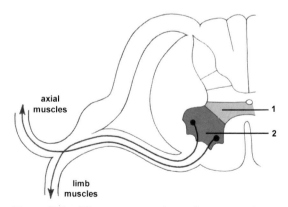

Figure 2.5   Efferent neurons leave the anterior horn from either (1) the visceromotor area or (2) the somatomotor area. (Adapted from Delmas 1973,[2] with permission.)

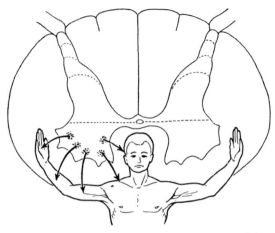

Figure 2.6 Somatotopic motor arrangement of the anterior horn at the cervical level. (Adapted from Delmas 1973,[2] with permission.)

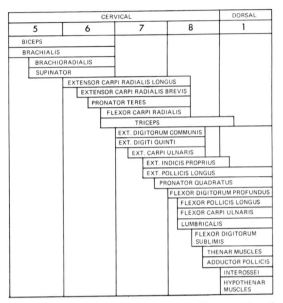

Figure 2.7 Metameric innervation of the muscles of the upper extremity according to Zancolli. (Adapted from Zancolli 1979,[5] with permission.)

is subdivided somatotopically; the most medial groups of cells supply the axial muscles (neck and trunk) and the lateral ones supply the limbs. The more lateral the cells, the more distal the muscles they supply in each limb. This configuration explains why some spinal cord injuries that infarct the central elements (central cord syndrome) more than the lateral elements lead to upper limb weakness but lower limb sparing.

In the cervical cord, the somatomotor area is widely expanded, with groups of cell bodies concentrated in so-called nuclei. The anteromedial nucleus gives rise to motoneurons that control the neck muscles, the anterolateral nucleus those for the shoulder girdle and upper arm, and the dorsolateral nucleus those for the lower arm and hand. Finally, the retrodorsal nucleus supplies the small muscles of the hand and fingers (*Fig. 2.6*). There is no true segmentation for individual muscles as there is for skin territories. Rather, these motor nuclei form longitudinal columns lying across several medullary segments. Each column can be viewed as the peripheral innervation center for a specific muscle. Each muscle therefore has its own motor center lying across several medullar segments.[3,4] *Figure 2.7* shows the longitudinal extent of the motor column for each muscle of the upper limb, as recorded by Zancolli from his own clinical experience with tetraplegic patients.[6] Another chart, based on Barthe's clinical experience (*Fig. 2.8*),[8] shows a few differences, mainly in the motor centers for the biceps, the triceps, the flexor carpi radialis, and the flexor carpi

ulnaris.[9] This anatomic arrangement explains why a muscle can be completely or only partially paralyzed according to the level of spinal cord injury. For instance, a spinal cord injury at the level of C6 (referred to as a C5 level injury) induces a complete paralysis of the extensor carpi radiales muscles (longus and brevis), whereas an injury at the level of C7 (referred to as a C6 level injury) leads to a partial lesion of the motor columns of these two muscles with residual and variable weak extension of the wrist.

Usually these motor columns extend across two or sometimes three spinal cord segments. However, a few muscles have a longer column and therefore motor innervation can arise from a larger area of the spinal cord. This accounts for variations in the clinical picture after a spinal cord injury. Such is the case for the triceps brachii, the motor column of which extends from C6 to T1. For the same level of spinal cord lesion, some patients will still have a functioning triceps, whereas in others it will be inactive.

Ascending and descending tracts (or longitudinal tracts)

The brain is connected to the rest of the body via fibers that run through the white matter. Ascending

	C2	C3	C4	C5	C6	C7	C8	T1
Trapezius								
Levator scapulae								
Diaphragm								
Rhomboids								
Serratus anterior								
Deltoids								
Biceps*								
Teres major								
External rotation								
Brachioradialis								
Extensor carpi radialis longus								
Internal rotation								
Extensor carpi radialis brevis								
Pectoralis major								
Pronator teres								
Triceps*								
Flexor carpi radialis*								
Latissimus dorsi								
Flexor carpi ulnaris*								
Extensor digiti communis*								
Extensor carpi ulnaris*								
Flexor digitorum superficialis*								
Flexor digitorum profundus								
Interossei*								
Opponens								

Figure 2.8 Metameric innervation of the muscles of the upper extremity according to Barthes.[4] Asterisks indicate differences from Zancolli's classification.[3] (Adapted from Tubiana 1991,[7] with permission.)

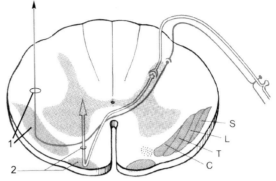

Figure 2.9 The lateral (1) and anterior (2) spinothalamic tracts. The afferent fibers terminate near or in the posterior horn. Then fibers of the tract arise and cross in the commissura alba, reach the opposite side, and ascend to the thalamus. Somatotopic arrangement: C, cervical; T, thoracic; L, lumbar; S, sacral. (Adapted from Kahle 1984,[1] with permission.)

fibers bring sensory information, and descending fibers transmit commands to the motoneurons.

Ascending tracts

Different areas of the white matter carry different types of sensation. The anterolateral column carries mostly nociceptive impulses, the lateral column carries mostly proprioceptive impulses, and the posterior column carries exteroceptive and proprioceptive impulses of epicritic sensibility.

The anterolateral column

Two tracts are identified in the anterolateral column, one lateral and one anterior. The lateral spinothalamic tract carries temperature and pain sensations. Nerve fibers reach the posterior horn, fibers from the tract

arise from these fibers, cross the cord transversally through the commissura alba to the opposite side, and reach the anterior column. The tract is divided somatotopically, with the cervical fibers located most ventromedially and the sacral fibers located most dorsolaterally (*Fig. 2.9*).

The anterior spinothalamic tract carries gross pressure and touch sensation. Impulses travel in the same manner and reach the anterior column. The tract is located ventral and medial to the anterolateral spinothalamic tract. Both tracts terminate in the thalamus.

The posterior column

The posterior column carries epicritic sensibility. Nerve fibers reach the posterior column, do not synapse, and do not cross, but rather ascend directly to the medulla oblongata where they synapse and cross. Two identifiable tracts are juxtaposed, the fasciculus gracilis of Goll medially and the fasciculus cuneatus of Burdach laterally. They are arranged somatotopically, with the fibers from C2 most lateral in Goll's fasciculus and sacral fibers most medial in Burdach's fasciculus (*Fig. 2.10*).

The lateral column

The lateral column carries principally proprioceptive (and some exteroceptive) impulses to the cerebellum. There is a direct tract located posteriorly (posterior

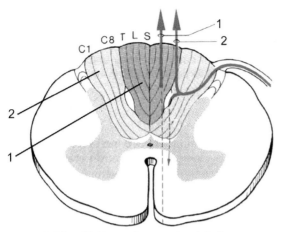

Figure 2.10 (1) Fasciculus gracilis of Goll, (2) fasciculus cuneatus of Burdach. Somatotopic arrangement: C1–C8, cervical fibers; T, thoracic fibers; L, lumbar fibers; S, sacral fibers. (Adapted from Kahle 1984,[1] with permission.)

spinocerebellar tract of Flechsig), and a crossed tract located anteriorly (anterior spinocerebellar tract of Gowers). Both of these tracts carry mainly thoracic, dorsal, and lumbar fibers (*Fig. 2.11*).

Descending tracts

A – The pyramidal or corticospinal tract carries voluntary motor fibers, which arise from the cortex. Most of them (80%) cross to the contralateral side in the medulla oblongata and travel in the lateral column as the lateral corticospinal (or crossed pyramidal) tract. The remaining fibers do not cross and travel in the anterior column as the anterior corticospinal tract (or direct pyramidal tract), finally crossing at the level of their termination. Both tracts thin as they travel distally, for they give off fibers all along the spinal cord.

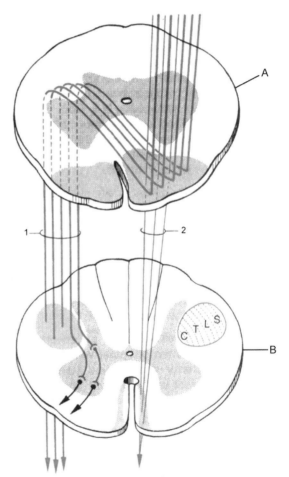

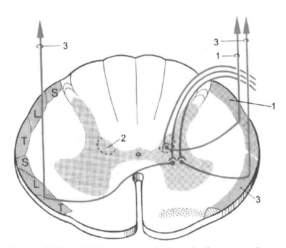

Figure 2.11 (1) Posterior spinocerebellar tract of Flechsig. The tract originates in the area of the dorsal nucleus of Clarke (2) and ascends on the ipsilateral side to the cerebellum. (3) Anterior spinocerebellar tract of Gowers. Fibers reach the same and the opposite side of the spinal cord, and ascend to the cerebellum. (Adapted from Kahle 1984,[1] with permission.)

Figure 2.12 The pyramidal tract: A, medulla oblongata; B, spinal cord. (1) The lateral corticospinal tract and (2) the anterior corticospinal tract. Somatotopic arrangement in the lateral tract: C, cervical; T, thoracic; L, lumbar; S, sacral. (Adapted from Kahle 1984,[1] with permission.)

These fibers reach the anterior horn either directly or via an interneuron, and transmit impulses of voluntary movement to the motor nerve fibers (*Fig. 2.12*). More than half of the pyramidal tract terminates in the cervical cord for the upper limb, whereas only a fourth terminates in the lumbosacral cord for the lower limb. There is a somatotopic arrangement in the lateral corticospinal tract, with lower limb fibers running on the periphery, and fibers for the arm running medially.

B – The extrapyramidal tract carries semi-voluntary motor fibers, which influence and control the motor system. They arise from the cortex and travel through at least six individualized tracts (*Fig. 2.13*):

- vestibulospinal tract, which controls balance and tonus;
- ventrolateral and lateral reticulospinal tracts;
- tegmentospinal tract;
- rubrospinal tract;
- tectospinal tract; and
- medial longitudinal fasciculus.

Both the rubrospinal and tectospinal tracts terminate in the cervical spine. All fibers from these tracts end around the motor cells in the anterior horn.

The vegetative tracts consist of poorly myelinated and unmyelinated fibers scattered in the substantia alba, which only rarely form compact bundles. The

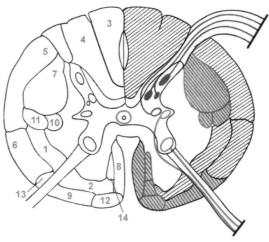

Figure 2.14 Topography of the white matter. Ascending tracts: (1) lateral spinothalamic tract, (2) anterior spinothalamic tract, (3) fasciculus gracilis of Goll, (4) fasciculus cuneatus of Burdach, (5) posterior spinocerebellar tract of Flechsig, (6) anterior spinocerebellar tract of Gowers. Descending tracts: (7) lateral corticospinal tract, (8) anterior corticospinal tract, (9) vestibulospinal tract, (10) reticulospinal tracts, (11) rubrospinal tract, (12) tectospinal tract, (13) olivospinal tract, (14) medial longitudinal fasciculus. (Adapted from Delmas 1973,[2] with permission.)

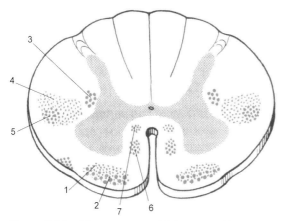

Figure 2.13 The extrapyramidal tract and its components: (1) vestibulospinal tract, (2) ventrolateral reticulospinal tract, (3) lateral reticulospinal tract, (4) tegmentospinal tract, (5) rubrospinal tract, (6) tectospinal tract, and (7) medial longitudinal fasciculus. (Adapted from Kahle 1984,[1] with permission.)

parependymal tract for genital function runs along both sides of the central canal. Förster's tract, which controls vasoconstriction and sweat secretion, runs ventral to the pyramidal tract and has the same somatotopic arrangement as the lateral pyramidal tract.

Although the tracts are not recognizable on a transverse section of the normal spinal cord, a global representation of all the tracts, ascending and descending, would roughly look like *Figure 2.14*.

Blood supply of the spinal cord

The spinal cord is vascularized from two sources: the vertebral arteries and the segmental arteries (intercostal and lumbar).

The vertebral arteries give off two posterior spinal arteries that run longitudinally along the posterior aspect of the cord and one anterior spinal artery that runs anteriorly, at the entrance of the anterior sulcus. The latter is widest at the cervical and lumbar

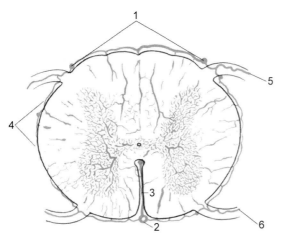

Figure 2.15 Vascularization of the spinal cord: (1) posterior spinal arteries, (2) anterior spinal artery, (3) sulcocommissural artery, (4) vasocorona, (5) posterior radicular branch, (6) anterior radicular branch. (Adapted from Kahle 1984,[1] with permission.)

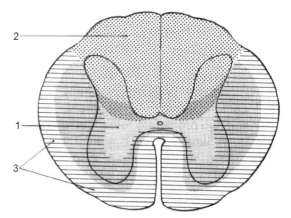

Figure 2.16 Areas of the spinal cord supplied by the different arteries: (1) anterior spinal artery, (2) posterior spinal artery, (3) plexus of the vasocorona. (Adapted from Kahle 1984,[1] with permission.)

enlargements, and thinnest in the midthoracic area. The anterior spinal artery gives off branches that penetrate the commissura alba, the sulcocommissural arteries, and branches that anastomose with the posterior spinal arteries to form a vascular ring (vasocorona) around the spinal cord. From this ring, vessels penetrate the white matter (*Fig. 2.15*).

Segmental arteries give off 31 pairs of spinal rami, which pass through the intervertebral foramina, then divide into an anterior and a posterior radicular branch, to supply the spinal roots and the meninges. Only a few of these radicular branches reach the spinal cord itself.

Topographically, the anterior spinal artery vascularizes the anterior horns, the most ventral part of the posterior horns, and most of the anterolateral funiculi. The posterior spinal arteries supply the remainder of the posterior horns and the posterior funiculi. The marginal zone of the anterolateral funiculi is supplied by the vasocorona (*Fig. 2.16*). As a whole, gray matter is much more richly vascularized than white matter.

Spinal cord syndromes

Complete transection

A complete transection of the spinal cord divides all the descending motor tracts, as well as all ascending sensory tracts. As a result complete paralysis occurs below the lesion. As stated above, muscles whose motor nucleus lies across the spinal lesion are only partially affected. If the damage occurs at the cervical enlargement and above, tetraplegia results, whereas lesions between the cervical enlargement and the lumbar enlargement result in paraplegia. All lesions above the sacral cord result in a loss of voluntary control of urination and defecation. Complete transection also produces a complete sensory loss below the lesion.

Incomplete transection

Incomplete transection of the spinal cord is most frequent at the cervical level,[11] and results in various syndromes according to the exact site and extent of the lesion. These incomplete syndromes are often much more ill-defined than the complete transection syndrome. However, three main syndromes can be recognized: central syndrome, anterior syndrome, and Brown–Sequard syndrome (*Fig. 2.17*).

Central (cord) syndrome

The central (cord) syndrome is the most frequent incomplete syndrome at the cervical level, and accounts for more than half of all incomplete syndromes.[12] It usually results from a hyperextension injury that occurs in a rigid, often osteoarthritic spine, which makes it frequent among older tetraplegic

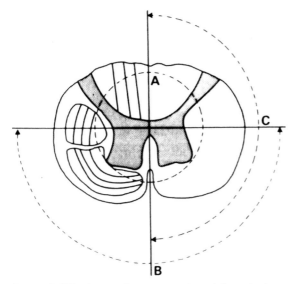

Figure 2.17 Incomplete transection of the spinal cord results: (A) central cord syndrome, (B) anterior syndrome, (C) Brown–Sequard syndrome. (Adapted from Barat and Arne1981,[11] with permission.)

patients. The cord lesion predominates in the gray matter, and extends variably into the white matter.

The clinical picture is dominated by a discrepancy between a severe motor loss in the upper limbs and a mild loss in the lower limbs. Clinical findings usually include:

- flaccid paralysis of the upper limbs, usually involving at least two medullary segments;
- spastic and moderate paralysis of the lower limbs;
- dissociated sensory loss, which predominates in the thorax and upper limbs, with a retained epicritic sensibility and loss of pain and temperature sensations (analgesia and thermoanesthesia); and
- retained control of urination and defecation.

When the spinal lesion is very limited, the clinical picture may be that of an isolated brachial diplegia. When the lesion is more extensive, the tetraplegia may be subtotal, with only sacral sparing.

Anterior syndrome

The anterior syndrome accounts for 25% of incomplete tetraplegias. Isolated by Abercrombie in 1843,[13] it can occur as a result of all types of injuries, with a slight predominance of flexion-induced fracture–dislocations of the spine and of those injuries that cause protrusion of the intervertebral disk. The trauma leads to a lesion of the anterior horns and the anterolateral tracts, with a possible division of the anterior spinal artery. The clinical picture includes:

- flaccid paralysis of the upper limbs, covering several segments;
- initially flaccid paralysis of the lower limbs, with a rapid return of motor reflexes; and
- dissociated sensory loss, disproportionate to the motor loss, with analgesia and thermoanesthesia, but retained epicritic and deep sensibilities, and with frequent infralesional paresthesias.

An isolated lesion of the sulcocommissural arteries results in ischemia of the anterior horns, with an isolated brachial monoplegia or diplegia.

Brown–Sequard syndrome

The Brown–Sequard syndrome follows a hemisection of the spinal cord. Very rarely pure, it is often either incomplete or mixed with other neurological symptoms. It is reported to account for 15–20% of incomplete tetraplegias. The causative spine lesion is usually a fracture and/or dislocation in hyperflexion. When pure, it includes:

- unilateral paralysis of the central type;
- ipsilateral loss of epicritic and deep sensibilities, and the retention of protopathic sensibility produces severe hyperesthesia;
- ipsilateral anesthetic zone above the lesion, resulting from destruction of the posterior root zone of entry at the level of the damage; and
- contralateral dissociated sensory loss, with analgesia and thermoanesthesia, but almost normal touch perception.

Usually, the Brown–Sequard syndrome is partial and mixed, is limited to a more severe picture on one side, has a rapid unilateral recovery; sensory disturbances remain more important on the side that is recovering. Brown–Sequard syndromes have the most favorable prognosis of all incomplete lesions, because in most cases patients recover the ability to walk and satisfactory bowel and bladder control.

References

1. Kahle W. Nervous system and sensory organs. In: Kahle W, Leonhart H, Platzer W, eds. Color Atlas and Textbook of Human Anatomy, Vol. III. 2nd edn. Stuttgart: Thieme; 1984:38–60.
2. Delmas A. Voies et Centres Nerveux. 9th edn. Paris: Masson; 1973:26–63.
3. Dejerine J. Sémiologie des Affections du Système Nerveux. Paris: Masson; 1926.
4. Kendall HO, Kendall FP. Muscle Testing and Function. Baltimore: Williams & Wilkins; 1949.
5. Zancolli E. Structural and Dynamic Basis of Hand Surgery. 2nd edn. Philadelphia: JB Lippincott, 1979.
6. Zancolli E, Zancolli E. Tetraplegies traumatiques. In: Tubiana R, ed. Traite' de Chirurgie de la Main. Paris: Masson; 1991.
7. Tubiana R. Paralyses of thumb. In: Tubiana R, ed. The Hand, Vol. IV. 2nd edn. Philadelphia: Saunders; 1991:221.
8. Barthes G. Contribution à l'étude de la métamérisation motrice médullaire [Thesis]. Université de Paris; 1964.
9. Audic B. The upper extremity and quadriplegia: medical aspects. In: Tubiana R, ed. The Hand, Vol. IV. Philadelphia: Saunders; 1973:529–540.
10. Guttman L. Spinal Cord Injuries. Comprehensive Management and Research. Oxford: Blackwell Scientific; 1973.
11. Barat M, Arne L. Les syndromes incomplets. In: Maury, ed: La Paraplégie. Paris: Flammarion; 1981:172–176.
12. Abercrombie J. Pathological and Practical Researches on Diseases of the Brain and the Spinal Cord. Philadelphia: Lee Blanchard; 1843.

3

Trauma to the cervical spinal cord

Incidence

In the USA, the prevalence of spinal cord trauma is calculated to be approximately 906 per million.[1] This corresponds to approximately 230,000 tetra- and paraplegics. The annual incidence is estimated at 40 new cases per million people, with motor vehicle accidents accounting for the great majority. Other prominent causes include falls, sports and recreational injuries such as diving accidents, and penetrating injuries such as gunshot wounds (see *Table 3.1*). The cervical and lumbar cord is most commonly affected, a consequence of the increased intervertebral motion at these levels. Of these types of injuries, 55% occur

Table 3.1 Etiology of spine injuries seen at the Acute Spine Injury Center of Northwestern University from 1972 to 1990*

Etiology	Number (%)
Automobile	1112 (31.79)
Fall	919 (26.27)
Gunshot	310 (8.86)
Diving	278 (7.95)
Other traumatic	254 (7.26)
Motorcycle	149 (4.26)
Other sports	142 (4.06)
Other medical	131 (3.74)
Pedestrian	94 (2.69)
Other	60 (1.72)
Unknown	49 (1.40)

*Adapted from Meyer (1995, p. 104).[2]

in patients who are 16 to 30 years of age, and males make up 80% of this group. Statistics from a large series of admissions for spinal cord injuries indicate that approximately 58% of all admissions were for cervical spine injuries, of which nearly half occurred at the C5–C6 or the C6–C7 level.[3] Of these, 60% were incomplete and 40% were complete. For the tetraplegic patient, the estimated lifetime cost, including yearly health care and living expenses, exceeds one million US dollars.[1]

Anatomy relative to pathology

The descriptive anatomy of the cervical spinal cord is reviewed in Chapter 2. On average, the cervical spinal cord compromises about 12 cm of the approximately 45 cm of the spinal cord. The cervical spinal cord is made up of eight segments. From these segments variable numbers of rootlets arise to form the spinal nerve of the segment. The cervical cord segments average 13 mm in length. The diameter of the cervical spinal cord is more than that of other areas.

The cervical spinal cord is encased within a bony ring formed from seven cervical vertebrae. The vertebral bodies of the first (atlas) and the second (axis) cervical vertebrae are fused developmentally to form the odontoid process. At this level, the spinal canal is relatively large compared to the diameter of the cervical spinal cord, with the cord occupying only one-third of the volume of the spinal canal versus approximately 50% at the C7 vertebral level. This increased volume of the canal relative to the cord diameter may account for the reduced incidence of neurological complications associated with bony injuries at the upper part of the cervical spine compared to other cervical levels (*Fig. 3.1*). The potential

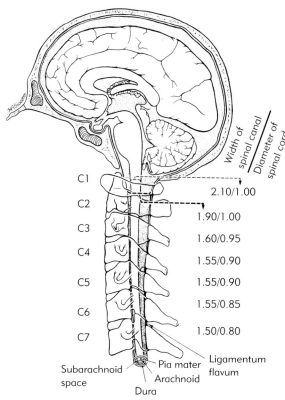

C1

C2

C3

C4

C5

C6

C7

Width of spinal canal

Diameter of spinal cord

2.10/1.00

1.90/1.00

1.60/0.95

1.55/0.90

1.55/0.90

1.55/0.85

1.50/0.80

Subarachnoid space

Pia mater

Arachnoid

Dura

Ligamentum flavum

Figure 3.1 The ratio of spinal canal to spinal cord at various cervical levels. (Adapted from Meyer 1989,[4] with permission.)

range of motion is greatest at the C5, C6, and C7 vertebral levels and the ratio of canal size to cord diameter is larger here (the cord reaches its greatest dimension relative to the spinal canal at about the C4 level). Therefore, it is through these segments that the greatest incidence of spinal cord trauma occurs.

Meyer et al. have conceptualized the lower cervical spine as constructed of three columns (*Fig. 3.2*).[3] The anterior column is formed from the anterior longitudinal ligament and the anterior two-thirds of the vertebral body. The middle column is composed of the posterior one-third of the vertebral body plus the posterior longitudinal ligament and the posterior annulus fibrosis. The posterior column (or vertebral arches) is composed of the facet joint and joint capsule, the spinous processes and the supraspinous and intraspinous ligaments. The facet joints allow flexion, extension, lateral bending, and rotation while serving to restrict translational movements between adjacent vertebral bodies through the disk space. It is through

this posterior column that unexpectedly excessive loads may pass, loads that may exceed the ability of these structures to resist translational movement.

Mechanisms of cervical cord trauma

The bony and ligamentous architecture of the cervical spine permits a significantly greater range of motion than in any other area of the spine. Unfortunately, these same features expose the enclosed cervical spinal cord to injurious forces greater than those experienced by other areas of the spine. The spinal cord may be injured directly by penetrating injuries from bullets or shell fragments or may be penetrated by a knife. However, most injuries occur from one of two primary sources. The first is from axial compression loading ventrally from vertebral body bone fragments following fractures or from herniated disk material. The vertebrae that protect the spinal cord may sustain injury from axial compressive loads that cause burst fractures. For example, burst fractures from closed injuries may drive vertebral body fragments or nucleus material into the spinal cord (*Fig. 3.3*).

The second is traction of the cord that occurs during translational movements between vertebral segments as ligaments are disrupted and the spine becomes unstable. The vertebrae that protect the spinal cord may sustain injury from flexion, extension, lateral bending, or rotational loads that exceed the tolerances of hard and soft tissues. Flexion and rotational forces may cause either unilateral or bilateral facet dislocations. A unilateral facet dislocation (*Fig. 3.4*) causes a twisting of the adjacent vertebral bodies and a compromise of the spinal canal. Bilateral facet dislocation leads to an anterior shift of the adjacent segments, which both compresses and stretches the spinal cord (*Fig. 3.5*). If one facet is dislocated, the cross-sectional area of the spinal canal is reduced by about 25%. Bilateral facet dislocations result in a 50% reduction in the cross-sectional area of the canal. It is estimated that more than 50% of the canal needs to be compromised before spinal cord injury occurs.[5] The most common direction in which excessive loading leads to injurious translation movement and subluxation or dislocation of one or both facets is flexion. In descending order of frequency, the other injurious forces include vertical or axial

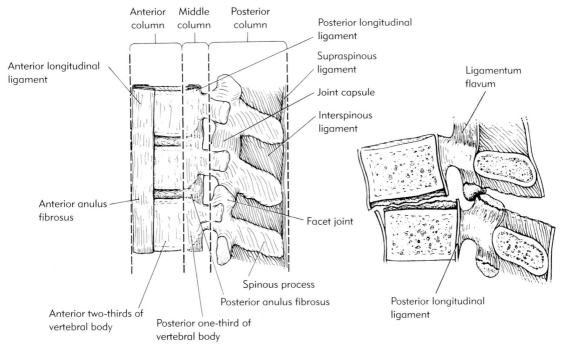

Figure 3.2 The 'three column' theory of vertebral disruption. Loss of any two results in instability. (Adapted from Meyer 1995,[3] with permission.)

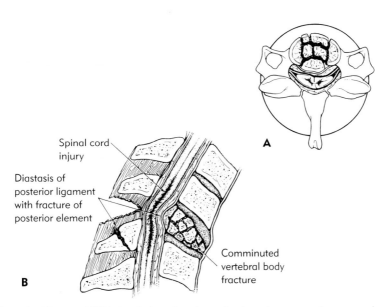

Figure 3.3 (A) Superior view and (B) lateral view showing spinal cord compression secondary to encroachment by elements of the fractured vertebral body. (Adapted from Meyer 1989,[4] with permission.)

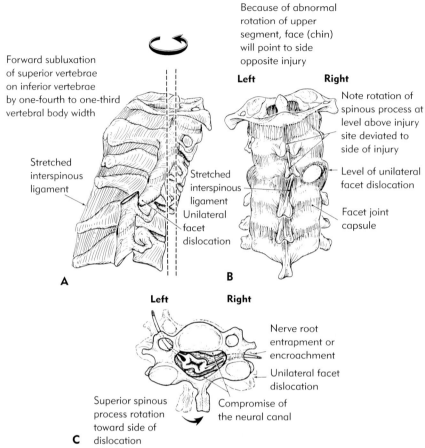

Forward subluxation
of superior vertebrae
on inferior vertebrae
by one-fourth to one-third
vertebral body width

Because of abnormal
rotation of upper
segment, face (chin)
will point to side
opposite injury

Left   **Right**

Note rotation of
spinous process at
level above injury
site deviated to
side of injury

Stretched
interspinous
ligament

Stretched
interspinous
ligament

Unilateral
facet
dislocation

Level of unilateral
facet dislocation

Facet joint
capsule

A

B

Left   **Right**

Nerve root
entrapment or
encroachment

Unilateral facet
dislocation

Superior spinous
process rotation
toward side of
dislocation

Compromise of
the neural canal

C

Figure 3.4   Pathological consequences of a unilateral facet dislocation: (A) lateral, (B) posterior, and (C) overhead transverse views. (Adapted from Meyer 1989,[4] with permission.)

compression, rotation and extension, and lateral bending. High-speed injuries usually produce some combination of these forces.

At one large center, 44% of cervical spine injuries occurred as a consequence of either an axial load or a combined flexion load injury.[3] The radiographic picture is either a wedge compression fracture or a 'teardrop' fracture of the vertebral body. Within this group of cervical spine injuries, almost 50% sustained either a complete or partial neurological injury. While injuries from either axial or torsional loading may be associated with observable fractures, their significance may be as indicators of ligament disruption.

Injury can occur to any level of the cervical spine. Odontoid fractures represent the superior-most types of injuries.[3] Injury at the higher levels, such as C2, may cause subluxations or rotational injuries, but these injuries are not typically associated with neurological findings because of the larger diameter of the spinal canal relative to cord size (discussed above). In one large series of odontoid fractures, between 70 and 75% of patients had no neurological consequences, 20% an incomplete injury, and only 5% a complete neurological injury.[3]

Histopathology of spinal cord trauma

Trauma to the spinal cord leads to a well-studied series of cytochemical and histologically identifiable events. The histological events can be separated into three basic phases, an acute reactive stage that lasts 2–3 weeks, a reparative stage that lasts for a variable period of time, and a stage of chronic scarring.

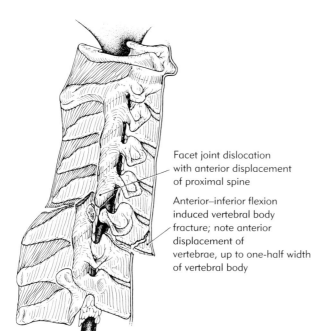

Facet joint dislocation with anterior displacement of proximal spine

Anterior–inferior flexion induced vertebral body fracture; note anterior displacement of vertebrae, up to one-half width of vertebral body

Figure 3.5 Pathological consequences of a bilateral facet dislocation. (Adapted from Meyer 1989,[4] with permission.)

Phase 1: immediate consequences

Contusion or frank laceration of the spinal cord disrupts the axonal pathways, destroys cell bodies within the zone of injury, and generates reactive exudates. Initial hemorrhage and rapid loss of dendritic integrity occurs as the injured axons and their myelin sheaths begin to disintegrate. Blood clots that form are eventually replaced by connective tissue scar. Neuronal cell bodies may be disrupted immediately by the force of injury or undergo cytopathological changes associated with disruption of their dendritic processes, referred to as central chromatolysis.

Following the initial hemorrhage, leukocytes move into the area and edema develops, which causes additional swelling of the spinal cord, identified on imaging studies as a change from the normal oval to a more rounded appearance. This further reduces the free space within the vertebral canal. The cord in the injured area becomes tense, with obliteration of subdural spaces, and develops a characteristic spindle shape, with a fusiform region of cord softening and typically a central area of necrosis in the posterior portion of the cord.

Phase 2: the reparative stage

The acute events subside over the initial 2–3 weeks. Acute inflammatory cells are replaced by phagocytory cells, a period referred to as reactive astrocytic gliosis. These cells ingest lipid debris from the breakdown of axons and cells. In the areas of greatest trauma, even the glial cells are destroyed and in this area only fibroblastic derived, connective tissue scar forms. Surviving neuronal cells are characterized by central chromatolysis, eccentric nuclei, and swollen cytoplasm, changes that persist for years.

Phase 3: stage of chronic scar

If post-injury survival is sufficiently long, the injured tissues are replaced by dense acellular connective tissue scar that fixes cord to meninges. For at least one segment above and below the zone of major injury, the parenchyma of the cord is characterized by an intense astrocytic fibrous gliosis.

Late changes

Many months or even years after the injury, long after neurological stability has been achieved, the patient may begin to experience a deterioration of previously surviving or recovered functions as a consequence of upward extension of the injury. The signs are exactly those associated with the development of primary syringomyelia, the pathological basis of which is a progressive spinal cord cavitation. The central portion of the cord is most affected, with the gray commissure and one or both posterior horns destroyed. The wall of the cavity consists of a glial connective tissue layer. The process can extend as far rostrally as the medulla. While most of the effect is proximal, the cavitation can extend distally as well, although this extension is typically neurologically silent.

Neurophysiology of spinal cord injuries

Spinal cord trauma that produces paralysis over a very short time course typically causes what is termed 'spinal shock', which is characterized by areflexia, atonia, and lack of response to plantar stimulation. These characteristics are presumed to be the sequelae of the withdrawal of descending facilitative influences from higher centers.

The bulbocavernosus reflex returns most rapidly, while tendon reflexes and muscle tone return more slowly, over several weeks, only to become exaggerated. This hyperactivity of either lower or both lower and upper extremity reflexes is seen in essentially all patients after cervical cord injury.

As opposed to the diffuse effects of most diseases that affect the spinal cord, such as multiple sclerosis, focal lesions affect the spinal cord in a much more clear-cut fashion. Characteristic abnormalities exist just above and at the level of the lesion and equally characteristic effects are seen below the lesion.

Findings at the level of injury

Very obvious sequelae of spinal cord trauma are seen at and below the lesion. These are best recognized by electrophysiological analysis of muscle innervated just above the lesion. Studies indicate that many physiological parameters are altered in what seem to be muscles of normal strength.[6] These include abnormal motor-unit firing patterns and rates. It is postulated that these effects may result from altered sensory inputs to motor axons or from alterations in the feedback from paretic muscles. More recently, studies using focal magnetic stimulation techniques that permit noninvasive stimulation of areas of the cortex demonstrated cortical remodeling as a consequence of spinal cord injury.[6]

At the level of the injury, trauma causes the death of a region of cells. This region is termed the 'injury zone'. Depending on the trauma, one or more segments may suffer death and, within a single segment, injury may be complete, partial, or patchy. Immediately following injury, the electromyogram (EMG) obtained from muscles innervated by cells within the injury zone is not revealing. The signal is devoid of voluntary motor units and there are no signs of muscle denervation.[7]

Within 2–3 weeks signs of denervation are apparent. Commonly seen are fibrillation potentials and positive sharp waves, which result from a motor axon losing contact with its parent cell body. Paraspinous muscles exhibit these abnormalities before the more peripheral muscles.

Where the lesion is incomplete, signs of reinnervation may be seen within one to several months. The earliest findings include increasing numbers of prolonged polyphasic motor units. The increase in numbers and size of motor units is frequently associated with gains in muscle strength. Improvement in strength of previously paralyzed muscles may be a consequence of terminal sprouting of surviving motor axons, as opposed to regeneration of new fibers from the zone of injury. This sprouting may lead to dysfunctional motor activity, such as arm–diaphragm synkinesis following high cervical cord injury.

Even clinically complete spinal cord lesions may still have some surviving motor axons, which are recognizable on EMG analysis, within the injury zone. The EMG data also suggest the loss of motor axons over multiple spinal cord segments (at least three to four myotomes) distal to the zone of injury. A reduced number of axons will innervate a greater than normal number of muscle fibers. These findings, which show the loss of motor neurons from two to five spinal levels below the zone of injury, have important consequences for the usefulness of various functional electrostimulation techniques (see Chapter 17). The true zone of injury and alteration is clearly much more extensive than previously assumed.

Other studies indicate differences in the ability of ventral and dorsally located cells to survive injury.[6] Sensory and motor levels from ventral primary rami correlate reasonably well with the radiographically apparent bony injury. In contrast, motor activity is seen in dorsal primary rami innervated paraspinous muscles two to three segments distal to the site of bony injury. Sensory function in the distribution of dorsal primary rami is preserved from one to six segments below that seen in anterior primary rami innervated dermatomes.

Findings below the level of injury

With a complete lesion of the spinal cord there is no voluntary activity in muscle caudal to the lesion. However, as there is continuity of motor cell, axon, and muscle fiber, there are no fibrillation potentials on EMG analysis to suggest denervation. Motor and sensory conduction should also be normal.

Exceptions to these expected findings occur and may be caused by such things as the development of, or in circumstances of pre-existing (to spinal cord injury), peripheral nerve entrapments. Extensive evidence demonstrates a high incidence of focal peripheral nerve lesions in the spinal cord injury population, with up to 36% of patients with cervical cord injury demonstrating abnormal upper extremity potentials.[6,7]

Autonomic dysfunction

With complete cervical cord injury, the autonomic nervous system is totally cut off from communications with the brain. This isolation from higher centers may be relevant to such occurrences as autonomic dysreflexia. Studies indicate a reduced level of spontaneous activity of sympathetic fibers in spinal cord injury patients. On the other hand, greatly prolonged (over normal) sympathetic responses to stimuli have been observed. These prolonged discharges are often coupled discharges of motor axons to skeletal muscles. The consequence is an inability of the sympathetic system to provide a specific and time-limited response below the level of injury.

Post-injury patterns

Electromyographic analyses of individuals following spinal cord injuries demonstrate characteristic features depending on whether the injury is partial or total. Muscles innervated proximal to the zone of spinal injury exhibit electrophysiological parameters,

including some reduction in the numbers of voluntary motor units, possibly as a consequence of the proximal effects of the spinal cord injury on proximally located motor axons. However, EMG recordings are otherwise relatively normal. Muscles innervated by motor horn cells at the zone of injury exhibit EMG evidence of a lower motor neuron palsy, including positive sharp waves, fibrillation potentials, and absent or very greatly reduced voluntary motor potentials. Muscles innervated distal to the zone of complete injury show EMG characteristics of an upper motor neuron paralysis, including the absence of voluntary motor units, the absence of fibrillation potentials in the presence of positive sharp waves, and spontaneous discharges.

Upper limb muscle recovery following cervical cord trauma

Using manual muscle testing, Ditunno et al.[8] and Waters et al.[9] studied recovery rates of several key muscles of the upper limb following cervical cord trauma, including the biceps, wrist extensors, and triceps. Only one-third of those with Medical Research Council (MRC) Grade 0 muscles at 1 month achieved a strength equal to or greater than Grade 3 at 4–6 months post-injury. However, in these muscles, motor recovery was seen as late as 24 months following injury, even in patients with MRC Grade 0 at 1 month.

With the exception of the triceps, all upper limb muscles with an initial strength of MRC Grade 1 recovered to at least Grade 3 at 1 year following injury. For example, Waters et al. reported that 97% of wrist extensors with an initial strength of MRC Grade 1 recovered to at least Grade 3 at 1 year following injury.[9] Of those patients with some muscle function at 1 month, 80% eventually reached MRC Grade 3, with the median strength of the patients studied reaching MRC Grade 4 during the first 4–6 months. If the muscle's strength was greater than MRC Grade 1 at 1 month post-injury, the median time to full recovery was about 6 months. Most muscle recovery occurred within the first 9 months (*Table 3.2*).[9]

Only 10% of patients with complete tetraplegia at 1 month following injury convert to an incomplete status.

Table 3.2 Prediction of upper extremity motor recovery

Manual muscle strength at 1 month*	Functional strength >3/5 at 1 year (%) Complete tetraplegia	Incomplete tetraplegia
0/5	20	24
1/5	90	73
2/5	100	100

*American Spinal Injury Association key muscles.

Other types of spinal cord pathology

Ischemia

The spinal cord is more resistant to the effects of ischemia than the brain. Animal studies indicate that the cord can be ischemic for periods up to 30 minutes without deleterious effects. However, when ischemia occurs, it affects primarily gray matter of the cord, the metabolic requirements of which are 3–5 times those of white matter. The effect is infarction of the central gray matter leading to motor paralysis and, frequently, sensory sparing since the long tracts survive the ischemic insult.

Cervical spondylolysis

Spondylolysis is defined as a nontraumatic or traumatic subluxation between two adjacent vertebral bodies. Posterior displacement may compromise the cord. There may be a vascular ischemic etiology to paralysis associated with cervical spondylolysis.

Degenerative arthritis

The effects of degenerative arthritis of the spine are more prominently manifest at those areas that exhibit the greatest range of motion, as is the case with trauma to the cervical spine. Osteophytes may protrude into the central canal, which effectively narrows the canal. There may be rupture of posterior ligamentous support and protrusion of nuclear material, and so the cord is further compromised. The spinal canal may be congenitally narrowed, especially in stocky individuals. These events may result in a canal with a normal anterior–posterior diameter of 17–18 mm becoming one with a diameter of only 9–10 mm. A fall onto an extended neck in an individual with a canal compromised by congenital or acquired stenosis of the spinal canal may result in tetraplegia. These injuries typically result in a syndromic incomplete tetraplegia, as discussed in Chapter 2.

References

1. Center NSCIS. Spinal cord injury: facts and figures at a glance. J Spinal Cord Med 2000; 23(2):153–156.
2. Meyer PR. Spinal cord injury. In: Young R, Woolsey R, eds. Diagnosis and Management of Disorders of the Spinal Cord. Philadelphia: WB Saunders; 1995:104.
3. Meyer PCG, Rusin J, Haak M. Spinal cord injury. In: Woolsey RM, Young RR, eds. Disorders of the Spinal Cord. Neurologic Clinics; Vol. 9. Philadelphia: WB Saunders; 1991:671–678.
4. Meyer PR. Surgery of Spine Trauma. New York: Churchill Livingstone; 1989.
5. Bedbrook G. Some pertinent observations on the pathology of traumatic spinal paralysis. Paraplegia 1963; 1:215–227.
6. Shefner JM, Tun C. Clinical neurophysiology of focal spinal cord injuries. In: Woolsey RM, Young RR, eds. Disorders of the Spinal Cord. Neurologic Clinics; Vol. 9. Philadelphia: WB Saunders, 1991:671–678.
7. Berman S, Young R, Sarkarati M, et al. Injury zone denervation in traumatic quadriplegia in humans. Muscle Nerve 1996; 19:701–706.
8. Ditunno JF, Stover S, Freed M, et al. Motor recovery of the upper extremities in traumatic quadriplegia: a multicenter study. Arch Phys Med Rehabil 1992; 73:431–436.
9. Waters RL, Adkins R, Yakura J, et al. Motor and sensory recovery following complete tetraplegia. Arch Phys Med Rehabil 1993; 74:242–247.

4

Initial protection of the upper limbs

Introduction

The major objective of the initial treatment of patients with acute spinal cord injury is preservation of the functional and anatomic continuity of the spinal cord. In a similar sense, preserving the health of the upper limbs must become a top priority in the acute post-injury and early rehabilitation period. Typically, the tetraplegic patient arrives at the acute care facility with uninjured, normal upper limbs. Left unattended, the joints rapidly become stiff, swollen, contracted, and painful and, once limb pathology becomes established, an inordinate amount of time and effort will be required to regain upper limb health. This adds considerably to the rehabilitative burden to be faced by the patient, family, and health care providers. However, a review of protocols from several spinal cord injury facilities indicates that far more attention is paid to such issues as bowel and bladder care than to concerns for the upper limbs. As mentioned in the Preface, however, tetraplegic patients would prefer to have upper limb function restored more than lower limb or sexual function.[1]

The acute injury period (0–6 weeks)

The initial care involves many disciplines, including physicians, psychologists, and occupational and physical therapists. The initial upper limb evaluation usually falls to the therapist, who assesses and records the status of the patient's upper limbs in terms of residual muscle power, joint range of motion, and sensation. If the patient has suffered a concomitant upper extremity injury or arrives at the acute care facility with a pre-existing condition, such as degenerative arthritis or rotator cuff pathology, the exact nature of the injury, the treatment already given, and any exercise restrictions secondary to injury and treatment must be transmitted to the therapist.

The initial treatment plan differs according to the level of injury; however, the principal therapy goals for all upper limbs in the initial weeks to months following injury include:

- preventing and treating hand edema;
- maintaining supple joints; and
- controlling pain and spasticity.

Prevention and treatment of edema

Edema of the hands and arms occurs to some degree in all tetraplegic patients. One of the significant components of neurogenic shock is the loss of sympathetic tone. This loss of autonomic innervation leads to abnormalities in vasomotor control characterized by a marked increase in arteriovenous shunting, an increase in capillary and venous pressures, and venous dilatation. Proteins of high molecular weight leak across endothelial basement membranes and stimulate the extracellular transudation of plasma fluids. This sympathetic-mediated edema fluid cannot be returned easily intravascularly, because the normal pumping action of the skeletal muscles is absent in the paralyzed limb. These protein-rich fluids are deemed to be the precursors of periarticular and peritendinous fibrosis.

Hand elevation

'... care being taken that the hand be not lower than the elbow, but a little higher, so that the blood do not flow toward the extremity ...' Hippocrates

Unless the hands are positioned well above heart level, the increased venous pressure that attends the

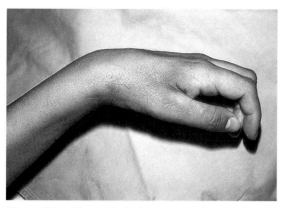

Figure 4.1 The pathological posture frequently assumed by the injured or paralyzed hand is one of wrist flexion and metacarpophalangeal joint extension.

dependent upper limb will magnify the edema. Therefore, one of the major tenets in the initial management of the acutely injured tetraplegic patient is to elevate the hands above heart level, either on pillows, during the period of bed-rest, or in some type of overhead support. Controlling the position of the wrist plays an important role in preventing edema. The major venous and lymphatic drainage from the digits and hand is via veins and lymphatic ducts that pass across the dorsum of the hand, which is why the dorsum of the paralyzed hand is the site of the most significant swelling. The paralyzed and unsupported hand frequently assumes the posture illustrated in *Figure 4.1*. Gravity causes wrist flexion, tightening of the extensor tendons, and metacarpophalangeal joint hyperextension. However, if the wrist is held

A

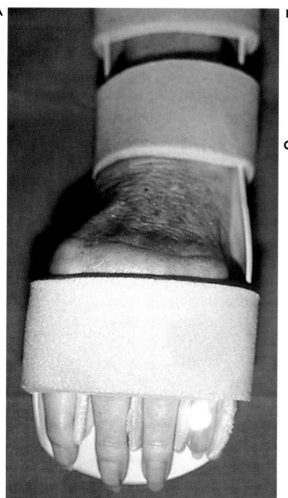

B

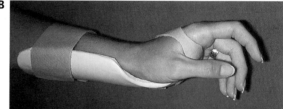

C

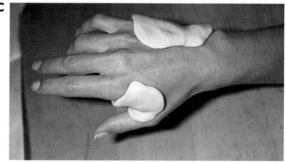

Figure 4.2 Several different types of splints useful in the acute injury period are illustrated. (A) Full hand resting splint that stabilizes the wrist in an extended position and the fingers in some flexion, (B) a long opponens splint that leaves the fingers free, and (C) a short hand splint that maintains the normal palmar arch of the hand.

extended, the viscoelastic properties of the flexor muscles of the fingers automatically flex the fingers at the metacarpophalangeal joint, which tightens the dorsal soft tissues and increases interstitial pressure enough to reduce extravascular fluid extravasation (edema). This position is best achieved with an orthosis individually fitted to both hands as soon as feasible by the physical or occupational therapist.

Splinting

Early application of a resting hand splint that maintains the wrist in near full extension and the metacarpophalangeal joints in near full flexion seems to provide protection against the development of edema. The therapist should determine whether the patient would benefit from a full or a short resting hand splint (*Fig. 4.2*). If wrist extension is less than Medical Research Council (MRC) Grade 3 or the wrist muscles are spastic or contracted, then a full resting hand splint is fabricated. Otherwise, a short resting hand splint is adequate. The initial splint requires frequent adjustment so that pressure points do not lead to skin ulceration. The splints are intended for use at night, but also during the day when the patient is not undergoing other therapy measures such as joint ranging, etc.

A recommended schedule for night-time use involves the patient wearing the splint for 2 h on the first night. The splints are removed and skin integrity evaluated. If any skin problems are noted, the splint is discontinued until adjustments are made. The therapist modifies the splint accordingly and then supervises a trial of splint wearing to make sure the pressure area is relieved. Wearing time is increased by increments of 1 h each night until the patient is able to tolerate the splint all night. It is useful for the therapist to post a schedule for night-time splinting at the patient's bedside.

Massage, compression, and exercise

If edema is present, developing, or persisting despite proper positioning and splinting, the patient may benefit from the application of an elastic compression glove. The risk that compression gloves may cause harmful levels of pressure requires frequent monitoring of the skin under the gloves.

Retrograde massage, combined with exercise, assists in moving edema fluids from interstitial to intravascular spaces. The role of exercise in pre-

venting and treating edema is discussed below in the context of preventing joint stiffness.

Maintaining supple joints

Stiffness and contracture are terms that are frequently, but incorrectly, used interchangeably. Stiffness is defined as increased resistance to movement and contracture is defined as an inability of a joint or muscle to be moved, either actively or passively, through its typical range of motion. Stiffness and contracture are unfortunately accepted by many clinicians as an unavoidable consequence of spinal cord injury. These dysfunctional deformities are multifactorial in etiology.[2] In the tetraplegic patient, normal muscles and muscles that suffer either an upper or lower motor neuron paralysis may suffer contracture. In lower motor neuron paralysis, also termed flaccid paralysis, the muscle itself undergoes major morphological alteration with loss of elastic muscle elements and replacement by inelastic fibrous tissue. The upper motor neuron paralyzed muscle is spastic to a greater or lessor degree, with its activity uncontrollable except by indirect measures such as pharmacological antispasmodic agents. Even the remaining normally innervated muscles may become pathological deformers because their actions are unrestrained by proper antagonists.

Positioning in bed

For most patients, positioning in bed should be designed to counter the tendency for the limbs to assume abnormal postures, which if untreated interfere with rehabilitation goals. For example, the acutely injured patient typically lies in the supine position on a soft mattress for long periods of time. The supine position is desirable for many reasons including ease of nursing, feeding, bathing, and catheterization. However, in this position, the trunk sinks into the mattress, the scapulae are pushed forward into antepulsion, and the pectoralis and serratus muscles rapidly undergo contraction. This contracture compromises shoulder motion and increases the risk of shoulder pain (*Fig. 4.3*).

When the recently injured patient lies supine, a soft pillow or wedge should be used to support the spine. This prevents the shoulders from rolling forward and places the pectoralis muscles under some stretch. Periods of time spent in the prone position

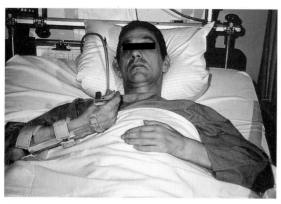

Figure 4.3 The patient should not lie for long periods with the arms across the chest, as this pulls the scapulae forward and increases the risk of the development of stiff, painful shoulders. The position also accentuates elbow flexion, which increases the risk of elbow flexion contracture.

are useful since, in this position, the shoulders are forced into a position of retropulsion. However, this position is difficult for the acutely injured patient to maintain because of the additional labor of respiration. The patient who wears a halo or cervical collar requires special efforts to achieve proper limb position and support.

Avoiding abnormal upper limb postures

Proper positioning in bed must also take into account the level of spinal cord injury and an understanding of the etiology of the abnormal resting postures of the upper limb, which differ according to the level of medullary injury. Spasticity-induced abnormal limb postures increase the risk of developing edema, with stiffness leading to contractures, pain, and spasticity.

For injuries above the C5 level, the arms are typically held adducted at the shoulder and the forearms are held in pronation. For such injuries, the arms should be positioned in some abduction and the forearms in supination, at least in the initial stages.

Injury at the C5 segment spares some innervation of the levator scapulae and rhomboid muscles. The trapezius muscle is fully innervated. The action of these shoulder elevators is unopposed because all the shoulder depressor muscles are paralyzed and the shoulder may be very elevated. Some innervation of the supra and infraspinatus muscles may also be spared and thus some abduction and external rotation

of the arm may be seen. However, because of paralysis of the deltoid and biceps muscles, the arms typically lie motionless and adducted aside the body. The arms should be positioned in some abduction and supported by pillows. Shoulder elevation is difficult to counteract until the patient begins to sit (*Fig. 4.4*).

Injury primarily at the C6 segment results in a very characteristic posture of the upper limb. The unopposed activities of the shoulder elevators (trapezius, levator scapulae), the external rotators and abductors of the arm (supraspinatus, deltoid), and the flexors of the elbow (biceps) cause the shoulders to be elevated, the arm abducted, and the elbow held in flexion. Injuries at the C6 level are at risk for the development of abduction contractures of the shoulders and flexion contractures of the elbows. The patient should lie with the shoulders adducted, with the arms extended by the side (*Fig. 4.4*) as opposed to lying across the chest (*Fig. 4.3*).

Injury at the C7 segment spares some shoulder depressors and elbow extensors. Therefore, while the posture of the arm may still be one of abduction at the shoulder, the action is somewhat better balanced than that in the C6 level injury. The elbow may still be held somewhat flexed, but less so since some triceps innervation may be present. However, the wrist extensors are strong and unopposed and the hand and wrist, and perhaps the fingers, are held extended or hyperextended. Very early, wrist splints should be fitted to maintain the wrist in 20–30° of extension to prevent excessive wrist extension. Extension of the wrist helps maintain the fingers in some flexion.

Injuries at the C8 segment are not typically associated with abnormal arm posture. However, clawing of the fingers may be evident since the finger extensors are unopposed by the intrinsic muscles of the hand.

Proper limb positioning during the acute immobilization period forms one of the four cornerstones to the prevention of stiffness and contracture. The other cornerstones are early passive ranging of paralyzed joints, education and persistent care until maximum recovery is obtained.

Exercise

'It should be kept in mind that exercise strengthens and inactivity wastes' Hippocrates

A

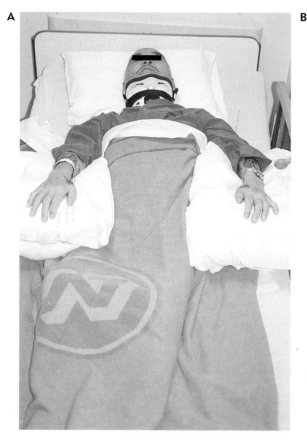

B

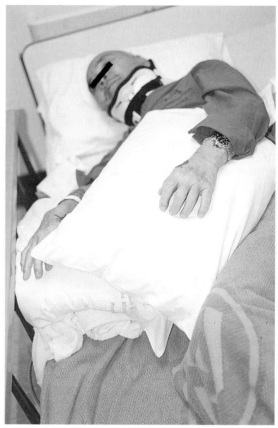

C

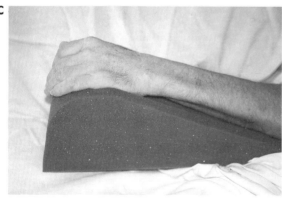

Figure 4.4 Proper supine bed positioning (A) during the acute post-injury period involves using pillows to prevent forward flexion of the shoulders, maintain the arms elevated, and support the wrists and hands. (B) The proper position for side-lying. (C) A commercially available foam support for the paralyzed arm and hand.

An immobilized joint undergoes degeneration over time, even in the absence of local injury. To prevent edema, stiffness, and joint degeneration, a systematic passive exercise protocol based on the extent of neurological injury should be developed for each patient. Even passive movement of the hands and arms moves interstitial fluid intravascularly. Early exercise may lessen the possibility of the patient developing profound bone demineralization, termed Sudek's atrophy,[3] which may be found in up to 20% of tetraplegic patients.

Early, and on a regular basis, splints should be removed and all the joints of the upper limb moved through as complete a range of passive motion as pain and edema allow. This is one part of the early treatment that can be taught to family members and others so that the responsibilities for therapy do not fall solely upon therapists and nursing staff. Some practitioners believe that moving a joint through its range once a day is sufficient to prevent contracture, although more frequent exercise seems ideal.

Education

Early education of the patient and family focuses on teaching passive range of motion exercises, how to put on and take off night splints, and checking for pressure areas. The therapist should demonstrate the proper technique for ranging joints and positioning pillows and have the family practice under supervision. Once the family demonstrates the proper technique, they are encouraged to perform the exercises. The patient is also educated to provide clear verbal instructions regarding care, and encouraged to be an active participant.

Pain and spasticity

Pain

Pain immediately following spinal cord trauma arises from injury to hard and soft tissues as part of the fractures and dislocations and from nerve sources, such as injured nerve roots and damage to the cord.[4] This pain from the acute injury usually resolves within weeks to months of the injury. In addition to the acute pain suffered by all patients, about 90% of spinal cord injury patients complain of the delayed onset of a different and troublesome pain. However, more than two-thirds of these indicate that the pain eventually stablizes and is controllable by conservative measures. For the remaining one-third, this secondary pain persists and magnifies the disability.

Several categories of pain have been identified. Root (peripheral nerve/segmental) pain is typically described as sharp, stabbing, or shooting, falls within neurological segments, and may be aggravated by light touch. Treatment may include cervical traction, analgesics, tricyclic agents, nerve blocks, or even rhizotomy. Central spinal cord (deafferent) pain is usually described as burning, squeezing, and continuous. It may be perceived at the level of injury (segmental) or below (phantom). Interestingly, cervical cord injuries have the lowest probability of developing chronic pain syndromes, for reasons as yet undetermined.

In the early post-injury period, if upper limb pain interferes with proper positioning, splint wear, or

exercise, an integrated, comprehensive approach to pain management is ideal. This includes a careful examination for the source of pain, such as an overlooked wrist or shoulder injury, or a concomitant brachial plexus injury. Electromyography (EMG) and magnetic resonance imaging (MRI) may be appropriate. Once the likely cause of persistent pain has been established, then an orderly trial of non-pharmacological strategies should begin. These include transcutaneous nerve stimulation, traction (where spinal stability is not an issue), acupuncture, massage, and prudent use of mobilization techniques. If unsuccessful, pharmacological measures are needed. An analgesic 'ladder' for malignant pain, as proposed by the World Health Organization, has merit. The lowest 'rungs' of the ladder include nonopioid analgesics, such as nonsteroidal anti-inflammatory drugs, followed by mild opioid agents such as codeine. Adjuvants, including tricyclic antidepressants (such as amitryptyline), selective serotonin re-uptake inhibitors (such as paroxitine), or anticonvulsants (such as gabapentine or tegretol) may be beneficial. Sympathetic or peripheral nerve blocks are of limited benefit in this population.

Spasticity

Fortunately, the upper limbs are often less prone to debilitating spasticity than the lower limbs. Spasticity is more common and problematic in incomplete versus complete cord injuries (e.g., in central cord type lesions). Uncontrolled upper limb spasticity developing in the acute or early rehabilitation period interferes with rehabilitation and must be treated aggressively. However, the management of problematic generalized spasticity is a therapeutic challenge. Initially, nonpharmacological physical modalities, including heat, cold, massage, manipulation, and electrical stimulation, should be tried. If unsuccessful, oral medications include such γ-aminobutyric acid 'B' agonists as baclofen or gabapentin, long-acting benzodiazepines such as clonazepam, or anticonvulsant agents. These same agents may be administered intrathecally by injection or by indwelling catheters and drug pumps.

In contrast, if one or more specific upper limb muscles are affected by significant spasticity, such as the elbow flexors or the intrinsic muscles of the hand, they may be selectively targeted for motor nerve or motor-point injections of various agents. Phenol[5,6] and alcohol have long been used. These are not reliably reversible and should be used with great discretion and only following a therapeutic trial with a long-acting local anesthetic agent such as bupivacaine. Their use in incomplete spinal cord lesions may lead to impaired recovery and diminished ultimate function. In addition, the long-term response is suboptimal. Braun *et al.* report that only four of 15 patients had an acceptable long-term response to phenol blockade.[7]

The bacillus *Clostridium botulinum* produces an exotoxic protein that causes a subtotal flaccid paralysis of muscles by interfering with acetylcholine release at the neuromuscular junction. It binds rapidly with axon terminals and little escapes the intramuscular injection site to cause systemic effects. It has gained wide use as a means of controlling spasticity since its effect is essentially completely reversible within 2–3 months of injection. It has been used with success in C5/C6 tetraplegia to block spastic forearm muscles.[8,9]

The early rehabilitation period

Once the spinal injury has stabilized sufficiently, the patient is allowed to sit in bed and eventually to sit upright in a wheelchair for increasing periods of time. Treatment becomes more focused on rehabilitation. If acute upper limb care has been diligently performed and the limbs maintained supple and pain-free, the patient can move forward toward the goal of greater independence. On the other hand, upper limb pathology caused by neglect must be overcome before the patient can progress toward rehabilitation goals.

Overcoming stiff, spastic, or painful joints

Joints that become painful and stiff restrict the patient from rapid rehabilitation. Frequently, a newly injured patient is transferred to the spinal cord center from the acute care hospital, where he or she has spent weeks to months lying supine in bed with the arms draped across the chest (*Fig. 4.3*). In such cases, the abnormal limb postures discussed above will have become painful, fixed deformities.

In general, slow static stretching may be the most effective and safest immediate treatment. The goal is to obtain some increased range of motion at each

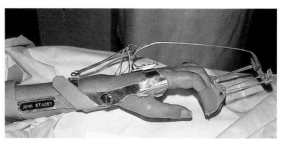

Figure 4.5 A rubber-band powered extension outrigger can be attached to a long opponens splint to overcome contracted fingers.

therapy session and then protect the gain in range with appropriate splinting between sessions. Prolonged traction (*Fig. 4.5*) may be used to slowly stretch a contracted joint, but it carries the risk of causing pressure sores. Other measures include nerve blocks or surgery.

Any neglected joint becomes stiff, contracted, and painful. Several predominate, but all must be treated if all rehabilitation goals are to be met.

The shoulder

Shoulder pathology is a significant problem in the tetraplegic patient population. Silverskiold studied a population of spinal cord injury patients and determined that 78% of tetraplegics experienced some shoulder symptoms during the first 6 months following injury.[10] By 18 months, the percentage had decreased, but these were significantly symptomatic patients in whom shoulder pain interfered with function. Overuse problems are very common sources of reduced function.

Campbell's findings in 24 tetraplegic patients followed during the acute period recognized the following as etiologies of shoulder pain:[11]

- capsular contracture and/or capsulitis;
- rotator cuff pathology and instability;
- osteonecrosis; and
- osteoarthritis.

Capsulitis and contracture

Unless proper positioning is employed soon after injury and vigorous passive range of motion exercises are performed the glenohumeral joint quickly becomes contracted in internal rotation. At best, this pathology limits upper limb mobility when the patient reaches the point of being able to sit in a wheelchair. More often, this contracture is associated with acute shoulder pain. Once shoulder stiffness becomes even minimally established, attempts at therapy typically trigger a second pathological feature, spasticity of parascapular and other upper motor neuron injury muscles. Shoulder pain then becomes a formidable deterrent to the rehabilitation goals.

Treatment for the stiffening and acutely painful shoulder is a rapid and aggressive response to the earliest signs of difficulty. This includes pain control modalities, anti-inflammatory, anti-spastic, and anti-adrenergic pharmacology, and gentle but persistent therapy. This can be a major challenge for the patient and rehabilitation team.

Rotator cuff pathology and instability

Without a full complement of shoulder-stabilizing muscles, as the patient begins to sit and move into the wheelchair he or she experiences instability; the principal direction of instability depends upon which muscles remain well innervated. Anterior instability predominates, followed by what is termed multi-directional instability. This is associated with pain as the muscles and ligaments become overstretched. Tears of the rotator cuff, perhaps antecedent to spinal cord injury, complicate the picture.

For the tetraplegic patient, most surgeons are reluctant to perform the common procedures developed to stabilize the unstable shoulder in ambulating patients. In the tetraplegic population, the results of stabilizing procedures are unpredictable, the post-surgical rehabilitation time is long, and the therapy arduous. For the rare patient with very high medullary lesions, a severely painful unstable shoulder might even require early (prior to 1 year) fusion to allow the patient to move forward with rehabilitation.

Osteonecrosis

Currently, essentially all victims of spinal cord trauma receive massive doses of corticosteroids within hours of injury. A small percentage develop osteonecrosis of the humeral head, characterized by pain, radio-lucency, and (in a significant number) collapse of the humeral head. Such unfortunate patients cannot bear weight, which curtails many rehabilitation plans. Various treatments have been advocated, including core decompression and placement of vascularized bone grafts. As yet, insufficient numbers of treated

patients have been followed to determine the best course of treatment.

Osteoarthritis

Once the patient begins to transfer, perform weight shifts, and push the wheelchair, the acromion assumes the role of the acetabulum of the hip, with the development of painful synovitis and, ultimately, rotator cuff attrition, as well as osteoarthritis of the glenohumeral joint. This is typically a problem that develops over time rather than during the early rehabilitation period.

The elbow

In the tetraplegic patient the elbow assumes significant weight-bearing roles in such activities as pressure relief and transfers. With the elbow extended, the olecranon is seated in the fossa, the anterior capsule is taut, and the joint is stable regardless of ligament muscle balance. However, as the elbow flexes, maintenance of this flexed posture under axial load depends on ligament competence and isometric muscle balance. The tetraplegic patient who lacks triceps innervation relies on the ability to lock the elbow in extension to perform transfers or weight shifts, important goals in early rehabilitation. Severe spasticity or flexion contracture of even one arm interferes with this ability to lock the elbow, an ability required for the patient to learn and perform weight-bearing activities safely.

Morrey *et al.* determined that most activities are performed within a 100° range (30–130°), and a pronation–supination arc of 100°.[12] Grover *et al.* blocked elbow extension with a brace to fix the elbow at various angles in a group of patients with and without triceps function.[13] They found that a flexion contracture of 25° or more prevented assisted or sliding board transfers in those patients who lacked triceps function. A flexion contracture of 50° or more compromised transfer functions in those patients with active triceps.

Spastic elbow flexor muscles

Effective splinting of the arm to prevent the development of a contracture in the presence of severe spasticity of the elbow flexors is difficult to achieve. Regaining passive elbow extension by passive stretching exercises is equally difficult once the elbow has become contracted. These realities make early attention to the spastic elbow and rapid institution of anti-spasticity measures all the more important. Anti-spasticity treatments should include the usual measures of systemic medication, such as baclofen, local use of heat or icing of the spastic biceps and/or brachialis muscles, and electrical stimulation of the triceps if the muscle responds to stimulation. These general measures are discussed above. If spasticity of the elbow flexor muscles cannot be controlled by the usual methods, then more aggressive treatment is indicated during the early rehabilitation phase. This includes the injection of botulinum toxin into the spastic muscle, phenol or alcohol injections into the musculocutaneous nerve (usually guided by electrical stimulation), or even surgical exposure and directly crushing the nerve. These latter methods are essentially self-reversible over time. The treated muscle will regain its innervation, but occasionally it will be less spastic upon recovery.

The most important benefit from such procedures is that the immediate reduction in flexor spasticity allows the therapist to be more effective in overcoming muscle shortening and early contractures. We have, on occasion, by preliminary EMG analysis, identified the biceps as spastic but the brachialis muscle much less so. In such cases, botulinum toxin injection into the biceps muscle eliminates functionally troublesome elbow flexor spasticity, yet does not significantly weaken elbow flexion. This allows the patient some useful elbow flexor strength with which to pursue rehabilitation goals.

Contracted elbow flexors

The unopposed action of the normally innervated elbow flexors and/or the spasticity induced by the upper motor neuron injury of abnormally innervated segments of the biceps and brachialis muscles lead to a fixed elbow flexion contracture. Conservative correction is difficult, especially if contracture is associated with severe biceps spasticity. Various therapy measures can be attempted, including attaching rubber-band traction from a wrist cuff to the foot of the patient's bed, serial casting, or dynamic elbow extension orthoses. All involve some risk of skin ulceration in the insensate arm and most fail if the contracture is firm.

One of the few indications for upper limb surgery in the early rehabilitation period is a fixed elbow flexion contracture that cannot be managed by conservative means. This may apply in several circumstances:

- the patient with no triceps activity who has already developed a fixed flexion contracture of the elbow greater than 25°;
- the biceps continue to be very spastic in spite of all reasonable conservative measures; and
- despite adequate conservative care, a progressive contracture is occurring.

Surgery might consist of one of the following procedures:

- standard anterior release, which might include biceps lengthening and anterior capsule release; or
- release of contracture and immediate biceps to triceps transfer.

We have operated on the elbow in the early post-injury or early rehabilitation period in only eight patients over a 25 year period. These patients usually had developed elbow flexion contractures greater than 60° and were resistant to conservative measures. However, many more patients with less severe deformities might benefit from the early release of flexion contractures, especially in light of the work of Grover et al.,[13] who documented the functional consequences of even limited flexion contracture of the elbow in the patient who does not recover triceps function.

The forearm

All tetraplegic patients with injuries at the C5 and C6 levels and most with C7 injuries experience imbalance of the rotator muscles of the forearm. The forearm may become stiff or contracted in either supination (more common) or pronation (less common). A supination contracture is usually the more functionally disabling.

Patients with C6 and C7 injuries maintain innervation of the biceps, which is both an elbow flexor and a strong supinator of the forearm. The supinator muscle may also remain innervated. The brachioradialis (BR) muscle assists in returning the supinated forearm to a position of neutral rotation, but does not effect pronation beyond this position. Patients with C8 level injuries retain some control of the pronator teres and are typically not at risk for developing supination contractures of the forearm.

For the C6 and C7 level injuries, the forearm naturally assumes a supinated posture. If the biceps muscle undergoes sufficient shortening as a consequence (or cause) of elbow flexion contracture, it causes a supination contracture of the forearm. Early care of spasticity of the biceps is an important factor in preventing the development of a forearm fixed in supination. In the acute injury period, it is beneficial to position the arms of the bed-confined patient in pronation. During passive exercise periods it is important to extend the elbow passively, and then, with the elbow fully extended, to pronate the forearm fully. This passively stretches the biceps and fully stretches the BR and the extensor carpi radialis longus (ECRL) muscles, since both of these muscles arise proximal to the elbow joint.

The surgical treatment of dynamic or fixed supination deformities is discussed in Chapter 11.

The wrist

Positional deformities at the wrist are common consequences of inattention to detail in early management. Great spasticity in the C5 and C6 injury patient may result in a flexed wrist, since finger and wrist flexors are more powerful than finger and wrist extensors. Where innervation of the wrist extensors is spared, as in injuries below the C6 level, the deformity is one of wrist extension and radial deviation, since the ECRL, an extensor and radial deviator, is more proximally innervated than the extensor carpi radialis brevis (ECRB). The ECRL may also become contracted secondary to a persistent flexion contracture of the elbow, as discussed above. Whatever the cause, if the ECRL becomes contracted, the wrist automatically extends as the elbow is extended. Wrist flexion may be possible only when the elbow is flexed, since this position loosens the tight ECRL. A contracted ECRL makes it difficult for the patient to reach out in space and position his or her hand around objects in preparation for a passive grasp using any existing tenodesis effect of the paralyzed flexor muscles of the fingers.

Contractures of the wrist are essentially always preventable by the appropriate initial management, including splinting of the wrist in slight extension and neutral radioulnar deviation. Frequent passive ranging into full flexion and extension must begin early post-injury. Even a relatively firm contracture can usually be overcome by vigorous stretching exercises. However, in this circumstance, the ECRL is more of a deforming force than a beneficial functional resource. On several occasions, we have lengthened a contracted MRC Grade 3–4 ECRL by releasing its

tendon in the distal forearm and then attaching the tendon of the ECRL to the tendon of the ECRB, retaining its wrist extensor function.

The fingers

In many centers, current recommendations for early splinting and range of motion exercises for the hand paralyzed by injury to the cervical spinal cord above the C8 level are directed at assisting the development of a passive 'tenodesis' grip between the fingers and palm or between thumb and fingers. The fingers, hand, and wrist are splinted in a position that favors some tightening (contracture) of the flexors of the thumb and fingers. Passive ranging is performed with this goal in mind, that is the fingers and wrist are not ranged simultaneously into full extension.

Better definition of the indications and outcomes of surgical procedures to improve grasp have led many clinical investigators to reassess the common goals of early splinting and therapy for the tetraplegic hand.

Functional splinting in the early rehabilitation phase

'All mechanical contrivances should either be properly done or not be done at all, for it is a disgraceful and awkward thing to use a mechanical means in an unmechanical way.' Hippocrates

Splinting the tetraplegic hand is an accepted practice among occupational therapists, although no studies validate the effectiveness of the many splinting regimens in the medical and therapy literature. As mentioned previously, splinting is an important method to prevent deformity and to promote a functional hand position.[14] The goal of splinting and therapy of the hand during the immediate post-injury and early rehabilitation period should be individualized according to the level of spinal cord injury and the expectations regarding the ultimate level of neurological recovery. There is no uniformity among spinal cord centers, either in terms of design or indication. We recommend the following as a philosophy to guide splinting in the early rehabilitation phase.

Weak wrist extension

In the early post-injury phase, these patients exhibit MRC Grade 1–3 wrist extension. If only active wrist extension is anticipated after neurological stability, the finger flexors should be permitted purposefully to become somewhat shortened. These patients typically must depend on wrist extension to effect a grasp, either by a natural passive or a surgically created tenodesis. Such patients should be fitted initially with a splint that maintains the wrist in some extension and should spend some time at night and when resting with their fingers taped into flexion, termed tenodesis splinting. Tenodesis splints are controversial because if they are incorrectly applied or worn for too long the patient may develop a fixed flexion contracture, which may compromise the use of specific grip patterns later. Proponents believe that their use hastens the development of a functional tenodesis grasp, which aids the patient in achieving early rehabilitation goals. If these splints are used, fingers must be carefully monitored and stretching exercises performed to prevent the development of fixed joint contractures. The tenodesis splint should be discontinued when the tendons have shortened enough to allow a tenodesis-type grasp.

Stronger wrist extension, forearm pronation, and some wrist flexion

In contrast, patients who are expected to regain some active forearm pronation and wrist flexion should be considered differently. For these patients, the goal of the initial hand splinting and therapy should be the maintenance of normal balance between paralyzed flexors and extensors. Since the paralyzed finger flexors are far more powerful than the finger extensors, extra effort must be expended to keep the flexors from contracting. For these patients there is the possibility of ultimately undergoing surgical procedures to assist them in opening their hands to grasp and firmly grip an object, independent of any passive tenodesis forces. As they progress through their initial rehabilitation, such patients may benefit from the early fitting of a dynamic wrist-extension, finger-flexion orthosis, or simple rubber-band driven adaptive devices to assist their gripping of objects.

Finger extension

For the patient who will ultimately regain control of the finger extensors, every effort should be directed at maintaining an absolutely supple hand during the initial post-injury and early rehabilitation phase. This requires the therapist and patient to be inventive with rubber-band devices to assist the patient in grasping

light objects during post-injury rehabilitation.[15] For such patients, the early fitting of a wrist-extension and/or finger-flexion orthosis may be indicated, since tendon-transfer surgery is usually not performed before 1 year post-injury.

Beginning weight-bearing – protecting the hand

This phase begins once the spine is judged adequately stable and the patient can begin to be out of bed for extended periods. At this point, the patient begins to learn how to manage his or her life within the confines of the wheelchair. During the previous weeks, the patient will have learned how to assist with range of motion exercises, either using the opposite upper limb as the therapist, or using various devices to assist in these goals. Rehabilitation begins with sitting protocols at the edge of the bed. If the patient is able to use the upper limbs to help balance at the edge of the bed, the therapist works with the patient on how to position his or her hands with the fingers in flexion to protect against overstretching the finger flexors and losing the tenodesis effect of conjunct wrist extension and finger flexion.

Initial rehabilitation education includes self-feeding with adaptive devices, performing light hygiene in bed or light hygiene at the sink using adaptive devices, and communication skills. Appropriate adaptive devices are issued to the patient and, as the patient progresses, he or she will be weaned off the devices if possible.

During this early rehabilitation period, the patient begins instruction in performing the activities of daily living (ADLs). Each facility usually has protocols that specify the curriculum and time course for ADL training. The scope of the ADLs that the patient learns is determined in part by the expectations for ultimate functional outcome. Many outcome studies have been carried out to generate guidelines for clinical practices (see Appendix VIII).

Of the ADLs taught to the tetraplegic patient, several deserve analysis because of the potential to cause harm to the upper limb. Improper technique leads to more rapid breakdown of unprotected joints and ligaments, and the development of pathological joint postures and dysfunctional stiffness and pain.

These ADLs include:

- methods of transfers and weight shifts, and
- methods to propel the wheelchair.

All involve the patient using the upper limbs in lieu of the paralyzed lower limbs. All involve axial loading across the multiple joints of fingers and wrist. The joints of the upper limb are not designed to bear large axial loads, such as the weight of the body, for prolonged periods or in a repetitive pattern. Yet for the tetraplegic patient, their upper limbs represent their only resource by which to accomplish these activities

with any semblance of independence. Therefore, the tetraplegic patient should be taught only the most mechanically sound and least injurious techniques consistent with his or her level of neurological injury and associated circumstances, such as the level of attendant care, etc.

Transfers and pressure relief

Many tetraplegic patients are taught to perform transfers by first locking the elbow in full extension and then using the flattened palms of their hands to

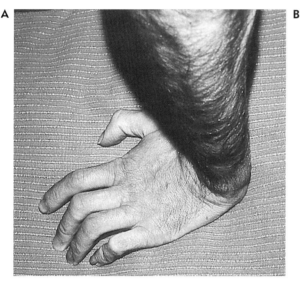

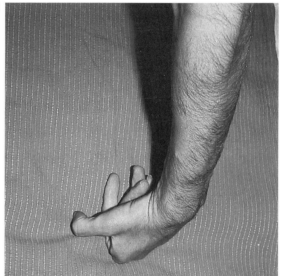

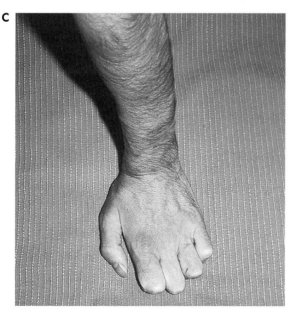

Figure 4.6 (A) A stable but injurious method of flat-hand transfer or weight shift. The metacarpophalangeal joints are hyperextended. With constant weight bearing, their collateral ligaments will break down and these joints will become unstable. The thumb is forcefully fully radially adducted and, with time, the ligaments supporting the carpometacarpal joint will be overstretched and this joint also will become unstable. (B) A more protective hand posture for transfers. The transfer is performed on the closed hand with pressure over the proximal phalanges. (C) In another satisfactory method the metacarpophalangeal joints are extended but not hyperextended. Weight is better distributed.

support their body's weight on the fully extended wrist. In this position, the thumb is pushed into retropulsion and the fingers are fully extended or even hyperextended at the metacarpophalangeal joint (*Fig. 4.6A*). This position may be one of stability, but over the long term will cause the ligaments that support the carpometacarpal joint of the thumb and the metacarpophalangeal joints of the fingers to elongate and thus these joints to become unstable.

This hand and wrist position for transfers is also incompatible with a good outcome for essentially all of the surgical procedures that might possibly be considered for improving hand function. For example, a commonly recommended procedure to restore stable pinch between the thumb and index finger involves surgically anchoring the tendon of the flexor pollicis longus to the volar surface of the radius. When the patient extends the wrist, the tenodesis is tightened and the thumb is pulled into flexion. However, this tenodesis becomes overstretched with time if the patient bears weight on the fully extended wrist and flattened hand, so the beneficial effect of the surgery will be lost.

If the patient retains the ability to stabilize the wrist, a more protective method of transfer involves rolling the fingers into near full flexion, as if forming a closed fist, and using the dorsal surface of the flexed proximal phalanges as the platform for weight bearing (*Fig. 4.6B*). If the patient lacks the ability to stabilize the wrist, a less protective maneuver, but one still better than a flat-hand transfer, is accomplished by the patient rolling the fingers into flexion

and performing the transfer as shown in *Figure 4.6C*. In this circumstance, the body's weight is more evenly distributed over the surfaces of the palm and fingers.

If there is no triceps strength, the therapist must teach the patient how to rotate the arm externally so he or she can maintain the arm extended at the elbow.

Pushing the wheelchair

Patients whose level of injury allows them to use a manual wheelchair must be instructed in pushing techniques that preserve their hands. Pushing directly on the tires leads to skin abrasions and injuries from sharp objects that penetrate the rubber of the tires. Push-gloves are very important since they protect the hands and also provide friction against the push-rim of the wheelchair.

The therapist should review with the patient how to position the hands on the rim. The patient may tend to wedge his or her thumb between the tire and the rim. Over time this can cause laxity of the thumb. The therapist should also evaluate the stroke pattern used to propel the wheelchair, as well as how the patient stops the wheelchair.

Techniques that expose the extended thumb to heavy loads are relatively incompatible with long term thumb stability and, more importantly, absolutely incompatible with most of the tenodesis or tendon transfer procedures developed to improve function. The patient should neither be taught nor encouraged to use the thumb to push so-called 'quad-knobs'

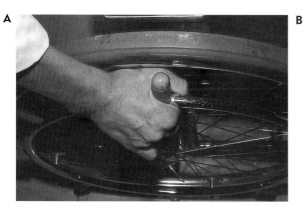
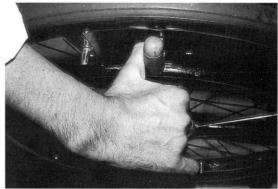

Figure 4.7 So-called 'quad knobs' are frequently used to assist the tetraplegic patient in propelling a manual chair. The patient must be instructed to push the knobs with either the heel of the hand or (A) with the knob deep within the thumb web, rather than (B) pushing with the thumb hooked about the knob.

(*Fig. 4.7*) directly or to push the rims of the chair with the thumb only.

Functional splinting

The early introduction of protective positional splinting is discussed above. Static orthoses are prescribed in the immediate post-injury and the early rehabilitation periods to:[14]

- prevent overstretching of ligaments;
- maintain functional position;
- prevent deformity (e.g., a claw deformity); and
- protect and stabilize flail joints.

Functional orthoses become more important for the tetraplegic patient when he or she begins to assume various aspects of self-care, such as hygiene and feeding.

Essentially, all tetraplegic patients with injuries above the C8 level benefit from the use of some type of functional orthoses during their initial rehabilita-

tion. Almost all use a static device; others may also use a dynamic orthosis.

Static functional orthoses

The type of static functional orthosis employed depends primarily on the neurological level of injury, the patient's needs and desires, and, more specifically, on whether or not the patient has sufficient muscle activity to stabilize his or her wrists.[14] For the patient who lacks antigravity power in the wrist extensors, the orthosis must assume this function. The most commonly employed orthosis for such a patient is termed a long opponens splint (*Fig. 4.8A*). These take many forms, including a simple wrist support that keeps the wrist from falling into flexion under the influence of gravity. Others are made specifically by an orthotist after measurements of the patient's hands and wrists have been taken. Typically, the hand and arm with the greater residual power is chosen to have the splint fitted. However, the patient's desires play a role in this choice. Even rubber bands may be used as

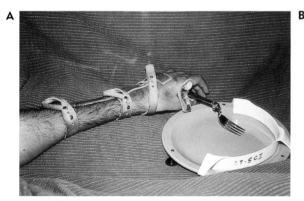

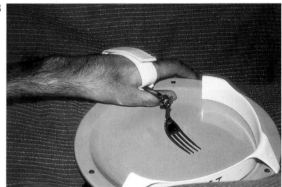

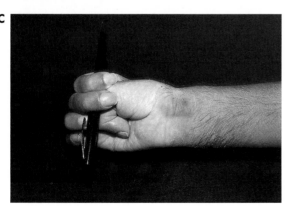

Figure 4.8 Various (A) long and (B) short opponens splints with different terminal (adaptive) devices. (C) Patients make use of different finger postures to assist in performing ADLs.

an external assistance device to provide simple grip for quadriplegic patients.[15]

Several types of end devices may be attached or built into the orthosis, including a slot into which the handle of a fork or spoon can be placed (*Fig. 4.8A*), or a rolled wire spring into which a pencil, pen, or typing stick can be wedged. Occasionally, if the wrist is stabilized by the splint, the patient can learn to place or have placed a fork or spoon into an interlocking finger grip such as that illustrated in *Figure 4.8C*.

If the patient is able to maintain a stable wrist against the effects of gravity and against some additional force, a smaller and more easily donned orthosis can be prescribed. This is usually termed a 'short opponens' splint. One type is illustrated in *Figure 4.8B*.

These orthoses are fastened to the arm either with velcro fasteners or with straps and rivet-like attachments (*Fig. 4.8*). Which type is employed depends upon the patient's abilities and therapist's and orthotist's preference. In donning the orthosis, the patient is taught to use the opposite hand, with or without the assistance of his or her teeth as an additional helping 'hand'.

Many, but not most, tetraplegic patients continue to use various functional orthoses following discharge from the rehabilitation facility.

Dynamic orthoses

The possibility of using a dynamic orthosis to allow better hand function is usually introduced during the early rehabilitation period. Many creative devices have been designed to provide a mechanical means of restoring grasp to the paralyzed hand. Various sources of power to open and close the orthosis have been proposed, including:

- shoulder harness[16] (similar to that used by an upper limb amputee to control a Dorrance-type hook prosthesis);
- gas powered devices;[17]
- electrically driven devices controlled by a shoulder position sensor;[18] or
- variations of myoelectric devices designed for amputees.[19,20]

Most found little favor and have been abandoned.

Wrist-driven, flexor-hinged orthosis

Less complicated devices that provide some ability to grasp and release objects have been employed more successfully. Most use the flexion and extension movement of the wrist to open and close the fingers and thumb, and are referred to as a wrist-extension/finger flexion or wrist-driven/flexor-hinge orthosis (WDFHO) or splint (WDFHS). They were introduced in the 1950s[21] and are still the most widely prescribed dynamic orthoses in the USA, even though the basic design has remained unchanged in nearly 40 years (*Fig. 4.9*). They are less commonly prescribed in other countries and are viewed by some as relics from the past.

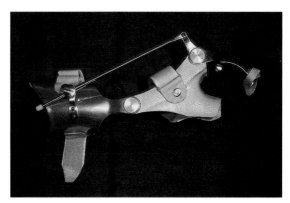

Figure 4.9 The most commonly prescribed dynamic orthosis is this wrist-driven splint designed to provide a 'three-jaw' chuck pinch. The three elements (an arm piece, a hand piece, and a finger piece) are hinged at the anatomic axis of the wrist and metacarpophalangeal joints. The fourth essential element is a connecting rod that transfers a reciprocal torque from the wrist to the digits. The device uses two levers and two joints located at the precise axis of wrist flexion and extension and the axis of metacarpophalangeal flexion and extension. The thumb is enclosed within the device so that it becomes an immobile post, with its projection one of maximum palmar abduction and carpometacarpal joint flexion. Other parts of the orthosis stabilize the interphalangeal joints of the index and middle fingers in predetermined positions of flexion. Parallelogram arrangements of push rods and interaxial linkages link the mobile wrist axis with the metacarpophalangeal axis so that as the wrist is progressively moved into extension, the levers push and/or pull the metacarpophalangeal joints into progressive flexion, and vice versa.

Prerequisites include the ability to sit in a wheelchair and pronate the forearm (since gravity is used to open the hand) and passive flexibility of the wrist. The ideal candidate has MRC Grade 4 or higher wrist extensor power. The device must be constructed from precise measurements made for the individual patient. It has to fit exceedingly well to be most useful. Most WDFHSs come with an actuating lever that allows the individual to adjust the flexion–extension arc of motion. In one setting, the opening favors grasping an object of large diameter. The other setting favors grasping objects of smaller diameter. This actuating lever is operated by the patient's unsplinted hand. Garrett *et al.* state that 75% of wrist extensor power is transferred to the fingertips with the WDFHS.[22]

If there is only a weak or even an absent active wrist extension torque, the splint can still be used, although much less efficiently. In such cases, the patient (using the opposite hand) pushes on the locking lever to open it and either allows gravity to flex the wrist or uses the opposite hand to push the splinted hand into flexion at the wrist. This causes the space between the mobile index and middle fingers and the post-like thumb to increase, and allows the patient to position the object to be grasped within the space between thumb and index. The patient then uses the opposite hand to push the splinted hand into extension at the wrist, thus closing the thumb and fingers around the object. As the opposite hand pushes the splinted hand into greater flexion, the grip is tightened. The ratcheted locking device permits action in the one direction, but prevents motion in the other direction. When the patient ceases pushing with the opposite hand, the device stays locked and the fingers stay gripped about the object until the patient unlocks the ratchet to release the object held.

Modifications of the basic wrist-driven flexor-hinge splint include a finger piece designed to eliminate rings for the middle and distal segments. Instead, the fingers are held by narrow straps. The actuating lever can be made adjustable and the actuating rod can be mounted dorsally. A C-bar can be added to keep the splint from slipping proximally. The forearm piece can be shortened and truss studs have been added for attachments, using straps attached on the radial side and with plastic rings on the straps. A rubber-band extension aid for prolonged activities reduces fatigue. A pencil holder can be added.[23]

Variations of the design have been introduced,[17,24–27] including external power with carbon dioxide or electric motors, and a shoulder-driven hand orthosis (mentioned above). Other variations include making the four-bar linkage adjustable by means of a telescoping connecting rod, or increasing the angle between the palmar and wrist pieces, which allows handling of differently sized objects, but increases the complexity of the device for the patient and manufacturer. This also decreases motion at the metacarpophalangeal joint, but it does allow grasp at linkage positions of higher pinch force.

The long-term acceptance of functional orthoses is relatively low. The device has many shortcomings. The thumb is mostly covered by the metal of the device, but it is usually the digit with the best sensibility in this population of patients. The device is difficult to self-don. Anything that leads to poor fitting reduces efficiency. The device is expensive to obtain and it is difficult to find sources for maintenance. Studies show that the functional outcome depends on three factors:[28]

- patient selection;
- objectivity of evaluator; and
- meticulous care in application and follow-up.

Its use other than at selected centers in the USA is very limited.

In summary, the long-term post-discharge use of orthoses is suspect. In multicenter studies, Garber[29] and later Ditunno *et al.*[30] found that of 56 tetraplegic patients discharged with 250 devices, only 36% of the devices were still in use after 2 years.

References

1. Hanson R, Franklin W. Sexual loss in relation to other functional losses for spinal cord injured males. Arch Phys Med Rehabil 1976; 57:291–293.
2. Guttman L. Spinal Cord Injuries. Oxford: Blackwell Scientific, 1973.
3. Andrews LG, Armitage KJ. Sudeck's atrophy in traumatic quadriplegia. Paraplegia 1971; 9:159–165.
4. Sie I, Waters R, Adkins R, et al. Upper extremity pain in the postrehabilitation spinal cord injured patient. Arch Phys Med Rehabil 1992; 73:44–48.
5. Khalili AA, Harmel MH, Forster S, et al. Management of spasticity by selective peripheral nerve block with dilute phenol solutions in clinical rehabilitation. Arch Phys Med Rehabil 1964; 45:513–519.

6. Wainapel SF, Haigney D, Labib K. Spastic hemiplegia in a quadriplegic patient: treatment with phenol nerve block. Arch Phys Med Rehabil 1984; 65:786–787.

7. Braun RM, Hoffer MM, Mooney V, et al. Phenol nerve block in treatment of acquired spastic hemiplegia in upper limb. J Bone Joint Surg 1973; 55:580–585.

8. Cromwell SJ, Paquette V. The effect of botulinum toxin A on the function of a person with poststroke quadriplegia. Phys Ther 1996; 76:395–402.

9. Richardson D, Edwards S, Sheean G, et al. The effect of botulinum toxin on hand function after complete spinal cord injury at the level of C5/6. Clin Rehabil 1997; 11(4):288–292.

10 Silfverskiold J, Waters R. Shoulder pain and functional disability in spinal cord injury patients. Clin Orthop Rel Res 1991; 272:141–145.

11. Campbell CC, Koris MJ. Etiologies of shoulder pain in cervical spinal cord injury. Clin Orthop Rel Res. 1996; 320:140–145.

12. Morrey B, An K, Chao E. Functional evaluation of the elbow. In: Morrey B, ed. The Elbow and its Disorders. Philadelphia: WB Saunders, 1985:73–91.

13. Grover J, Gellman H, Waters R. The effect of a flexion contracture of the elbow on the ability to transfer in patients who have quadriplegia at the sixth cervical level. J Bone Joint Surg 1996; 78A:1397–1400.

14. Krajnik S, Bridle M. Hand splinting in quadriplegia: current practice. Am J Occup Ther 1992; 46:149–156.

15. Pham H, Noble C, Hentz V. Rubber band as external assist device to provide simple grip for quadriplegic patients. Ann Plast Surg 1988; 21(2):180–182.

16. Dollfus P, Oberlé M. Technical note: Preliminary communication, a tridigital dynamic orthosis for tetraplegic patients. Paraplegia 1984; 22:115–118.

17. Stenehjem J, Swenson J, Sprague C. Wrist driven flexor hinge orthosis: linkage design improvements. Arch Phys Med Rehabil 1983; 64:566–568.

18. Patterson R, Halpern D, Kubicek W. A proportionally controlled externally powered hand splint. Arch Phys Med Rehabil 1971; 52(9):434–438.

19. Grahn EC. A power unit for functional hand splints. Bull Proset Res 1970; 2:53–57.

20. Janovsky F. Myoelektrisch gesteuerte Handorthese, ORTHOMOT OM 1. Biomed Tech 1973; 18(5): 172–175.

21. Bisgrove J, Shrosbree R, Key A. New functional dynamic wrist extension – finger flexion hand splint – preliminary report. J Assoc Phys Med Rehabil 1954; 8:162–163.

22 Garrett A, Perry J, Nickel V. Traumatic quadriplegia. J Am Med Assoc 1964; 187:107–111.

23. McCleur S, Conry J. Modifications of the wrist-driven flexor hinge splint. Arch Phys Med Rehabil 1971; 52(5):233–235.

24. Engen TJ, L Ottnat L. Upper extremity orthotics. Orthop Prosthet Appl J 1967;:112–127.

25. Engen T. Lightweight modulare orthosis. Prosthet Orthot Int 1989; 13:125–129.

26 Nickel V, Perry J. The flexor hinged hand. J Bone Joint Surg 1958; 40A:971–979.

27. Nickel V, Perry J, Garrett A. Development of useful function in the severely paralyzed hand. J Bone Joint Surg 1963; 45A(5):933–952.

28. Kay H. Clinical evaluation of the Engen plastic hand orthosis. Artif Limbs 1969; 13(1):13–26.

29. Garber SL, Gregorio T. Upper extremity assistive devices: assessment of use by spinal cord-injured patients with quadriplegia. Am J Occup Ther 1990; 44:126–131.

30. Ditunno JF, Stover S, Freed M, et al. Motor recovery of the upper extremities in traumatic quadriplegia: a multicenter study. Arch Phys Med Rehabil 1992; 73:431–436.

5

The tetraplegic patient and the environment

L Floris, C Dif, and MA Le Mouel

Introduction

Over the past dozen years, progress in the rapid transport of patients with spinal cord injuries, improved effectiveness in resuscitation following trauma, and their very rapid transfer to specialty rehabilitation centers have led to improved survival rates and an increased life span for patients who suffer cervical spinal cord injuries.

The benefits afforded to patients in these specialty centers occur in two phases:

- the first is devoted to re-education to diminish the deficits associated with the spinal cord lesion; and
- the second is to enable psychosocial adaptation, the goal of which is to assist the individual's re-entry into his or her environment thus reducing the handicap brought about by the impairment.

The therapeutic plan is developed on the basis of the anticipated level of recovery. The new international classification of handicaps, defined by the World Health Organization (WHO) in 1990,[1] provides a conceptual framework for our methodology. It differentiates between an 'impairment', a 'disability', and a 'handicap':

- impairment describes the effects on an organ or organ systems and (in relation to spinal cord injuries) reflects the level of the spinal cord lesion;
- disability describes the limitations encountered in daily life, and corresponds to the functional consequences of the problem;

- handicap reflects the difficulties that result from the 'disability' or the 'impairment', and is itself linked to the environment and to social and cultural factors.

The impairment scale established by the American Spinal Injury Association (ASIA) in 1982 standardized the analysis of the motor and sensory levels. Evaluation of the disability in the tetraplegic patient is based essentially on the presence or absence of prehension, since this function determines independence. Evaluation of the handicap is more complicated, because it takes into account the characteristics of the environment of the patient, at the individual (personal), material, and structural levels, and of the patient's lifestyle (the values and central interests of the patient). This evaluation helps to limit the effect of the handicap through appropriate initial care and subsequent rehabilitation.

The therapeutic plan is developed over the course of several meetings. These include not only the patient, but also the mix of different professionals (physicians, occupational therapists, physical therapists, nurses, psychologists, and sociologists) who come together to define the short- and mid-term objectives that mark the stages of treatment of the patient.

Among these different professionals the occupational therapists occupy a central place, and intervene in all the stages of rehabilitation that benefit the tetraplegic patient. From the moment of admission, they work to minimize the circumstances of the handicap with respect to the management of the patient's environment, principally the hospital room. In the phases of retraining they work to minimize the effects of the handicap through the development of directed activities. Finally, in the phase of rehabilitation they seek to diminish the functional consequences of the handicap by developing compensatory and assistive techniques. Occupational therapists also help to organize the return home of the patient, and take into account the patient's lifestyle to diminish the circumstances of the handicap at home.

Environment of the patient with spinal cord injury during the period of rehabilitation

This stage takes place in a medical environment imposed by consequences of the tetraplegic condition, but in keeping with the norms of treatment and rehabilitation. For the patients, this is a novel environment, far removed from their usual one.

In this period of evaluation assessments of the patient's needs are made, and the means and techniques of rehabilitation are put into place. This evaluation helps monitor the patient during his or her medical, functional, and psychological evolution, and

helps establish the necessary compensations and different adaptive devices.

This stage is designed to allow the patient to realize the maximum independence, assuaging the dependence on the nurturing circumstances of the hospital room, since in this facility there is access to automatic functions, technical devices, and human assistance. It is designed also to increase the patient's ultimate level of independence in the outside world and to assist him or her in utilizing all the possible compensatory skills and mechanisms.

The admission

At the time of admission, the initial treatment takes place in the patient's hospital room. The principal ergonomic goal is to allow the tetraplegic patient to signal the nursing staff or attendants, which strengthens the patient's sense of security. These patients have a motor deficit of greater or lesser significance that affects the upper limbs and necessitates adaptation of the existing calling devices, adaptations that can be activated by the upper limb or by the patient's head (*Fig. 5.1*).

The principal requirement of the patient and his or her family is to be able to use the telephone. How the telephone should be adapted depends upon

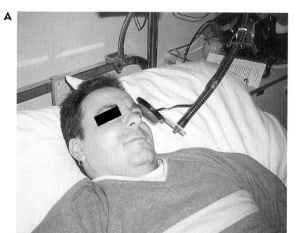
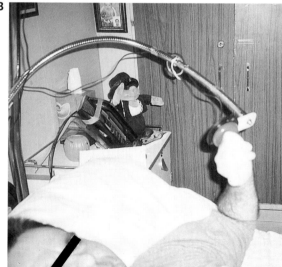

Figure 5.1 (A) A call-button on a flexible support to alert the nurse, controlled by the head. (B) A flexible call-button, hand controlled.

the specific motor circumstances of the patient: from a simple hand-held model to the utilization of a 'hands-free' telephone with keypad modifications to the use of an infrared controller.

Such an infrared system permits control of all aspects of the room's environment, including the telephone, television, radio, multimedia, lights, other electrical apparatus, window shades, and doors, and can also be used to signal the nurse. It consists of a programmable command system that recognizes the infrared codes of each function of the different devices mentioned above. The patient uses a contact switch attached to the head or upper limb or a voice command.

During this period in bed, the patient's other needs become prioritized, including access to reading materials, adapting simple command consoles, placing an adaptation on the upper limb to turn pages, or using more sophisticated devices such as an electric page-turner.

Moving toward independence

One must consider that a tetraplegic patient faces the difficulties of daily life (everything that happens from getting out of bed in the morning until going to bed in the evening) imprisoned within a wheelchair, with precarious balance, spasticity to a greater or lesser degree, the upper limbs weak, and little or no grasp. Even at night in bed the patient must worry about urination and protecting the skin by turning.

During this early stage of rehabilitation, the patient must understand that already, in the hospital, the goal is to achieve the maximum daily independence. Every possible assistance is given to the patient in this journey, in particular for movement and the elementary activities of daily life. Several modalities are offered:

- development of functional possibilities;
- adaptative and technical devices; and
- human assistance.

Mobility

Depending on the level of injury, tetraplegic individuals can acquire some level of independence in their mobility. An appropriate choice of wheelchair allows patients to enlarge their environment, and to move about on the ward and within the facility:

- an electric wheelchair is suitable for the high-level tetraplegic; and
- a manual wheelchair is suitable for the lower level tetraplegic (*Fig. 5.2*).

Table 5.1 describes the characteristics of the chairs, and the arrangement of the patient according to the functional level of the tetraplegic individual.

Basic activites of daily living

Drinking

It is very important for the tetraplegic patient to understand the notion of protecting his or her

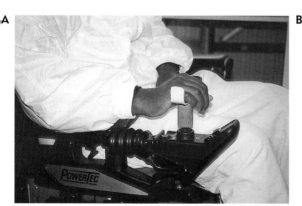 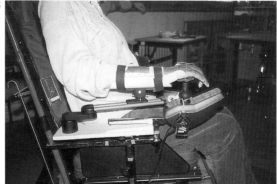

Figure 5.2   (A) Adaptation of a joy-stick controller to drive an electric wheelchair. (B) Driving using a mobile arm support.

Table 5.1 Wheelchairs for tetraplegic patients

Level of injury	Type of chair	Seating in chair	Control and propulsion	Transfers
C4	Electric	For trunk balance, high back and head support	Head command, occipital or chin	Third party and a lift
		For arm support, adaptable armrests	Access to all electric chair functions by electronics	
C5	Electric	For trunk balance, high back and head support	Hand command with adaptations for facilitating arm movements (mobile arm support) and adaptive joystick	Third party and a lift
		For arm support, adaptable armrests		
C6	Electric	Normal back support	Electric hand command with adaptive joystick	Transfer device with sliding board and third party, rarely alone
	Manual	Light manual chair	Hand propelled	
			Adaptive hand devices: non-skid rims, push gloves	
C7, C8	Manual	Light and sport model	Normal propulsion	Transfers alone, with or without sliding board

kidneys. No matter the circumstance (in bed or in the wheelchair), the patient must be able to obtain a drink when alone. If the patient cannot use his or her arms, the adaptation used is usually a flexible device, or a straw and support bottle. If the difficulty in gripping is only minimal, the patient can use an adaptive glass and bottle.

Eating
Independence in self-feeding is only really possible for the C6 level (and more able) tetraplegic patient in whom the deltoid and biceps are functional. A simple adaptive device, termed a metacarpal cuff (Universal or 'U' cuff), holds a fork or spoon, and can be adapted according to the motor potentials of each patient (*Fig. 5.3*). Such devices may be fitted to an orthosis that stabilizes the wrist when the wrist motors are weak or absent. The details of these adaptive devices deserve a case-by-case analysis for activities such as cutting meat, pealing fruit, opening a package, and arrangement for the patient at the table.

For the patient injured at the C5 level, the learning process is very lengthy. Its application is a function of

the strength of shoulder elevation, elbow flexion, and elbow release, and of the position of the arm and hand, particularly the extent of persistent forearm supination. Patients may be able to utilize an arm suspension or a mobile arm support. Patients injured at this high level will never be totally independent.

Hygiene and dressing
The ability to perform these activities is associated essentially with tetraplegic patients injured at the C6 level (those with functional deltoid, biceps, and radial wrist extensor muscles). The learning process is progressive and the progress becomes apparent as the patient acquires skills through sports, physical, and occupational therapy. Three identifiable activities include care of the face, body hygiene, and dressing.

Care of the face
The problems encountered by the patient include positioning him- or herself in front of the washbasin, access to the environment, gripping, and using objects. Difficulties in using the water faucets can be reduced by installing the type that automatically

A

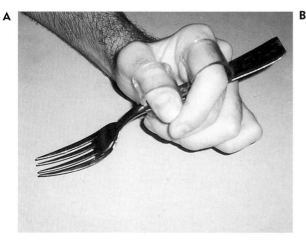

B

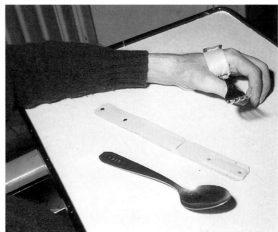

C

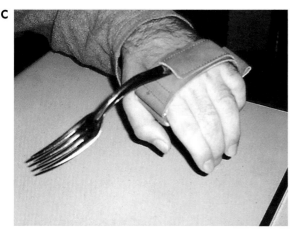

Figure 5.3 (A–C) Technical assistive devices for mealtimes, adapted according to the motor level of the patient.

mixes hot and cold water. Grasping hygienic devices (such as toothbrushes, toothpaste, hair brushes, razors, and makeup), can be facilitated by various adaptive devices, including universal cuffs, or rings, or by using different types of grips such as a bimanual grip (*Figs 5.4* and *5.5*).

For C5 patients who are essentially totally dependent, teeth brushing can be accomplished by combining an adaptive device with an orthosis that stabilizes the wrist, but some human assistance is necessary.

Personal hygiene

Personal hygiene may take place in bed or on the commode chair. In bed this necessitates turning over and sitting (which is achieved using a motorized bed), and the installation of an overhead frame, support, or sling. Nevertheless, the problems of preparing the basic requisites, such as a basin, water, and towels, must still be solved.

On a commode chair the prerequisites include:

- sufficient balance;
- sufficient flexibility to lean the torso to reach the different areas of the body and the possibility of returning the torso from this leaning position;
- practical organization of the working area to reach the necessary objects; and
- ability to hold these objects (e.g., bath gel, shampoo, flannel) made easier by adaptive devices.

Dressing

In dressing, the upper part of the body is the most accessible when using supple clothing. Such things as buttons, snaps, or zippers present difficulties, which may be obviated with the use of Velcro closures.

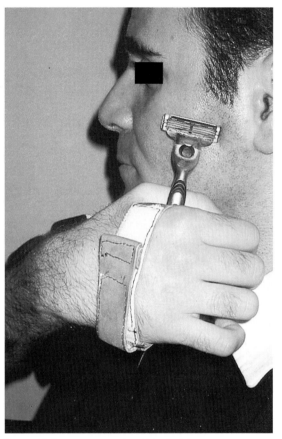

Figure 5.4 A universal cuff for holding a razor.

Dressing the lower part of the body is a skill more applicable for the C7 and C8 tetraplegic patient who can expect to gain near complete independence. The C6 tetraplegic patient is very inconvenienced by an insufficiently strong or unstable tenodesis, limited sensation in the hand, and an absent triceps.

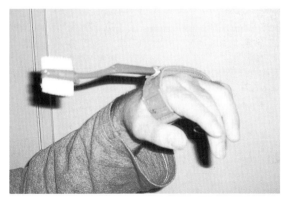

Figure 5.5 Adaptive tooth brush.

Inspection and prophylaxis

The patient must learn how to inspect him- or herself and to anticipate cutaneous and orthopedic complications (by giving appropriate attention to cushions, anti-bedsore mattress, padding pressure points, good chair condition, etc.). The daily environment of the patient can be modified in certain ways to increase comfort and safety. For example, preventing burns is emphasized in the bathroom by installing a combination faucet that controls the temperature of the water and, for the patient who smokes, by adopting different techniques for lighting a cigarette.

Sphincters

Emptying the bladder

The goal is to permit the tetraplegic patient to achieve self-catheterization, recognized as the best method of emptying. For some male patients, the occupational therapist works with the patient to find adaptive devices that facilitate the preparation and appropriate mechanics: adaptive aids to hold pants in the proper position, adaptive zippers, special mirrors, and technical aids to help grasp the catheter. For female patients, transfer from the chair to bed remains a significant obstacle to total independence in self-catheterization.

If there is no possibility of improving prehension, and thus being able to perform these activities, the tetraplegic individual will need to depend on another person.

Emptying the bowels

For the majority of tetraplegic individuals, this activity cannot be performed alone and therefore requires nursing assistance.

Transfers

Training in transfers is progressive:

- A strong, athletic C7 tetraplegic patient can recover to the same level as a paraplegic, in terms of bed mobility, self-care and hygiene, chair commode use, and driving a car.
- The C6 tetraplegic patient can achieve complete independence in transfers from the bed to chair. This requires compensating for the absence of triceps function by hyperextending the elbows and

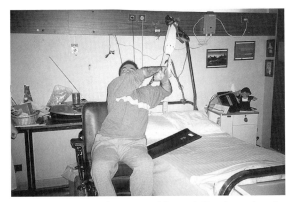

Figure 5.6 Transfer assisted by a sliding board and an overhead sling (C6 tetraplegic patient).

careful balance. A transfer or sliding board facilitates this movement and lessens the risk of falling (*Fig. 5.6*). An aid may be needed for certain more difficult transfers, such as in and out of the car or the bathtub. Such instruction must be given on an individual basis.

Communication

Every method of communication should be studied and learned:

Handwriting
Handwriting should be possible using different writing implements adapted to the condition of the digits or, similarly, held in the mouth in patients with severe upper limb deficits. One example is a large felt

pen held with two rings, one for the thumb and one for the index with the pen gripped between these fingers (*Fig. 5.7*). This does not allow normal handwriting, but it does permit the tetraplegic patient some independence in signing his or her name.

Manual or computer keyboard
Use of these devices is facilitated by different accessories, such as a mouth-held typing 'stick' for high-level tetraplegic patients, a universal or 'U'-cuff with an attached typing stick, a mobile arm support to enlarge the reachable area, or voice recognition systems (*Fig. 5.8*).

A

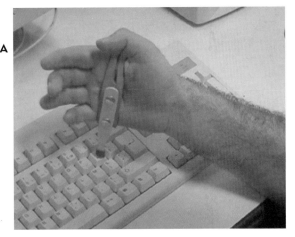

B

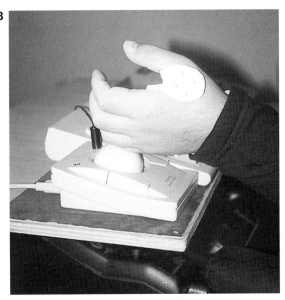

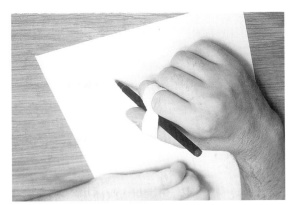

Figure 5.7 Adaptive writing aid (C6 tetraplegic patient).

Figure 5.8 (A) Access to the keyboard of a computer. (B) Using a 'track-ball' to control a computer.

Telephone

A number of telephone designs are available, including 'hands-free' models, infrared command models, portable hands-free models, and a number of possible adaptations for holding the handset and dialing the number. Access to the Internet greatly facilitates communication for the tetraplegic patient.

Adjustment phase

The adjustment phase, termed 'readjustment', focuses on the patient's future plans for life, and is developed with the patient and his or her caregivers and family. The plan is based not on the circumstances of the care facility, but on the realities of the patient's future circumstances (in the place where the patient will actually live), relevant aspects of his or her past life, and the organization of treatment. This return to the usual social, family, and even professional structure hinges on different factors related to:

- coming back home and organization of the household;
- family relationships;
- social relationships;
- work (or school) and cultural interests, including the ability to move about in the outside environment.

The effort at readjustment is based on a careful evaluation of the acquired independence, outside conditions (e.g., the family, social, and work milieu), economic status, and the patient's habits. The circumstances of disability, as defined by all these elements, are more or less important; they determine the type of aids that must be put in place for different activities. The proposed solutions must take into account the patient's financial and personal considerations.

Organization of the home

Personal aids

The personal aids needed depend on the levels of family support and help from neighbors and on the level of assistance to which the person has access on a daily basis (nursing support, domestic support, meal preparation, and outside help). These aids apply to all the daily activities, including those related to the body (such as personal hygiene, dressing, feeding, sphincter activities) and also to domestic activities (such as meal preparation, doing the laundry, developing budgets, etc.).

Material assistance

Material assistance includes not only the material and technical aids needed by the patient, but also those needed by the patient's attendant. Material assistance includes a hospital bed, anti-pressure sore mattress and cushion, washbasin, wheelchair, lifting hoist, sliding board, and so on.

Adjustments

All the elements in the individual's environment that represent obstacles to independence should be listed (doors too narrow, steps too high, slippery floors, inaccessible storage space, and unreachable light switches). Areas and items that may require adjustment include:

- access to the property, apartment, or house;
- hallway space in the domicile;
- work-space too high or too low (not enough space below for the legs);
- sanitation facilities (location, plumbing fixtures, access); and
- furnishings.

Animal aids

After training, a dog can accompany a tetraplegic person and can respond to some commands, such as fetch an object from the floor, open a door, sound an alarm, etc.

Moving about outside the hospital

In the course of readaptation, the tetraplegic individual will seek activities other than the usual routine and may turn toward the outside environment, including leaving his or her house to visit shops, banks, offices, and move about the sidewalks and streets. The individual's maneuverability in the outside environment should be sufficiently adapted such that he or she experiences the maximum independence. There are multiple obstacles, such as high sidewalks, uneven ground, more or less significant inclines, and dangerous walkways and streets.

Using a personal automobile or public transport, such as train, bus, subway, or plane, can augment moving over distances.

Public transport

Tetraplegic individuals often encounter many difficulties in terms of accessibility and human assistance: steep inclines, stairways, distances too great, height of the ticket counter, etc.

Personal automobile

Only tetraplegic patients at the C7/C8 level are truly able to drive an automobile with complete independence in transfers and in storing the wheelchair in the

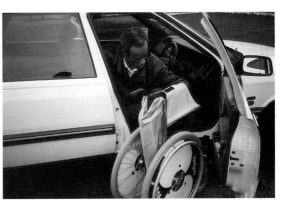

Figure 5.10   Storing the wheelchair in the vehicle (C7 patient with surgical rehabilitation).

vehicle (*Figs 5.9* and *5.10*). A C6 tetraplegic individual with good function of the upper limbs (or surgical rehabilitation of upper limb function) can expect to drive a vehicle. *Table 5.2* describes the different adaptations and aids necessary for function according to the level of the tetraplegia.

When the individual cannot drive, he or she is transferred onto the passenger seat (either a personalized seat built into the vehicle or by using a pivoting seat). The individual can also stay in the wheelchair, for which a 'van'-type vehicle is needed

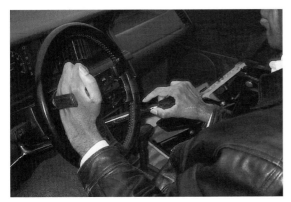

Figure 5.9   Adaptive driving using a fork on the steering wheel and a brake–accelerator lever.

Table 5.2   Vehicles for tetraplegic patients

Level of tetraplegia	Transfer into vehicle	Storing the chair	Driving
C7–C8	Accomplished alone, with or without sliding board	Performed by the patient with or without robotic arm adaptation	Automatic transmission
			Assistive steering and braking
			Fork or ball on the steering wheel compensates for prehension deficit
C6	Accomplished with human help and adaptive aids (e.g., sliding board or seated pivot and lift)	Accomplished by another person in the case of a transfer onto the seat of the vehicle	Brake and accelerate with hand control
	Installation to allow driving in the electric wheelchair		Satellite steering wheel or voice command for turn-signals, lights, horn, windshield-wipers, etc.

and a system with an elevated track or rail facilitates the tetraplegic's entry into the vehicle.

Leisure activities

Leisure activities deserve very careful study. The goal is to make leisure activities accessible, according to the level of the handicap. The occupational therapists must prepare many adjustments to leisure activities since the individual's return to work is more difficult or even impossible. Leisure activities are practical inside or outside the home. At home, leisure activities might include reading, watching television, games, music, and handicrafts. Outside the home, a number of activities are possible, including meetings, conferences, and cultural events such as the theater, cinema, museums, libraries, and art galleries. Sports activities are possible, through special sporting federations and associations. Sporting equipment needs to be accessible (e.g., gyms, swimming pools, and stadiums). In a similar sense, tourism is organized by special associations, and includes cruises, leisure clubs, amusement parks, and so on.

Associations

It is often the case that at the time of discharge from the rehabilitation facility, the handicapped individual and his or her family feel isolated for the first time. Paraplegia Associations facilitate meeting other paralyzed individuals and offer many benefits, including counseling and information, an exchange of experiences, materials and equipment, organized activities, vacations, and management of specialized services.

School and work activities

The most important condition necessary for professional or scholarly reintegration is the resolution (by different means) of the problems associated with the handicap, including difficulties in bodily activities, care, and movement.

School activities

When the schooling of an adolescent in the traditional manner is incompatible with the handicap, the funding or administrative agency may enable a change to a boarding school or day care in a specialty center

(offering both school and medical services). These offer schooling and a continuation of rehabilitation and care.

After 16 years of age, several solutions are available to the young person who cannot attend normal schools:

- continuing studies at a secondary school;
- going on to university; and
- pursuing an apprenticeship.

If the organization of daily affairs and accommodation can be assured, the adolescent can integrate into specialized structures such as advanced or professional schools.

Work activities

Resuming work is not possible unless there is:

- compatibility between the duties of the job and the individual's functional capacity; and
- the possibility of resolving specific management issues, such as accessibility, set-up of the work place, organization of daily care, and achieving the required freedom of movement.

The opposite circumstances necessitate a change helped by:

- a change of position within the same work environment; or
- job retraining and reclassification.

This can take place in a professional rehabilitation center or in the form of an apprenticeship at the employer's work place. In each case, patient motivation remains the determinant factor in the success of such projects.

About 'computers'

For the tetraplegic patient, the computer is a means of easy access to:

- leisure activities (games, culture, meetings, and discussions over the Internet);
- organizing the home; and
- organizing school and work.

The interface must be carefully chosen:

- computer mouse directed by head movement;
- adapted keyboard; and/or
- voice recognition.

References

1. World Health Organization. International Classification of Impairment, Disabilities, and Handicaps: a manual of classification according to the consequences of disease. Geneva: World Health Organization; 1990.

Bibliography

Detraz M. Ergotherapie. In: Encyclopedia de Medicine et Chirurgie, 26-150 A10. Paris: Elsevier; 1992:20.

Le Gall M, Ruet J. Evaluation et analyse de l'autonomie. In: Encyclopedia de Medicine et Chirurgie, 26-030 A10 Kinesitherapie, reeducation fonctionnelle. Paris: Elsevier, 1996:8.

Minaire P. La mesure d'independence, historique, presentation, perspectives. J Readaptation Med 1991; 11:168–174.

Thoumier P, Thevenin L, Jossel L. Reeducation des paraplegiques et tetraplegiques adultes. In: Encyclopedia de Medicine et Chirurgie, 26-460 A10. Kinesitherapie, reeducation fonctionnelle. Paris: Elsevier, 1995:15.

6

Upper limb evaluation in the stabilizing patient

Introduction

At some point in the course of rehabilitation, as neurological recovery begins to plateau, the rehabilitation team examines the patient specifically to determine whether upper limb functional reconstructive surgery or long-term bracing would be beneficial. Several formats have been useful when upper limb reconstructive surgery or long-term functional bracing is being considered. Appendix III includes several examples of examination formats designed to capture important details of the patient's pre-injury history, current functional status, and the key elements of the current motor and sensory resources that remain to the patient. Equally important information regarding less easily measured factors such as motivation, intelligence, psychological well-being, and patient goals completes the scope of the evaluation. Most of the critical information about these intangible factors is best gained through discussions with the many caregivers who have knowledge of the patient, including therapists, nursing staff, psychologists, social workers, rehabilitation physicians, and, occasionally, other patients. The hands-on part of the examination is best conducted together by the therapists and surgeon.

General evaluation of the potential candidate

Those criteria that identify suitable candidates and the indications for upper limb reconstructive surgery or orthotics are discussed in detail in Chapter 8. The discussion here of the general aspects of the upper limb examination omits details, albeit important ones, regarding assessment of the psychological status of the patient and his or her motivation and intelligence. Lack of complete psychological stability, while a strong contraindication to upper limb surgery to restore lost function, is not a contraindication to the team examining the patient's upper limb. From the perspective of defining and identifying ideal prospective candidates for upper limb rehabilitation, a complete upper limb physical and functional examination may be extremely beneficial in identifying issues of motivation, intelligence, and goals. Once issues that conflict with successful rehabilitation are identified, the team is better able to plan further strategies.

Adequate time must be provided for the examination and the examination should be performed at a time when the patient is not fatigued from prior therapy or testing. All the essential elements of the examination should be carried out.

Past history of injury or afflictions involving the upper limbs

The general examination should include questions regarding any past injury to the shoulders, arms, and hands, and specific questions as to whether the patient suffered injury to the upper limbs as part of the events that caused spinal cord trauma. Several pre-existing conditions, such as chronic afflictions of the rotator cuff of the shoulder, may predispose the patient with cervical cord injury to functionally limiting pain once more vigorous physical rehabilitation begins. In older patient, chronic osteoarthritis may have caused pre-injury joint stiffness. Pre-existing joint contractures do not respond readily, if at all, to therapy to improve range of motion.

Injuries to upper limb structures may occur simultaneously with the cord trauma. Common are glenohumeral joint injuries (such as subluxation or dislocation), injuries to the nerve elements of the brachial plexus, and other more distally located fractures or dislocations, particularly to the wrist. These pre-existing entities must be sought by direct questioning and by obtaining suitable imaging studies where history, examination, and clinical suspicion dictate.

Current functional status

The patient's current functional status should be analyzed in the light of such parameters as neurological level and type of injury, and the time since injury. The analysis of current function must be conducted with the patient sitting in his or her wheelchair. Little is to be learned by performing this examination while the patient is confined to bed because of the need to heal a pressure sore or during recovery from bladder infection.

It is necessary for the patient to bring all currently used orthoses and adaptive devices, such as typing sticks, adaptive forks, and spoons. Objects that are used for feeding, self-grooming, wheelchair mobility, driving (if the patient is able to drive), and communication should be examined in the context of how they are used by the patient. By examining the common objects that the patient has found helpful, the rehabilitation team can gain perspective regarding how the

individual patient has learned to adapt to his or her new environment. How the patient currently uses his or her hands in performing tasks must be closely observed. Important information is learned by observing what type of grip the patient adopts to enable any use of the hands (*Fig. 6.1*). What may, at first glance, seem unusually complex or inefficient coping mechanisms or tools may actually be a crucial window into how the patient perceives his or her environment. If the patient uses a manual wheelchair, special attention should be paid to how the hands are used in propelling the chair. Similarly, observations of how transfers and weight shifts are performed are important. The goal is to identify the suboptimal habits of locomotion or transfers, especially those incompatible

A

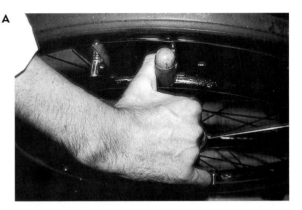

B

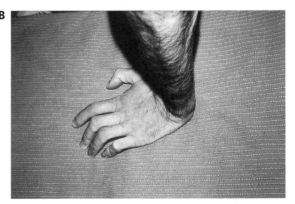

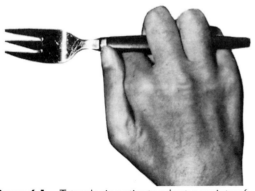

Figure 6.1 Tetraplegic patients adopt a variety of unusual but functionally effective hand postures to allow them to grip common objects and perform ADLs. Forks or pens may be woven through fingers in an attempt to increase stability of grasp. (Reproduced from Moberg 1978,[5] with permission.)

Figure 6.2 The hand positions used by the patient for (A) wheelchair mobility and (B) transfers must be evaluated. If the patient uses (B) a flat hand for transferring or (A) pushes quad knobs with an extended thumb this must be recognized and the patient must be instructed in methods that are compatible with a good surgical outcome.

with preserving normal structure and stability in the long term or those habits that will lead to poor results following surgery, such as transfers on hyperextended thumbs and fingers (*Fig. 6.2*).

Subsequent surgery or splinting may make it difficult or impossible for patients to use their hands in the way that they have become accustomed. Unless the new are far superior to the old ways, the patient may be displeased with the outcome of surgery or the expensive new brace.

It is useful to develop a standardized list of functions of daily living to be evaluated. Appendix VIII is an example of one format.

The patient frequently may bring up points of view regarding functional aspects that may differ considerably from those of the therapist or surgeon. The way the patient thinks may be very different from the way the surgeon thinks. The examining team should avoid the temptation to visualize as the ultimate objective only a hand that closely resembles a normally functioning hand.

The global functional status can be assessed using one or more of several now standard schemes such as the Functional Independence Measurement (see Appendix III and also Chapter 18).[1,2]

The upper limb physical examination

Passive and active joint range of motion and joint stability

The passive and the active range of motion of all the joints of the upper limb should be measured and

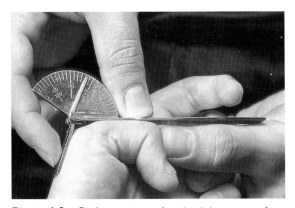

Figure 6.3 Both passive and active joint range of motion should be measured and recorded.

recorded (*Fig. 6.3*). Functionally significant joint contractures or instabilities should be highlighted on the chart. A number of charts or diagrams are available to assist in the examination and recording of the data (*Fig. 6.4*). Any pain that occurs with either passive or active joint movement should be recorded. The wrist is actively and passively flexed and extended and the patient's digital posture examined to assess the current tenodesis tone. Abnormal digital postures that will compromise the outcome of any surgery are identified (*Fig. 6.5*).

Joint stability should be assessed by stress testing. Key joints include the carpometacarpal and metacarpophalangeal joints of the thumb and the metacarpophalangeal joints of the other fingers. Extreme joint laxity of one or another of these key joints guides the choice of treatment. For example, excessive laxity at the paralyzed thumb's carpometacarpal joint is evidence of overstretching of the supporting ligaments. Such an unstable joint might best be fused as part of a plan to restore strong grasp.

Active motor systems

Every muscle of each upper limb should be tested by standard manual motor-testing techniques. Special attention is paid to key muscles such as the several parts of the deltoid, the triceps, and the wrist extensors. The data are recorded in a flow chart so that progress over time can be appreciated easily. Of necessity, tetraplegic patients learn quickly to perform substitutions or adaptive 'trick' maneuvers. Some experience is required to perform an adequate test.

Several key muscles are more difficult to evaluate effectively than are others.

Deltoid

To test the muscle, the patient must be able to sit in the wheelchair, as it is difficult to test the deltoid muscle reliably with the patient lying or reclining in bed. The patient is asked first to horizontally abduct both arms to 90° of abduction (*Fig. 6.6A*). Most patients almost automatically flex the elbow nearly completely as they abduct the arm at the shoulder. In this position, the general strength of both deltoid muscles can be assessed. Next, the observer should stand behind and slightly beside the arm to be tested. The patient is advised to loop the elbow of the

Hand Surgery Evaluation (Tetraplegia)

Hospital:

Patient's name: _____

Date of examination:

_____

Examiner's signature:

_____

Born: Sex:

Home address: Telephone
                                 number:

Ward: Doctor:

Occupation before accident:
Occupation now, if any:

Date of injury: Type of accident: Car accident
Level of skeletal injury: Diving
Leading arm-hand before: Gunshot
Leading arm-hand now: _____

Use of wheelchair: Handdriven   Can raise seat in wheelchair?
                      Electric   Can turn over in bed without help?
                      Other   Can transfer without help from bed to wheelchair?
                                    Can transfer without help from wheelchair to car
                                    and back again?

Functional C level: Eating with?   Grip?   Tools?

Right   Left   Method of grooming? (Shaving, make-up)

                 Method of writing?

                 Stabilization in wheelchair?

Contractures?
Previous amputations?
Unusual lack of joint stability?

Group: Right   Left

          [O] [Cu] : [ ]   [O] [Cu] : [ ]

          Tr [ ]   Tr [ ]

Delete as necessary.

Name:

Spasticity (significant)   Shoulder   Wrist

                           Elbow   Hand

Muscles available:
(Highets scheme)

	Right	Left
Trapezius		
Latissimus dorsi		
Deltoid		
Serratus anterior		
Rotators out		
Rotators in		
Pectoralis muscles:		
Sternoclavicular part		
Costal part		
Triceps		
Biceps + Brachialis		
Brachioradialis		
Radial carpal		
extensors (together)		
Pronator		
Finger extensors		
Long thumb abductor		
Thumb extensor		
Flexor carpi radialis		
Flexor pollicis longus		
Extensor carpi ulnaris		
Finger flexors		
Intrinsics		
Passive range of flexion		
Thumb metacarpophalangeal		
joint in degrees:		

    R   L

Patient's understanding:

Cooperation expected:

Sensibility: (only two-point discrimination
test with paperclip of value;
includes proprioception)

	R.	L.
Thumb pulp		
Index		
Middle		
Ring		
Little		
Dorsal radial area		
Dorsal ulnar area		

Unusual features and remarks:

Patient's main hand and arm problems:

Suggestions for improvement by splinting or
surgery:

Figure 6.4   A sample format to guide and record the findings of the upper limb evaluation.

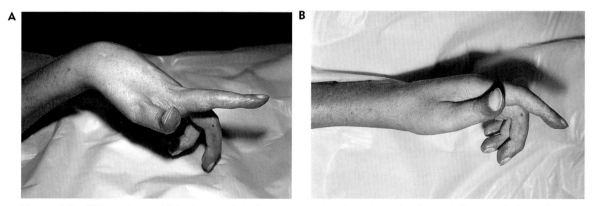

Figure 6.5   This patient exhibited a spastic index extensor that kept the index finger fully extended whether the wrist was (A) bent or (B) extended. This abnormality must be corrected for this patient to become a good candidate for restoration of key pinch (see Chapter 12).

A

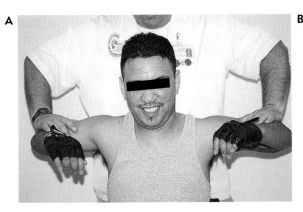

B

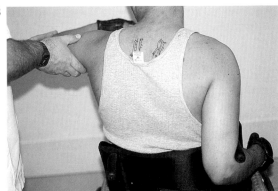

C

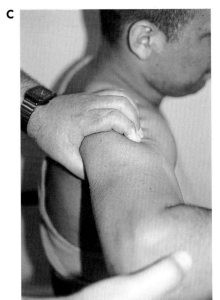

D

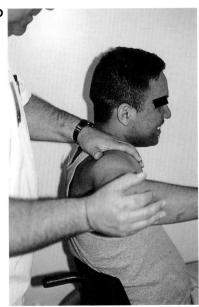

Figure 6.6 Evaluating the strength of (A) the deltoid and (B)–(D) the posterior half of the deltoid (see text).

opposite arm around the handle of the wheelchair, if such exists, to stabilize the trunk (*Fig. 6.6B*). If the chair lacks a handle, then some other maneuver must be performed to effect trunk stabilization. For example, another individual may serve the same purpose as the wheelchair handle by allowing the patient to loop his or her arm through the second observer's tensed arm. The observer places the palm of one hand against the posterior surface of the patient's humerus. The fingers of the free hand grasp the posterior half of the deltoid muscle. This is most easily achieved by inserting the thumb into the interval between the posterior edge of the deltoid and the long head of the triceps muscle (*Fig. 6.6C*). The patient is asked to push his or her arm and shoulder as hard as

possible against the flat of the examiner's other hand. The tension and bulk of the posterior half of the deltoid is assessed by the observer's opposite hand as the patient makes a maximal effort (*Fig. 6.6D*).

Another useful method to examine the strength of the posterior deltoid is to have the patient lie prone with the arm to be examined allowed to hang off the side of the bed. The patient is asked to abduct the shoulder from this position while the examiner resists this motion and, at the same time, palpates the muscle mass of the posterior deltoid.

Pectoralis major

The patient is asked to press the palms together as forcefully as possible while the examiner palpates both pectoralis muscles to assess their bulk and resistance to displacement.

Brachioradialis

In performing its normal function as an accessory flexor of the elbow, the brachioradialis (BR) cannot be isolated from the effects of the primary flexors of the elbow, the biceps, and brachialis. Experience has shown that its strength can only be estimated. This is best accomplished by first positioning the forearm of the patient in about 90° of flexion at the elbow and the forearm in neutral rotation. Next, the patient is asked to try to forcefully further flex the elbow while the examiner resists greater flexion with one hand and palpates the contracting BR muscle with the other (*Fig. 6.7*). By grasping the contracting muscle, the examiner can appreciate its bulk. By trying to displace the contracting muscle to one side or the other, the examiner is able to assess its relative strength. A muscle of small volume that is easily displaced from its normal straight line of pull is probably too weak to perform much functionally significant work if surgically transferred.

A

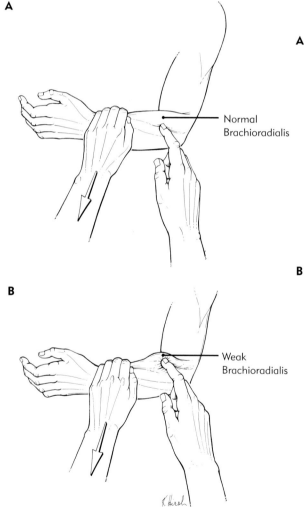

B

Normal Brachioradialis

Weak Brachioradialis

Figure 6.7 (A) A strong brachioradialis (BR) muscle has increased bulk and is not easily displaced when it is contracting. (B) A weak BR muscle is easily displaced laterally even when the muscle is being maximally contracted.

A

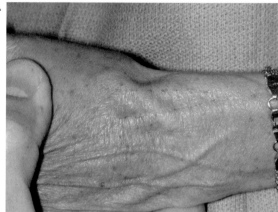

B

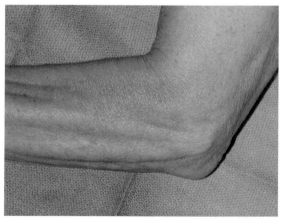

Figure 6.8 If both radial wrist extensors are contracting strongly, the observer may appreciate the formation of a 'V-shaped' notch directly in line with the second metacarpal. If both extensor carpi radialis longus (ECRL) and extensor carpi radialis brevis (ECRB) are contracting strongly, one may appreciate a groove or depression near the lateral epicondyle.

Extensor carpi radialis longus and brevis

Several techniques have been described to assist the examiner in determining whether one or both radial wrist extensors are strongly contracting. The extensor carpi radialis longus (ECRL) is typically innervated by slightly higher spinal segments than the extensor carpi radialis brevis (ECRB). Its insertion is on the radial side of the base of the second metacarpal. If this muscle is contracting, one can usually palpate the tendon coming under some tension by first resisting wrist extension efforts and then placing a finger over the course of the tendon, at the distal margin of the extensor retinaculum. The tendon of the ECRB inserts on the radial side of the base of the third metacarpal. If both the ECRL and ECRB contract, both tendons become tense. In the thinner wrist, this may result in the formation of a hollow or depression, or a 'V'-shaped notch just distal to the edge of the extensor retinaculum, with the apex of the 'V' pointing proximally (*Fig. 6.8A*). Just below the lateral epicondyle, the observer may appreciate an indentation forming at the juncture of these two muscles. When both are contracting, it is impossible to reliably estimate the strength of one relative to the other (*Fig. 6.8B*). This determination may need to be made at the time of any surgery that proposes to transfer one or the other of these muscles. Several intraoperative techniques are discussed in Chapter 13.

Standard manual muscle testing is adequate to determine the residual strength of the other commonly preserved forearm muscles.

Sensory examination

The typical sensory modalities, such as light touch and temperature sensation, are tested in a general manner for each spinal segment using the commonly described anatomic areas (*Fig. 6.9*). Other indirect evidence of retained sensation is sought, such as evidence of sweating. Sensory evaluation of the hand should also include testing for retained proprioception. Moberg has championed the use of two-point discrimination tests as a measure of retained proprioception and finer discrimination.[3] This is a simple, inexpensive and easily performed evaluation.

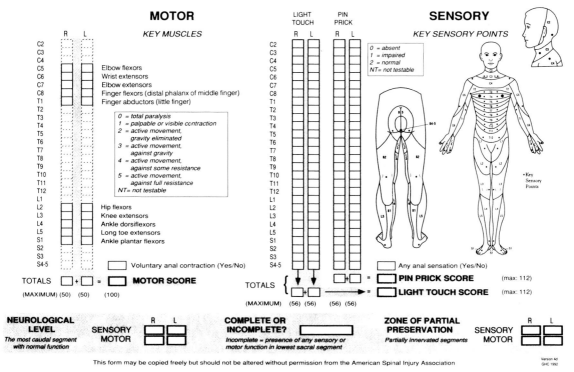

Figure 6.9 A sample chart for determining neurological classification. (Courtesy of the American Spinal Injury Association.)

Moberg's two-point discrimination test

While several commercially available tools can be used to perform this test, the least expensive and most readily available tool, as Moberg advised, is a straightened paperclip folded into a 'U' shape. Accuracy with this testing method requires a gentle application of either one point or both points of the tool to the skin (*Fig. 6.10*). The patient is asked to look away from the finger being tested and to tell the observer whether he or she perceives one or both points touching the skin. The subject is advised not to merely guess, but to state that he or she can not tell any difference if that is the case.

The observer may begin with the two points of the tool separated by 15 mm. If the patient cannot distinguish the difference between a single point and two points separated by 15 mm that touch the skin, there is no need to further test this digit. The two points of the tool are bent progressively closer together in 1–2 mm increments until the patient can no longer distinguish one from two points. The final distance between the two points becomes the recorded measurement. Usually, two to four trials at the closest discernable interval are advised to be certain that the patient is not merely guessing at the response. The normally innervated digit can determine two points at an interval of 2–3 mm. Moberg believed that proprioception was retained in a digit still capable of discrimination of two points 12–15 mm apart. Given the usual metameric patterns of innervation and injury, it may not be necessary to test all digits equally care-

fully. The C5 injury patient is able to tell the observer that one or another digit is anesthetic.

Other tests have been proposed to determine the presence or absence of proprioception.[4] For example, the finger to be tested is placed in one position or another and the 'blindfolded' patient is asked to determine whether a joint (e.g., the proximal interphalangeal joint) is flexed or extended. The 'common-objects test' involves placing a series of different but common objects on the fingers to be tested and asking the blindfolded patient to identify which object is placed. All these tests may be reliable, but the two-point examination described above remains the simplest to perform and is the most commonly used.

Pathological features

The examiner must search for those pathological features most likely to compromise functional recovery from surgery of orthotics. These include such characteristics as hypersensitivity of one or more digits, static or dynamic flexion or extension contractures or laxity of any joint of the upper limb, and troublesome spasticity, as illustrated above. Hypersensitivity of the digits or hand may make it impossible for the patient to touch or hold objects. Contractures or laxity may interfere with either opening or closing the hand or digits around objects. Severe spasticity of the upper limb equally compromises function. Where these features exist, they or their causes must be analyzed to determine if they are treatable.

A
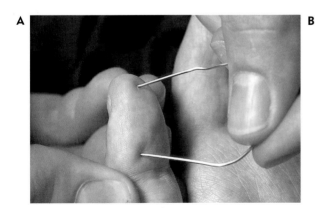
B
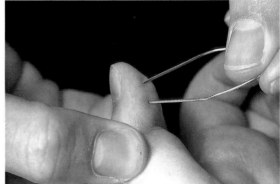

Figure 6.10 The points of the device should be pressed gently against the skin. The skin should barely blanch at the point(s) of contact. (A) Two-point discrimination is greater than 15 mm, so the finger lacks proprioception. (B) Two-point discrimination is about 7 mm, so this digit has preserved proprioception.

Some of these pathological features may be treatable and, if treated, the patient may become a much better candidate for functional upper limb surgery or orthotics. For example, upper limb spasticity may be brought under control by the addition of anti-spasmodic medication. A pathological contracture of a key joint may be treated by directed therapy, dynamic splinting, or even by a preliminary surgical procedure. Some pathological features seem to defy treatment, such as extreme hypersensitivity.

Conclusion

At completion of the basic examination, the evaluating team should have gained sufficient information to classify each limb according to the classification system introduced in Chapter 7 and to begin to formulate a specific treatment plan.

References

1. Whiteneck C. A functional independence measure trial in SCI model symptoms. ASIA Abstracts Digest 1988:48.
2. Schindler L, Robbins G, Hamlin C. Functional effect of bilateral tendon transfers on a person with C5 quadriplegia. Am J Occup Ther 1994; 48:750–757.
3. Moberg E. Criticism and study of the methods for examining sensibility in the hand. Neurology 1962; 12:8–12.
4. McCloskey D. Kinesthetic sensibility. Phys Rev 1978; 58:763–820.
5. Moberg E. The Upper Limb in Tetraplegia. Stuttgart: Georg Thieme Verlag; 1978: 73.

7

Classifying the surgical candidate: a system of classification for the tetraplegic based on residual limb power

Introduction

Several systems to classify spinal cord injury patients have been proposed and used by various professionals involved in the care of such patients. Some systems were based on the location of the bony injury as determined radiographically. Others were based on the evaluation of residual motor and sensory function, which could then be related to specific areas of the spinal cord itself. Still others were based on commonly recurring patterns of injury, such as the older Frankel and newer American Spinal Injury Association (ASIA) scales.

There are advantages and disadvantages unique to each classification system, and no single system satisfies everyone. Each system is (or was) most useful to the particular group of clinicians promoting the system. Surgeons interested in upper limb rehabilitation found the need to introduce yet another classification system, termed the International Classification, and discussed below.

History

50 years ago, the pioneers of surgical rehabilitation of the upper limb classified the level of tetraplegia according to the location of the vertebral lesion.[1] This classification, although helpful at the time, was not convenient because frequently the medullary level of the spinal cord damage does not correspond with the location of the bony lesion. In many circumstances, there was no visible bony injury. Also, a terminological disparity arose because there are eight medullar segments but only seven vertebrae.

Progressively, most physicians dealing with para- and tetraplegic patients started to classify them according to the level of the spinal (medullary) lesion. However, confusion soon followed because in English-speaking countries the injury level was designated by the last uninjured cord segment, whereas in several other countries, especially in Europe, it was designated by the first injured level. Another shortcoming of this classification was the lack of differentiation between the right and the left side of the body. In reality, approximately half the patients have differences between the two arms significant enough to indicate a separate classification. Finally, the motor level does not always coincide with the sensory level, especially true of higher level injuries. These deficiencies suggested the need for a system that separately classifies the type and level of injury for each patient and each limb. All these flaws were taken into account by ASIA, which in 1982 published standards for neurological classification of spinal cord injuries, which have thereafter been revised periodically.[2] The format recommended by ASIA and entitled *Standard Neurological Classification of Spinal Cord Injury – Version 4D, 1992* is reproduced in Appendix I.

The ASIA classification

The ASIA impairment scale is a modification of the Frankel scale and assigns patients with spinal cord injuries into one of five categories:

A Complete: no motor or sensory function is preserved in the sacral segments S4–S5.
B Incomplete: sensory but not motor function is preserved below the neurological level and extends through the sacral segments S4–S5.
C Incomplete: motor function is preserved below the neurological level, and the majority of key muscles below the neurological level have a muscle MRC Grade less than 3.
D Incomplete: motor function is preserved below the neurological level, and the majority of key muscles below the neurological level have a muscle grade greater than or equal to 3.
E Normal: motor and sensory function is normal.

In this classification, the neurological level refers to the most caudal segment of the spinal cord with normal sensory and motor function on both sides of the body. However, it is recommended not to use this as such (i.e., as a single level), because there may be differences between motor and sensory levels and sides of body. Instead, the recommendation is to use a sensory level (R-sensory and L-sensory) and a motor level (R-motor and L-motor).

The sensory level refers to the most caudal segment of the spinal cord with normal sensory function. It is determined by testing for presence or absence of pin prick and light touch in key points of the body. Pin prick is performed using a disposable safety pin, and light touch with a wisp of cotton wool. There is one key point for each of the 28 dermatomes on the right and on the left side of the body (see *Fig. 2.4*). For the upper limb, these key points include:

- C4, top of the acromioclavicular joint;
- C5, lateral side of the antecubital fossa;
- C6, thumb;
- C7, middle finger;
- C8, little finger; and
- T1, medial side of the antecubital fossa.

A scoring system has been added to the classification, permitting an enumeration of the patient's neurological progression over time. Pin prick and light touch are separately scored at each key point, according to

Table 7.1 Sensory scale for pin prick and for light touch

Score	Description
0	Absent
1	Impaired (including hyperesthesia)
2	Normal
NT	Not testable

the scoring system shown in *Table 7.1*. These scores are then summed across the dermatomes and sides of the body to generate two global scores, one for pin prick and one for light touch (maximum of 112 each).

The motor level refers to the most caudal segment of the spinal cord with (preserved) useful motor function. A key muscle (on the right and on the left side of the body) is tested in each of the 10 paired myotomes of the upper and lower limbs. For the upper limb, the key muscles are:

- C5, the elbow flexors [biceps and brachioradialis (BR)];
- C6, the wrist extensors [extensor carpi radialis longus (ECRL) and brevis (ECRB)];
- C7, the elbow extensors (triceps);
- C8, the finger flexors (flexor digitorum profundus, middle finger); and
- T1, the abductor digiti minimi.

Table 7.2 Muscle grading according to the Medical Research Council

Grade	Muscle function
0	Total paralysis
1	Palpable or visible contraction
2	Active movement, full range of motion (ROM) with gravity
3	Full active ROM against gravity
4	Full active ROM against moderate resistance
5	Normal (full active ROM against full resistance)
NT	Not testable

The strength of the muscle is graded on a six-point scale, according to Medical Research Council (MRC) recommendations (*Table 7.2*).[3]

The motor level is defined by the lowest key muscle that has a MRC Grade of at least 3, provided the key muscles above that level are judged to be normal (Grade 4 or 5). These scores are summed across myotomes and sides of the body to generate a single global motor score (maximum of 100).

The ASIA classification thus comprises one motor and one sensory level for each side of the body (R-motor, R-sensory; L-motor, L-sensory), as well as two sensory scores (one for pin prick and one for light touch) and one motor score (Appendix I, the ASIA Standard Neurological Classification of Spinal Cord Injury). This classification, which is now used world wide, has made possible accurate communication between clinicians and investigators, and also valid comparisons between past and future spinal cord injury data bases.

Surgical classifications

Even when accurately applied, the ASIA classification does not provide sufficient information about each muscle of the upper limbs in tetraplegia. As rehabilitative surgery of the tetraplegic's upper limb is based mainly on tendon transfers, required was a classification based on residual muscle power, with a specific focus on muscles of Grade 4 and above, that are suitable for transfer. Most surgical pioneers in this field introduced classifications based on this concept. Zancolli, in 1968, published a classification that con-

sisted of four groups based on the lowest functioning muscle group (*Table 7.3*).[4] However, he realized that these groups were too heterogeneous and chose to subdivide the lower three groups into subgroups (*Table 7.4*). Although he stated that the sensory level varied between one patient and another, he did not include any sensory component in his classification.

In 1972, Lamb and Chan published a classification system based on six groups (*Table 7.5*).[5] They included the presence of an active triceps within their classification system as Group 5. Lamb and Chan's lowest group, Group 6, included patients with preservation of the finger extensors, which implied that there was little or no need for surgery in patients with a lower level of injury. They stated that patients in Groups 3 to 6 could benefit from surgery. They did not find the need for an additional sensory classification, as all the patients in these four lower groups had sensation to light touch and pin prick on the radial side of the hand at least. They did not find Moberg's two-point discrimination (2PD) test to be of any value in the preoperative assessment of patients.

Table 7.3 Zancolli's classification

Group	Lowest functioning muscle group
I	Flexor of the elbow
II	Extensor of the wrist
III	Extrinsic extensor of the fingers
IV	Extrinsic flexor of the fingers and thumb extensor

Table 7.4 Zancolli's subgroups

Subgroup	Criteria
IIA	Weak extension of the wrist
IIB	Strong extension of the wrist
IIIA	Complete extension of ulnar fingers and paralysis of radial fingers and thumb
IIIB	Complete extension of all fingers and weak thumb extension
IVA	Complete flexion of ulnar fingers and paralysis (or weakness) of radial fingers and thumb; complete extension of the thumb
IVB	Complete flexion of fingers and thumb

Table 7.5   Lamb's classification

Group	Criteria
1	Shoulder shrug only
2	Group 1 + shoulder abduction + elbow flexion
3	Group 2 + wrist dorsiflexion, pronation, and supination
4	Group 3 + flexor carpi radialis
5	Group 4 + elbow extension
6	Group 5 + finger extension

Table 7.6   Freehafer's classification

Group	Voluntary function that remains
1	No voluntary function of the wrist and hand
2	Weak wrist extension
3	Useful brachioradialis and extensor carpi radiales
4	Group 3 + triceps, pronator teres, and flexor carpi radialis
5	Weakness of intrinsics
6	Exceptions

In 1974, Freehafer *et al.* published a similar classification in six groups (*Table 7.6*), and introduced the need for a group dedicated to exceptions.[6] In 1975, Moberg introduced his own classification, which included two sensory groups and eight motors groups.[7]

The International Classification

Improved awareness of the extent to which a tetraplegic patient can be rehabilitated and improvement in the quality of results after surgical reconstruction led to a formal gathering of experts in Edinburgh in June 1978.[8] This was to become the first of a series of International Conferences on Surgical Rehabilitation of the Upper Limb in Tetraplegia. At this first meeting, the foundation for a surgical classification was established, based on the classification developed by Moberg in 1975,[7] and the International Classi-

fication (IC) was finalized during the Second International Conference, held in Giens (France) in 1984.[9] This classification was later adopted by the International Federation for Societies for Surgery of the Hand (IFSSH) and revisited at subsequent International Conferences on Tetraplegia.

This IC does not include information about the status of muscles about the shoulder or elbow. It is a guide to the status of the forearm and hand only. In recognition of Moberg's strong emphasis on the benefits of elbow extension in the tetraplegic patient, the indications for its reconstruction, that is absence of triceps function, is stated separately.

The classification has sensory and motor components. Moberg introduced the sensory component in 1975.[7] He had noticed that tactile gnosis parallels proprioception, and can accurately be tested in the hand by the 2PD test, performed with a simple bent paperclip.[10,11] He eschewed special calipers and gauges for this task. Moberg forcefully argued that if the 2PD is greater than 10–12 mm in the thumb (C6 territory, see above), then the sensory input from this hand is inadequate to control grip.[12–14] In this case, vision becomes the only afferent resource available. The IC's sensory designation in this case is 'occulo', abbreviated to 'O'. If the 2PD is equal to or less than 10–12 mm in the thumb, sensation is adequate for proprioception and the hand is able to provide adequate afferent control of the grip. In this case the IC's sensory designation is 'cutaneous', abbreviated to 'Cu'. If both ocular and cutaneous afferent impulses are present, the IC's sensory designation is abbreviated 'O/Cu'.

The motor classification is based on residual motor function and includes only muscles that originate around or below the level of the elbow and are MRC Grade 4 or 5 strength. Group 0 includes cases in which no muscle below the elbow is suitable for transfer. A new muscle is added for each successive group until Group 9 (lack of intrinsics only), and group 10 includes all exceptions (*Table 7.7*). Each upper limb is considered separately, so there are two classifications per patient (R and L).

A few points must be stressed:

- Several muscles are difficult to test, namely the BR and the ECRB. However, it is mandatory to be able to quantify their strength. In the tetraplegic population, the BR is frequently a potentially

Table 7.7 International Classification

Group	Lowest muscle grade >4
0	No muscle below elbow
1	Brachioradialis
2	Extensor carpi radialis longus
3	Extensor carpi radialis brevis
4	Pronator
5	Flexor carpi radialis
6	Finger extensors
7	Thumb extensors
8	Partial digital flexors
9	Lacks only intrinsics
10	Exceptions

transferable muscle, and the result of surgery is unpredictable, if not failure, if it is initially a weak Grade 4 or a Grade 3. As for the ECRB, it frequently remains the only wrist extensor if the ECRL is transferred. If it is weak, this may result in considerable functional loss for the patient. Chapter 6 explains the most accurate ways to test these two muscles.

- The usefulness of the sensory component may be questioned, as most patients from IC Group 2 and higher have a thumb with adequate sensation (O/Cu). Arguably, its use might be restricted to IC Groups 0 and 1.

- This classification is merely a momentary 'snapshot' of the muscular status of the tetraplegic patient. In itself muscle strength is an inadequate indicator of successful surgical rehabilitation of the upper limbs. It is only one of the many elements that help the rehabilitation team decide whether or not to perform surgery, and which type of procedure is indicated for each individual patient.

Most surgeons who perform surgical rehabilitation for the tetraplegic upper limb adopt this IC. Its methodology is simple, reasonably intuitive, and easily learned. Chapters 11 (IC Group 0) through 16 (IC Group 10) are organized according to this system.

References

1. Lipscomb PR, Elkin EC, Henderson ED. Tendon transfers to restore function of hands in tetraplegia, especially after fracture–dislocation of the sixth cervical vertebra on the seventh. J Bone Joint Surg 1958; 40:1071–1080.

2. American Spinal Injury Association. Standards for Neurological and Functional Classification of Spinal Cord Injury. Atlanta: American Spinal Injury Association, 1992.

3. Medical Research Council. Aids to Investigation of Peripheral Nerve Injuries. 2nd edn. Medical Research Council War Memorandum No. 7. London: HMSO, 1943:1.

4. Zancolli E. Structural and Dynamic Bases of Hand Surgery. Philadelphia: Lippincott, 1968.

5. Lamb DW, Chan KM. Surgical reconstruction of the upper limb in traumatic tetraplegia. J Bone Joint Surg 1983; 65B:291–298.

6. Freehafer AA, Von Haam E, Allen V. Tendon transfers to improve grasp after injuries of the cervical spinal cord. J Bone Joint Surg 1976; 56A:951–959.

7. Moberg E. Surgical treatment for absent single-hand grip and elbow extension in quadriplegia. J Bone Joint Surg (Am) 1975; 57(2):196–206.

8. McDowell CL, Moberg EA, Graham Smith A. International conference on surgical rehabilitation of the upper limb in tetraplegia. J Hand Surg 1979; 4:387–390.

9. McDowell CL, Moberg EA, House JH. The second international conference on surgical rehabilitation of the upper limb in tetraplegia (Proceedings). J Hand Surg 1986; 11A:604–608.

10. Moberg E. Criticism and study of methods for examining sensibility in the hand. Neurology 1962; 12:8–19.

11. Moberg E. Nerve repair in hand surgery. An analysis. Surg Clin North Am 1968; 48:985–991.

12. Moberg E, McDowell CL, House JH. Third International Conference on Surgical Rehabilitation of the Upper Limb in Tetraplegia (Proceedings). J Hand Surg 1989; 14(A);1064–1066.

13. Hentz VR, House J, McDowell CL, et al. Rehabilitation and surgical reconstruction of the upper limb in tetraplegia: an update. J Hand Surg 1992; 17A: 964–967.

14. Moberg EA. Upper limb surgical rehabilitation in tetraplegia. In: McCollister Evans C, ed. Surgery of the Musculoskeletal System. New York: Churchill Livingstone, 1990:915–941.

8

Indications for performing surgical rehabilitation

Introduction

The goal of surgery or functional bracing is to move the patient toward a state of greater and greater independence. The indications for functional upper limb surgery or bracing for the tetraplegic patient have evolved (see Chapter 1) in keeping with the evolution of the overall care for these patients. And, just as the philosophy of care differs from one spinal cord facility or country to another, so do the surgical indications. Indications for surgery are based on many factors, including the past experience of the spinal cord unit's physician and therapy staff, their personal biases, and the interest, availability, and experience of surgical subspecialists. Some very well-respected spinal cord injury centers have a strongly positive bias toward promoting the possibility of upper limb surgery for their patients through early education and evaluation. Other equally respected centers have an opposite philosophical bias. Over the past two decades, indications have broadened because of the evolving sense of the importance of this area to overall rehabilitation. As mentioned in Chapter 1, the history of upper limb functional reconstructive surgery for the tetraplegic individual has been marked by periods of both high and low acceptance. In the USA, current circumstances have been influenced in part by governmental mandate. Today, one of the provisions necessary before a center can be designated a 'model' spinal cord injury center is access to upper limb reconstructive surgery. Questions regarding surgical rehabilitation are now commonly included in Physical Medicine and Rehabilitation in-service training and board examinations in the USA. Lectures on this topic are a regular part of the curriculum for Spinal Cord Injury Board Certification review courses.

Through exposure to physiatrist colleagues, many more surgeons have become increasingly knowledgeable about both the special conditions imposed by this devastating injury and the many reasons why the tetraplegic is so different from other patients who are candidates for upper limb functional reconstructive surgery. In addition, the surgeon's armamentarium has grown as additional procedures have been found to pass the test of time.

The rights of the disabled and their role in society have changed through such seemingly disparate events as the 'Special Olympics' or the 'International Paraplegia Games', initially championed by Europeans, and the American's with Disability Act (ADA), passed by the US Congress and signed into law by President Clinton in 1992. In much of the industrialized world, it has been realized that even the tetraplegic patient can contribute to society, and can be an asset rather than a societal liability through skillful physical and psychological rehabilitation and vocational education.

These trends strongly re-emphasize the contention expressed by Erik Moberg in his 1978 monograph that 'the possibility of improving the function of the hands and arms (of tetraplegics) would be an important contribution, as there is much truth in the saying that 'their hands are their life'.[1] Aside from the brain, tetraplegic patients' upper limbs represent their most important functional resource. In a survey of male patients, 75% rated restoration of normal function of arms and hands as more important than the return of normal bowel and bladder, legs, and sexual function.[2] Thus, while much has changed regarding the indications for surgical rehabilitation over the past 25 years, the tetraplegic patient's desire for improved function has not.

Timing of surgical interventions – achieving stability

The issue of timing for surgical rehabilitation is contentious. In general, there are few indications to perform functionally directed surgical procedures before the neurological picture has stabilized clearly (physical stability), the patient has come to accept the significance of the injury (mental stability), and the goals of rehabilitation have been clearly established (social stability.) However, there are clear indications for upper limb surgical intervention before the patient has attained these three areas of stability, although more often the immediate goal of such surgery is the correction of disabling deformity.

To achieve overall stability takes time, perhaps the oft-stated 1 year. Some issues that affect timing are very obvious. For example, surgical goals and thus indications cannot be accurately determined until the patient has achieved neurological stability. Others are less obvious, but equally important. Until the patient has come to accept that, more than likely, he or she will always be a tetraplegic, the patient will understandably be disappointed with almost any functional gain achieved through surgery or bracing. The functional outcome can never compare to normal, and until psychological stability is achieved, in his or her heart, normality is what the patient most desires and anything less is, by definition, less acceptable or, frequently, unacceptable. It must be clear to all concerned that the patient fully understands the limitations of surgical reconstruction and is able to accept the significant lower order of performance afforded by even the best planned and executed surgery, compared to normal function.

There are other very practical time-related considerations. The enormity of life's changes brought about by the injury is overwhelming for even the strongest psyche. The recently injured patient is faced with unprecedented functional challenges. Overcoming the obstacles associated with this injury requires huge expenditures of time and energy. Upper limb functional surgery must be secondary to the need to spend time and energy on more pressing tasks, such as how

to manage bowel and bladder, perform the activities of daily living (ADLs), and organize for life as a tetraplegic outside the confines of the acute care or rehabilitation facility. The patient must have adequate time to participate in the necessary pre- and postoperative exercise protocols.

There are both physical and psychological contraindications to upper limb functional surgery. It is important to recognize these. Once recognized and analyzed, it may be possible to overcome the obstacle to surgery by various forms of treatment, such as directed therapy or even preliminary surgery.

Surgical preparedness

As for most elective procedures, surgery should be carried out only when the conditions are ideal; however, to achieve ideal circumstances is more difficult for the patient with cervical spinal cord injury. The tetraplegic patient must be carefully prepared for surgery because the pre- and postoperative physical and emotional consequences are more significant than for almost any other class of patient. For these patients, the term 'immobilization', as in protecting the operated part in a cast, takes on an entirely new meaning.

Locomotion

Electing to undergo surgery requires the patient to accept a variable period of increased dependence on additional equipment and other people for basic needs. The patient who routinely uses a manual wheelchair must obtain a powered chair for postoperative locomotion, since he or she will probably not be able to push a manual chair for weeks to months following surgery. Often, the physical structure of the home or apartment may have to be modified to accommodate the increased width and weight of a powered chair. Patients may not be able to afford to rent a powered chair and may have no insurance to provide this. Even the patient whose routine locomotion is with a powered chair may need the chair controls to be switched to the opposite side and may need a period of training and adaptation before having surgery.

The patient who is able to drive a car or van preoperatively will more than likely not be able to perform this activity following surgery and immobilization.

Attendant care

The postoperative patient will require additional assistance in performing many ADLs, particularly those that require forceful use of the arms and hands, such as transfers, dressing, and hygiene. A family member, friend, or a paid attendant must be available to provide this extra support. As alluded to above, there may be strong economic barriers to surgical candidacy. Those who accept this additional responsibility must be educated as to any precautions that need to be observed in assisting the postoperative patient in transfers or other activities.

Additional adaptive devices

The temporarily one-handed postsurgical patient may need to adopt different strategies to carry out other ADLs. If he has been able to perform self-catheterization, for example, he may need to utilize another method of urinary drainage during the postoperative period.

In the immediate preoperative period, the tetraplegic's respiratory and urological systems require much more detailed attention and the patient should be free from pressure sores. Regional anesthesia rather than general anesthesia is preferable.

Prestability 'early' upper limb surgery for pathological conditions

The most common indication for upper limb surgery before neurological stability has been achieved is the development of pathological conditions that interfere with the patient's ability to progress toward the goals of rehabilitation. Such indications include the development of flexion contractures at the elbow, the development of a supination contracture of the forearm, or the presence of uncontrollable spasticity in upper limb muscle groups, such as the biceps. The principles and practical surgical management of these elbow and forearm disorders are discussed in Chapter 10.

A second though less common indication for early upper limb surgery is to correct pathology that either pre-existed the spinal cord injury or was incurred at the time of spinal cord injury.

Matching patient to procedure – general considerations

While the general goal of surgery is greater independence, the specific goals of any surgical plan are determined primarily by the level of function remaining and, secondarily, by the presence of pathological conditions, particularly contractures, hypersensitivity, uncontrolled spasticity, and uncontrolled regional pain pathologies. The specific goals then govern the choice of procedure when procedural options exist.

Almost every tetraplegic patient who retains active control over one or more forearm muscles (C5 or more distal) is a potential candidate for functional reconstructive upper limb surgery. For example, almost every tetraplegic patient, who retains good strength in the deltoid or biceps muscles is a potential candidate for surgical reconstruction of active elbow extension if this is absent.

Not every patient needs or will choose to undergo surgery, but essentially all tetraplegic patients who retain control of the shoulder and elbow could benefit from surgery. Within the potential controversy regarding who is a candidate lie certain dichotomies. The tetraplegic patient who lacks MRC Grade 3 wrist extension but who has a strong brachioradialis (BR) can, by surgical transfer of BR to the wrist extensor, achieve better than antigravity wrist extension. In itself, little that is measurable by dynamometer or manual muscle testing has been gained. However, this small gain in wrist extension strength may make it possible for the patient to use a wrist-driven, flexor-hinged orthosis and achieve useful grasp and release, or the patient may subsequently undergo surgical tenodesis of the tendon of the flexor pollicis longus to the radius (Moberg key-grip procedure) and achieve a functionally useful key pinch without the need for any external orthosis (see Chapter 12). This is an example of the old adage, 'When you have nothing, a little (gained) becomes a lot.' In such cases, a very small surgical change may yield a large (to the patient) measurable functional improvement. In fact, this small change may be all that is surgically possible for this patient, who lacks so much. However, experience has taught that a very weak patient who is many years post-injury will have learned many functional habits and substitutions, and such 'tricks' are deeply ingrained. Unless the outcome of surgery makes a dramatic functional improvement, and this is rarely possible in the weaker patient, the patient will have trouble learning different habits if major re-education is necessary to take advantage of the small functional gains. Such patients may be overwhelmed by the efforts at re-education and will be disappointed by the results of surgery.

At the opposite end of the spectrum are the IC Group 6 or 7 patients. These patients have many functionally strong forearm muscles under excellent central control, including flexion and extension of the wrist. Since they are so strong, these patients usually function, in comparison to IC Group 2 or 3 patients, at a relatively high level. When compared to normal, however, these patients' weak digital grasp and pinch pales in contrast. Upper limb surgery for such a patient may convert a hand that, in comparison to the hand of an IC Group 2 patient, is functioning 'well' to one with a truly dramatically increased function.

The IC Group 1 patient who is barely functioning may see little risk or inconvenience from surgery, since he or she is functioning at such a marginal level. This patient, who is far more dependent on others for care, may willingly accept a short period of even greater dependence in return for any functional improvement. In contrast, the IC Group 8 patient, who retains some active flexion of thumb and digits and who is already functioning at a much higher level than an IC Group 2 patient, may see things from the opposite perspective. This patient is far more independent and is less willing to give up his or her independence, even briefly, unless absolutely convinced of the value of the sacrifice. However, it is the patient who already functions at the higher level who will realize a far greater gain from a single properly selected surgical procedure.

Summary

The general indications, timing, and choice of procedure can be determined by asking and answering appropriately the following 10 questions:

1. Has the patient achieved neurological, emotional, and social stability?
2. What are the current levels of motor and sensory resources and function? The number and strength of muscles that remain under good voluntary control are the most important variables.
3. Are patient expectations realistic?
4. Does the patient possess the necessary intelligence and motivation? Some procedures require very little in the way of motivation to succeed. For example, a procedure such as an arthrodesis of a specific joint requires little in the way of patient motivation to be successful. In contrast, a complex set of muscle–tendon transfers requires a great deal of motor re-education for the patient to achieve an optimal result.
5. Does the patient have the necessary time to invest in obtaining a good result? The patient must be able to set aside the time necessary for postoperative immobilization in a cast or splint and the time necessary for therapy and re-education.
6. Are the necessary support services and personnel available and committed?
7. Have all the obstacles to success been considered and a plan developed to overcome any remaining ones?
8. Does the patient understand the potential complications as well as the potential benefits?
9. Can the patient and professional team tolerate a complication, failure, or suboptimal result? Both medical staff and the patient must be prepared for avoidable and unavoidable complications that lead to a suboptimal outcome or frank failure.
10. Is the patient's current health and well-being ideal?

Chapters 10 through 16 discuss the surgical procedures indicated for specific groups of patients classified according to the International Classification system introduced in Chapter 7. The specifics of matching patient and procedure are discussed in these subsequent chapters.

References

1. Moberg E. The Upper Limb in Tetraplegia. A new approach to surgical rehabilitation. Stuttgart: George Thieme, 1978.
2. Hanson RW, Franklin WR. Sexual loss in relation to other functional losses for spinal cord injured males. Arch Phys Med Rehabil 1976; 57:291–293.

Principles of tendon transfers, tenodeses, and fusions

Introduction

Surgical improvement of the tetraplegic upper limb involves a limited number of surgical procedures, three of which are the most commonly performed: tendon transfers, tenodeses, and fusions (arthrodeses). In this chapter these procedures are defined and described, including the general principles, technical concepts, relative indications and contraindications, and general postoperative requirements. A special emphasis is placed on tenodesis procedures and the so-called 'tenodesis effect.' These concepts are the foundations upon which the principles of rehabilitation of the hand in the tetraplegic patient are based. In the chapters that follow, those procedures favored by the authors for each specific International Classification (IC) group (see Chapter 7) are discussed in greater detail.

Tenodesis and the tenodesis effect

A tenodesis is defined as the automatic movement of a joint produced by the motion of another, usually more proximal, joint. The majority of tetraplegic patients belong to IC Groups 2 and 3, and by definition they have Medical Research Council (MRC) Grade 4 active wrist extension. For those in IC Group 2 this is through the extensor carpi radialis longus muscle (ECRL) and for those in IC Group 3 it is through both the ECRL and extensor carpi radialis brevis (ECRB), but all the muscles that normally move the fingers, whether extrinsic or intrinsic, are paralyzed. Therefore, these patients have no active flexion or extension of any joints of the fingers, and no active motion of the thumb. However, in the still supple hand, if they actively bring their wrist into a position of extension the flexion of the fingers and flexion and adduction of the thumb occur automatically. Together, these result in an automatic pinch-like movement between the pulp of the thumb and the radial aspect of the index finger. This is referred to as the 'tenodesis effect' (*Figs 9.1A* and *9.1B*). It is a consequence of the relative lengthening of the volar surface of the wrist as it is extended, which increases the tension on the digital flexors and simultaneously reduces the tension on the digital extensors, thus bringing the fingers and thumb automatically into passive flexion. If the wrist is supple and the patient can pronate the forearm, gravity flexes the wrist when the patient relaxes the ECRL and/or ECRB. This relatively lengthens the dorsal surface, which tightens the extrinsic extensor tendons and relaxes the flexor tendons. The fingers and thumb then automatically extend to some degree, which opens the hand (*Fig. 9.1C and D*).

This tenodesis effect is very helpful for these patients as it frequently provides them with a functional pinch, even though weak. In the absence of surgery, it is usually their only means of acquiring an object using one hand. (Patients who lack any tenodesis effect must grasp objects using both hands simultaneously, the bimanual grip.) As they also possess active supination of the forearm, using their biceps and/or supinator muscle, the tenodesis grip allows them to pick up, balance, and carry many light objects. However, they are able to carry light objects with the forearm in pronation only if they have a very tight tenodesis effect. To release the object, the patient must be able to pronate the forearm and relax

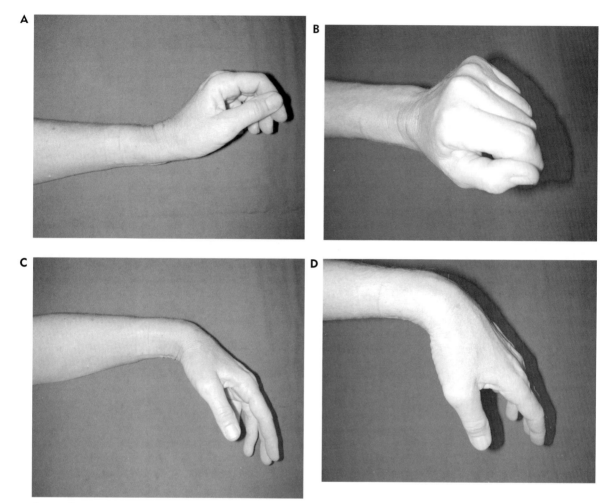

Figure 9.1 The tenodesis effect. As the wrist extends, the fingers and thumb automatically flex (A) and (B). Reciprocal finger extension occurs with wrist flexion (C) and (D).

the wrist extensor muscles so that gravity can flex the wrist. In IC Group 2 and 3 patients, the pronator teres (PT) muscle is paralyzed and the patient must use either shoulder abduction or other adaptive 'tricks' to effect pronation. If the forearm cannot be pronated, for example because of a supination contracture, the tenodesis effect is much less functional.

As discussed in Chapter 4, many post-injury splinting protocols are designed to encourage an exaggerated (beyond normal) tenodesis effect by allowing the digital flexors to undergo a degree of contracture. In the early phases of rehabilitation most patients are educated by the therapists to use this tenodesis effect.

With higher levels of injury, namely IC Group 1 patients, no useful active wrist extension exists. Moberg pointed out that, in such patients, the goal of surgery must be restoration of an automatic lateral tenodesis pinch,[1] which he termed a 'key grip or pinch'. He demonstrated that it can be achieved by directing the force of the brachioradialis (BR), typically the only surgically transferable muscle available, into the tendon of the ECRB muscle (see Chapter 12) to restore useful wrist extension. For this technique to provide a satisfactory pinch, other procedures must be added during the same stage (discussed in detail in Chapter 12).

In lower cervical levels of injury with preserved active wrist extension, the tenodesis effect (i.e., wrist extension–finger flexion and wrist flexion–finger extension) must be preserved. A flexible wrist enhances natural finger flexion and extension, and furthermore augments the effect of tendon transfers that run longitudinally over the dorsal and volar aspects of the wrist. For these reasons arthrodesis of the wrist should be performed with the utmost caution in the tetraplegic patient (see Chapter 11 for specific indications). It can be useful in other paralytic situations, where it may simplify the mechanics of the hand and wrist. If the wrist is stabilized by fusion, any flexor and/or extensor muscles of the wrist become available motors for tendon transfers. However, in tetraplegic patients who have wrist extension preserved, the loss of the tenodesis effect has far more impact than the gain provided by any additional motor for transfer.

Surgical tenodeses

Tenodeses can be achieved surgically, to create a new motion or reinforce an existing one without the need to transfer an active muscle. This motion is activated indirectly (automatically) by movement of a more proximal joint (passive tenodesis) or directly by an active muscle left *in situ* (active tenodesis). In the first case (passive tenodesis) the tendon is typically anchored to bone, or to tissues firmly fixed to bone, in such a way that motion of a proximal joint causes a force to be transmitted through the tendon. In the second case, the tendon is anchored to the tendon of either an active or even a paralyzed muscle. Activation of that tendon's muscle (in the case of the active muscle) causes a force to be transmitted through both the muscle's native tendon and the 'tenodesed' tendon. In the case of a passive tenodesis the motion and force that are produced at the distal joint by a surgical tenodesis depend on many variables, including the power of the muscle that moves the more proximal joint.

These procedures are indicated when there is no motor available to restore a specific motion by tendon transfer. Preoperative requirements include a complete (or near complete) passive range of motion of the involved joints (both the joint to be affected by the tenodesis and the proximal joint that activates the

tenodesis), and no spasticity of the affected muscles. If a passive tenodesis is to be performed, it can be activated either by gravity (see below) or by an active proximal muscle, which must be at least MRC Grade 3+ in strength. When performing an active tenodesis, the activating motor must be at least MRC Grade 4.

These procedures, which lead to an automatic motion, require little postoperative re-education compared to tendon transfer procedures. This type of tenodesis may even benefit a patient who is not well motivated or co-operative.

Passive tenodesis

The procedure involves fixing a paralyzed tendon (normally activating a distal joint) into some firm point proximal to a joint that can be moved by the contraction of a muscle still under voluntary control, but also proximal to a joint the motion of which depends on the effect of gravity. Many different passive tenodesis have been described as useful in restoring function in the tetraplegic hand. They can be classified according to the required functions of finger and thumb extension and flexion. Tenodeses that mimic the normal function of the intrinsic muscles of the thumb and fingers are termed intrinsic tenodesis.

Finger extension tenodesis

Finger extension tenodesis comprises fixing the tendons of the extensor digitorum communis (EDC) proximal to the flexion–extension axis of motion of the wrist joint. The extensor pollicis longus (EPL) is often tenodesed along with the EDC. In tetraplegic patients within IC Groups 1–3, and for many within IC Group 4, this tenodesis is usually activated through gravity alone; that is with the forearm in pronation, gravity causes the wrist to fall automatically into flexion, which brings the fingers (and thumb) into passive extension. In lower levels of tetraplegia (e.g., some IC Group 4 and 5 patients), it is activated by the flexor carpi radialis (FCR). This procedure is seldom utilized in the lower groups (IC Groups 6–10), as the finger extensors are active in these groups.

The classic procedure described by Zancolli consists of severing the EDC tendons several centimeters

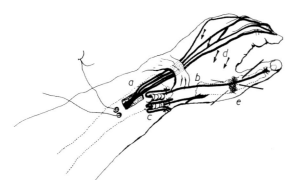

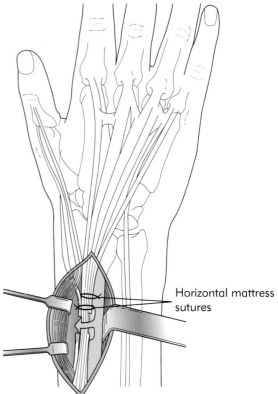

Figure 9.2 Zancolli's method of tenodesing the tendons of the EDC, EPL, and APL to the radius. (Modified with permission from Zancolli 1968.)[2]

above the wrist joint and fixing them into a bony window created on the dorsal aspect of the radius (*Fig. 9.2*).[2] Tension of the tenodesis must be such that the metacarpophalangeal (MP) joints of the fingers (and the two distal joints of the thumb) begin to extend in the early stages of wrist flexion, starting at neutral wrist extension. Other tendons besides the EPL may be included by simply suturing them to the EDC [e.g., the extensor digiti minimi or abductor pollicis longus (APL)]. Tendons can also be fixed onto the periarticular tissues (e.g., the dorsal retinaculum). Although much easier to perform, this type of fixation is prone to elongating over time because of the passive forces exerted on the juncture of the tendon and retinaculum.

An alternative technique is to preserve the continuity of the extensor tendons and reroute them under an arrow-shaped bony ledge, as suggested by Hentz *et al.*,[3] or into a horseshoe-shaped hole in the distal radius, as suggested by House *et al.* (*Fig. 9.3*).[4] This appealing technique is not easy to perform, as the cortical bone in that area is rather thick and difficult to carve precisely. Allieu described a perhaps easier technique that utilizes a simple plate and screws (*Fig. 9.4*).[5] The only flaw in leaving the extensor tendons in continuity is that the tension of the tenodesis is not as easily modified as when the tendons are divided.

A purely passive tenodesis provides the weakest force of extension, because activation is indirect and through gravity alone. However, it is usually sufficient for functional finger extension, an action that requires little if any strength.

Horizontal mattress sutures

Figure 9.3 Hamlin's method of dorsal extensor tenodesis.[4]

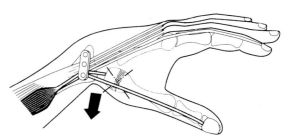

Figure 9.4 Allieu's method of dorsal extensor tenodesis. (Modified with permission from Allieu 1994.)[5]

Finger flexor tenodesis

Advocated by Bunnell[6] and Wilson,[7] tenodesis of the superficial or deep digital flexor tendons to the radius is seldom performed today, because the arc of finger motion that the tenodesis effect (wrist extension) provides is not very effective. The tension is either set too loose and the fingertips still remain away from the palm in wrist extension or it is set too tight and the fingers remain fairly flexed, even in wrist flexion. Either hand-closing or -opening is favored. In the past, the tenodesis was tensioned to favor grasp, but it seems that many patients were unhappy with this somewhat stiff, clawed hand.

What is occasionally used today is a tenodesis of the index flexor digitorum superficialis tendon, either alone or along with tenodesis of the superficialis tendon of the middle finger.[5,8] This procedure makes the index finger a better platform for the thumb to pinch against during a lateral (key) pinch between the thumb and the index finger (see Chapter 12). Another type of tenodesis of the flexor superficialis, the lasso procedure described by Zancolli,[9] is discussed along with other intrinsic tenodeses procedures in Chapter 13 and 14.

Thumb tenodesis

Initial tenodesis procedures aimed to restore thumb opposition, at a time when it was thought to be important to restore pulp-to-pulp pinch between thumb and index. This tenodesis, referred to by Curtis[10] as an 'opponodesis', was described by Bunnell in 1944.[11] A free tendon graft, either a flexor superficialis or the palmaris longus, was surgically anchored into the base of the proximal phalanx of the thumb, and routed subcutaneously across the palm to the distal ulna, where it was attached 4 cm (1.5 inches) proximal to its distal end. Extension of the wrist tightens the tenodesis, producing thumb opposition. Supination of the forearm further tightens the tenodesis. Today, most surgeons believe that thumb opposition is too ambitious a goal in most tetraplegic patients, and that restoration of a forceful lateral pinch is of primary importance.

Today the most commonly performed thumb tenodesis is that of the flexor pollicis longus (FPL) to the radius. Mentioned also by Bunnell,[11] it was popularized by Moberg.[1] The FPL tendon is approached at the wrist and tenodesed to the radius at the proximal edge of the pronator quadratus. The fixation is performed through a quadrangular window and two proximal holes (*Fig. 9.5*) or through two smaller quadrangular windows as preferred by Moberg,[1] the

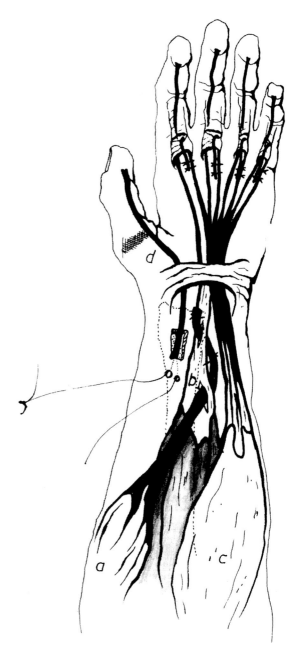

Figure 9.5 Zancolli's method of tenodesing the flexor pollicis longus to the radius. (Modified with permission from Zancolli 1979.)[12]

tendon passing into one and out the other (*Fig. 9.6*). Tension of the tenodesis must be selected carefully during the procedure with passive testing movements of the wrist. Too tight a tension results in premature flexion of the thumb's interphalangeal (IP) joint, which alters the grip by opposing the tip of the thumb instead of its pulp to the lateral side of the index. In contrast, too loose a tension results in an insufficient force of pinch and an inability to grasp necessary objects. Zancolli recommended that the tension be adjusted such that the thumb produces a lateral pinch against the radial side of the adjacent fingers as the wrist reaches near-full extension.

The original FPL tenodesis procedure was modified by Moberg to increase its strength and at the same time provide a more reliable contact between the thumb pulp and index finger.[1] To increase the force of pinch, Moberg recommended opening the annular pulley (A1) at the MP joint level, which permits the tendon to bowstring somewhat, and thereby increase the torque at this joint. To avoid the problem of premature flexion of the IP joint, he fixed it with a large threaded Kirschner wire. However, if the MP joint has a native wide arc of flexion, incision of the A1 pulley may lead to excessive flexion as the tenodesed FPL tendon tightens. This may cause the thumb to miss the lateral aspect of the index during an attempted pinch with wrist extension. Moberg recommended anchoring the extensor pollicis brevis (EPB) just proximal to the thumb's MP joint when passive flexion is too great (*Fig. 9.6*). Hentz *et al.* use a tenodesis of both EPL and EPB.[8] Stabilization of the

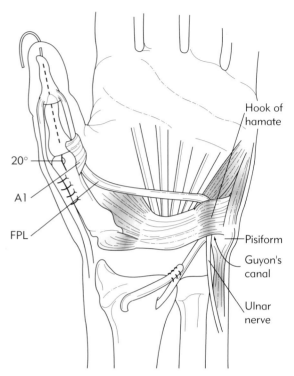

Figure 9.7 The Brand–Moberg modification of Moberg's original method of flexor pollicis longus (FPL) tenodesis (see text for details).

thumb's IP joint with a Kirschner wire has given rise to many inconveniences, and other authors have subsequently recommended more conventional fusions.

Moberg later modified his technique into a 'Brand–Moberg' tenodesis.[13] The FPL is divided as high as possible in the forearm, then delivered through a small incision at the thumb's MP level, and rerouted across the palm, deep to the flexor tendons and neurovascular bundles. The FPL tendon is passed proximally via Guyon's canal, to the volar surface of the radius, where it is anchored (*Fig. 9.7*). The tension of the tenodesis is deemed correct when the thumb pulp presses firmly against the radial side of the index with the wrist in the neutral position. This route of FPL transfer makes the release of the A1 pulley and dorsal EPL and EPB tenodesis unnecessary and, according to Moberg,[13] provides a more stable thumb action against the index finger. However, other authors, including Hentz *et al.*,[14] found it gave less power than the direct procedure, probably because of a slackening of Guyon's canal pulley. This procedure is described in greater detail in Chapter 12.

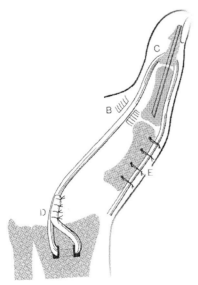

Figure 9.6 Moberg's method of flexor pollicis longus tenodesis. (Modified with permission from Moberg 1975.)[1]

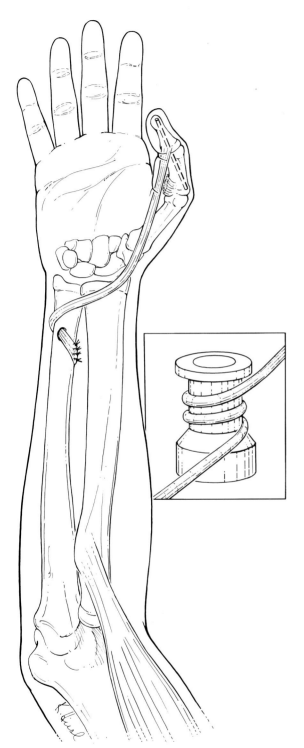

Brummer described another thumb flexor tenodesis based on the residual supinating action of the biceps (*Fig. 9.8*), sometimes referred to as the 'winch procedure'.[15] The FPL is divided proximally and fixed to the volar aspect of the distal ulna. When the biceps contracts, the forearm supinates at the same time as the elbow flexes. Forearm supination induces a passive extension of the wrist through gravity. Both active forearm supination and gravity-assisted wrist extension activate the tenodesis, which produces a weak lateral pinch. Such a pinch in supination of the forearm may not be the most satisfactory from a functional point of view, but it may be helpful in very high-level spinal cord injury patients. This procedure is illustrated in Chapter 11.

Tenodesis of the EPL can be performed together with the EDC (see above) or separately. In the latter case, the proximal fixation of the tendon can be carried out around the extensor retinaculum[12] or through the retinaculum around Lister's tubercle (*Fig. 9.9*).[16] The tendon can also be rerouted radially to add some abduction of the thumb, and thus widen the first web space.[17]

Tenodesis of the APL has been advocated to bring the thumb into mild antepulsion during a lateral pinch to favor a more distal pinch.[12] The tendon is severed proximally and split into two strips. One is passed around the FCR, and the other one is left in place, sutured to itself with median tension around its fibroosseous tunnel. Other authors use the APL tenodesis to maintain the thumb abducted during finger extension, to increase the opening of the first web.[16] The tendon is divided proximally, drawn out of its fibro-

Figure 9.8 Brummer's modification of the flexor pollicis longus tenodesis to obtain key or lateral pinch is illustrated (see text for details).

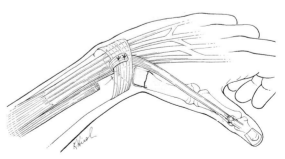

Figure 9.9 House's method of extensor pollicis longus tenodesis.

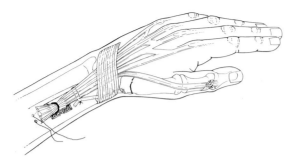

Figure 9.10 Tenodesis of extensor digitorum communis, extensor pollicis longus, and abductor pollicis longus to the radius.

osseous compartment, and joined, together with the EPL, to the EDC tenodesis (*Fig. 9.10*). These tenodeses are not very effective because their line of pull is so close to the flexion–extension axis of the wrist that there is very little change in tension through the tenodesis, whatever the position of the wrist.

Allieu has advocated a combined tenodesis of the FPL and the EPL (*Fig. 9.11*).[5] He creates a hole in the lateral aspect of the distal radius through which the tendons are passed in opposite directions, and sutured together. This technique facilitates adjustment of the tension of each tenodesis.

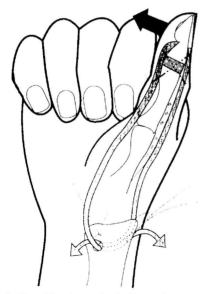

Figure 9.11 Allieu's method of tenodesing the flexor pollicis longus and extensor pollicis longus together. (Modified with permission from Allieu 1994.)[5]

Intrinsic tenodesis

Intrinsic muscles of the fingers are paralyzed in all the IC Groups, and all their complex actions cannot be replaced by tendon transfers because there are insufficient numbers of motors available. There is a tendency to hyperextension of the MP joints as the wrist is flexed in patients whose extensors have been allowed to contract, especially in those who have undergone surgical procedures to improve digital extension. If this occurs, the IP joints reciprocally flex and hand opening is compromised (*Fig. 9.12A*).

In higher levels of tetraplegia (e.g., Groups 1 and 2) reconstruction of a passive lateral or key pinch is frequently performed, so a tendency toward MP joint hyperextension interferes with achieving an effective pinch posture (*Fig. 9.12B*). Several procedures have

A

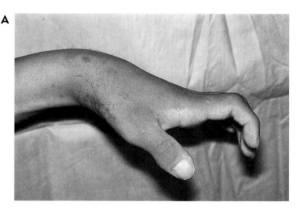

B

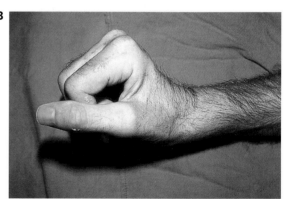

Figure 9.12 (A) Absence of intrinsic extension may lead to a claw-hand posture of the digits as the wrist is flexed. (B) The hyperextended digits cannot provide an effective platform for the thumb during attempts at pinch.

been developed to bring the index (and sometimes middle) finger MP joints into better flexion. Hamlin uses one of the two index extensor tendons, dividing the tendon at the level of the MP joint, passing it through the lumbrical canal, and fixing it to the A2 pulley.[3] When the wrist is flexed, the MP joints of the index flexes also, which brings the radial side of the index into a better position to face the thumb pulp.

House uses a free graft tendon sling that is taken around the head of the second metacarpal, through the lumbrical canals of the index and long fingers, and sutured distally to the extensor hood (*Fig. 9.13*).[18] As there is a tendency for the distal sutures to slacken, it is advisable to fix the grafts to the periosteum or through the base of the middle phalanx.[13]

In lower levels of tetraplegia (e.g., Groups 4–6), the tendency to hyperextension of the MP joints increases if active finger flexion is restored, and leads to a claw deformity that interferes with grasp. Fowler's intrinsic tenodesis followed the normal anatomical pathway of the finger interossei.[19] Free tendon grafts were fixed proximally to the dorsal retinaculum at the wrist, brought distally volar to the intermetacarpal ligament, and sutured to the distal tendons of the interossei. Technically demanding, this procedure has been supplanted by simpler ones. Zancolli initially described volar capsulodesis of the MP joints, but these slackened with time.[12] Later, he described the familiar 'lasso' procedure.[9] The para-

lyzed flexor digitorum superficialis (FDS) of each finger is transected at the level of its chiasm. The divided tendon is rerouted around the A1 pulley and sutured to itself just proximal to this pulley. The A1 pulley is anatomically fixed to the MP joint's volar plate, which in turn is fixed to the base of the proximal phalanx. Therefore, traction on the A1 pulley produces flexion of the MP joint (*Fig. 9.14*). In his initial description of the procedure, Zancolli recommended adjusting the tension of the lasso with the finger extended and the superficialis tendon under maximum distal stretch. In tetraplegia, as the FDSs are paralyzed, the tension should be set somewhat greater, as subsequently the system will slacken. Throughout the procedure, care must be taken not to touch the flexor digitorum profundi (FDPs) to avoid creating adhesions between FDP and FDS.

All these tenodeses require a period of complete immobilization in a cast for 3–4 weeks. The position of postoperative immobilization must be such that no tension is applied to the tenodesis. This is of particular importance as a tenodesis is often performed at the same time as other procedures, which may require a different position of immobilization. For example, if a transfer of the BR to the wrist extensors is performed at the same time as a tenodesis of the FPL to the radius, the wrist should not be immobilized in flexion. Therefore, the thumb must be protected by hyperflexion of both MP and IP joints.

Subsequent rehabilitation following these tenodeses procedures is neither long nor complicated. It is limited to restoring good movement of the proximal joints. No resistance should be exerted on the tenodesis until many weeks postoperatively, otherwise it will slacken and become less effective. It is absolutely critical that the patient be taught how to protect the tenodesis.

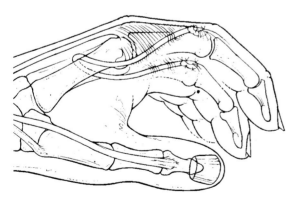

Figure 9.13 House described an intrinsic substitution procedure that uses a free tendon graft to checkrein the metacarpophalangeal joints against hyperextension and augment interphalangeal joint extension as the wrist is flexed. The technical aspects of this procedure are discussed in Chapter 13. (Modified with permission from House et al. 1976.)[4]

Active tenodesis

An active tenodesis consists of attaching a paralyzed tendon to an active one, usually performed by suturing these together. When the active muscle contracts, it exerts force simultaneously through its native and the tenodesed tendon, inducing primary motion at the native joint(s) and a secondary motion at the joint(s) normally affected by the tenodesed tendon. Preoperative requirements are basically the same as for a passive tenodesis, except that the motor muscle must

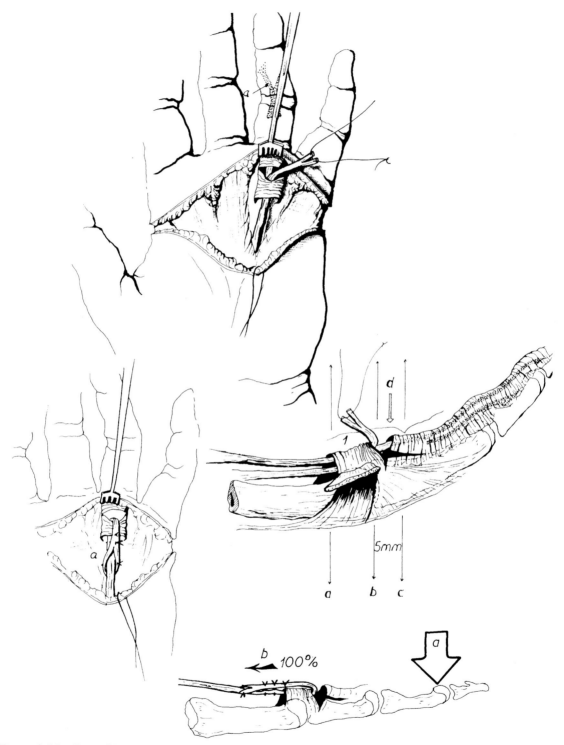

Figure 9.14 Zancolli's intrinsic substitution procedure, termed the 'lasso' procedure. The technical aspects of this procedure are discussed in Chapter 13. (Modified with permission from Zancolli 1979.)[12]

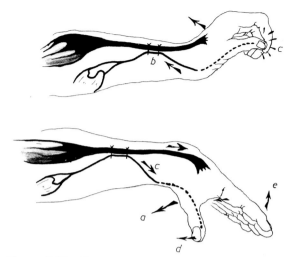

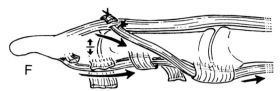

Figure 9.16   The split flexor pollicis longus to extensor pollicis longus transfer described by Mohammed et al.[21] serves to stabilize the interphalangeal joint of the thumb against excessive flexion.

Figure 9.15   Zancolli's 'active' tenodesis between the tendon of the paralyzed flexor pollicis longus and the active extensor carpi radialis brevis, to power the thumb in pinch. (Modified with permission from Zancolli 1979.)[12]

be MRC Grade 4 or above. In the tetraplegic patient, two active tenodeses are used mainly.

Active tenodesis of the flexor pollicis longus to the extensor carpi radialis brevis

Zancolli has described active tenodesis of the FPL to the ECRB for situations in which the still active ECRL is to be transferred to restore finger flexion, but no motor is available to restore thumb flexion.[20] The ECRB is left in place, and the FPL is brought side-to-side with it at forearm level, without interrupting its continuity, and sutured laterally to the ECRB over a few centimeters (*Fig. 9.15*). The tension is adjusted so that the thumb comes into contact with the lateral aspect of the index finger when the wrist reaches near maximal extension. The procedure is described in greater detail in Chapter 13. This is an elegant way of activating the thumb to provide pinch. However, in some cases it may decrease the range of active extension of the wrist, probably because of adhesions of the ECRB in the suture area.

Active tenodesis of the flexor pollicis longus to the extensor pollicis longus

Another active tenodesis is that of the FPL to the EPL, described by Mohammed *et al.* in 1992

(*Fig. 9.16*).[21] It is actually an 'activated tenodesis' because the paralyzed FPL is rehabilitated by a tendon transfer (usually from the BR) during the same stage. One-third to half of the FPL is split from the remainder, dissected distally, divided from its bony insertion, withdrawn from the distal pulley, and rerouted dorsally to the extensor tendon into which it is inserted. This tenodesis is very unique in that it does not induce a secondary motion, but rather stabilizes the thumb's IP joint by limiting its flexion. It was designed as an alternative to thumb IP fusion when the powerful BR was to be transferred to the FPL. Left unstabilized, the transfer frequently induced a functionally detrimental hyperflexion of the IP joint, which interfered with the lateral or key pinch. This procedure is described in detail in Chapter 12.

Suture of the extensor tendons

Suture of the extensor tendons to each other is a form of active tenodesis. It is performed when some of the tendons are active (usually the ulnar ones) and others are paralyzed or weak (usually the radial ones), a situation that is not infrequent in some patients intermediate between IC Groups 5 and 6. A direct lateral suture of all the tendons is performed so that the stronger ulnar tones assist the weaker radial ones in extending the fingers. Some authors recommend some superficial stripping of the synovial surface of the tendons before suturing, so as to create some adhesion between the tendons.

Tendon transfers

Tendon transfers are the most commonly performed procedures in surgical rehabilitation of the tetraplegic upper limb. Available transfers are few in number and rather standardized, as so few donor motors are available.

Principles

The general principles of tendon transfers set forth by Bunnell 60 years ago still apply.[11] They include considerations regarding the physiology of the donor muscle (such as its strength and amplitude), the condition of all the affected joints (e.g., passive ROM), and technical issues, such as how to optimally direct the force of the donor muscle to effect its new task. In addition, decisions regarding re-education of the transferred muscle must be based on sound principles.

The donor muscle

A muscle can be used as a donor only if it is sufficiently strong. Using the MRC grading system (see Chapter 7), it is possible to quantify muscle strength with reasonable consistency. It is generally agreed that a muscle usually loses at least half a grade of strength when transferred. Therefore, a muscle can be transferred reliably only if its strength is at least MRC Grade 4. However, the strength of the muscle ideally should be appropriate to its new task. For example, a muscle transferred to the finger flexors must be initially very strong (4+ or 5), whereas a muscle planned for transfer to finger extensors can be somewhat weaker (4 or 4-), as ultimately it is required to work only against gravity most of the time.

The choice of the donor muscle is of the utmost importance in tetraplegic patients. They have very few remaining active muscles, and it must be established with certainty that taking a muscle as a donor will not induce any functional loss. With this key principle in mind, use of the BR as a donor is fairly safe in complete tetraplegia, because if it is strong enough to be used as a donor, the other elbow flexors (which have a higher motor innervation in the spinal cord) are likely to be normal, and the elbow will retain strong active flexion. In contrast, the ECRL can be used only if the ECRB is strong enough to ensure powerful postoperative wrist extension, since active wrist extension is so important for these patients (see 'tenodesis effect' above).

Other considerations that affect the choice of a donor muscle include the anatomic length of the muscle and its tendon, and the contractile properties of the muscle, termed amplitude of excursion. If a proximally located muscle, such as the ECRL, is selected for a distal function (e.g., restoring finger flexion), its anatomic length may be insufficient to reach the normal anatomic site of insertion (e.g., the distal phalanx) to perform the new task. This length deficit may be overcome by using an intercalated graft, but this creates two potential weak points (the sutured junctures) instead of one and increases the potential for adhesions. If there is a choice between several potential motors, one that does not require lengthening with a graft is preferred.

Excursion of the donor must be appropriate to its new function. Effecting thumb opposition, for instance, requires much less excursion than finger flexion. For the tetraplegic patient in IC Groups 3 and below there is a possible choice between the BR and ECRL for restoring finger flexion. The ECRL, which has a much longer excursion, is better suited for this task.

The donor muscle must be assigned to only one task or function. It should not be transferred simultaneously to two tendons that possess different functional amplitudes of motion, for example to the EPL and APL because the former's amplitude is roughly twice that of the latter's. If this transfer is performed, the donor muscle preferentially performs the function of the tendon with the lower amplitude, and so is 'checkreined' in the process and thus unable to fully perform the function that requires additional excursion. In the example given, the transfer may effect strong and full thumb abduction, but only weak and incomplete thumb extension.

Finally, the donor muscle should, whenever possible, be synergistic with the movement to be restored. This greatly facilitates re-education and integration to its new function. For instance, it is much more appropriate to use a wrist extensor than a wrist flexor to restore finger flexion, since wrist extension and finger flexion are synergistic movements, as are wrist flexion and finger extension. In the example given above (the choice of BR versus ECRL to restore finger extension), this is another reason for choosing ECRL rather than BR for finger flexion. In the tetraplegic patient the potential donors are so few that this rule cannot always be followed.

If a transferred muscle is to perform a secondary distal action while still retaining its native function, the primary function at the proximal joint must be counterbalanced by an antagonist. In the tetraplegic patient this situation occurs every time the BR is used as a transfer to effect a more distal function. Its action as an elbow flexor must be balanced by the extensor action of the antagonistic triceps, so as to stabilize the elbow. Otherwise some of the power of the transferred BR is exerted at the elbow, and it is less effective distally. For this reason, the elbow must be stabilized by first restoring extension if the triceps is paralyzed, generally before restoration of grasp is considered (see Chapter 10).

The recipient site

If active motion of a joint is to be restored, there must be a full passive motion of that joint. If contractures have developed, they must be treated before tendon transfers are planned. This may require therapy, passive and dynamic splinting, and sometimes a preliminary surgical procedure to mobilize a stiff joint, termed arthrolysis, and/or an adhesed tendon, termed tendolysis.

Another local requirement is suppleness of the soft tissues through which the transferred tendon must ultimately glide. There should be no firmly scarred skin or skin graft along the proposed line of transfer, otherwise adhesions are likely to occur between the transferred tendon and the surrounding tissues, which will impede tendon gliding and limit function.

Technical issues

The same principles apply here as for any other tendon transfer. The tendons must be handled with care, preferably with sutures rather than sharp forceps, and continuously moistened. The course of the transferred tendon must be in a straight line, so it should be dissected far proximally, but without damage to its neurovascular supply. If a pulley is necessary be aware that it weakens the transfer because of added friction between the tendon and pulley.

There has been some discussion among experts regarding whether or not to resect some length of tendon proximal to the suture site. Moberg recommended resecting 7–8 cm (2.7–3 inches) of the recipient muscle proximal to the site of tendon transfer when it is completely paralyzed, as he believed that fibrous remnants of the denervated muscle become fixed to surrounding tissues, and thus prevent adequate excursion of the transferred musculocutaneous unit.[13] However, most authors do not perform his maneuver routinely.

Appropriate tensioning of the transfer at the time of surgery is one of the most difficult issues and to achieve the ideal tension requires experience. It is recommended, when performing a transfer, that a temporary stitch be placed and then, through passive joint movements, evaluate whether the tension is ideal.

The sutures between the recipient and the donor tendons must be strong, so as to avoid elongation or rupture. This is especially important if one of the two muscles is spastic and undergoes uncontrolled contractions. A strong tendon-to-tendon juncture allows early re-education and thus lessens the potential for adhesions. Interweaving the two tendons creates the ideal juncture, as described by Pulvertaft.[22]

Ejeskar recommends routine implantation in the donor and recipient tendons of stainless steel suture 'indicators' a standard distance apart on each side of the suture line and measuring their distance with regular radiography.[23] These measurements show accurately whether elongation has occurred or if the sutured juncture has ruptured; this enables early re-operation if necessary.

Postoperative regimen and re-education

After a tendon transfer, key joints are typically immobilized by casting the limb in positions that relatively relax the tendon junctures for several weeks. While recommendations differ, a period of 4 weeks is suitable for most of the procedures discussed herein. If the juncture is strong enough, isometric contractions can be initiated earlier. Electrical stimulation has also been advocated to reduce postoperative adhesions at the suture site. Following a period of enforced immobilization, active motion is initiated. Resisted motion should not be performed until several weeks later. In some cases (deltoid transfer to the triceps), full ROM is not allowed until many weeks later. Re-education after tendon transfer procedures requires much more compliance from the patient than does a tenodesis; active participation is mandatory. Preoperatively, the patient must have been given complete information regarding the surgery, its goals, and the functional improvement to be expected. Developing a good personal relationship with the therapist with whom the patient is going to spend many hours is essential. If such is not the case, it is probably wiser not to perform surgery until these conditions are met.

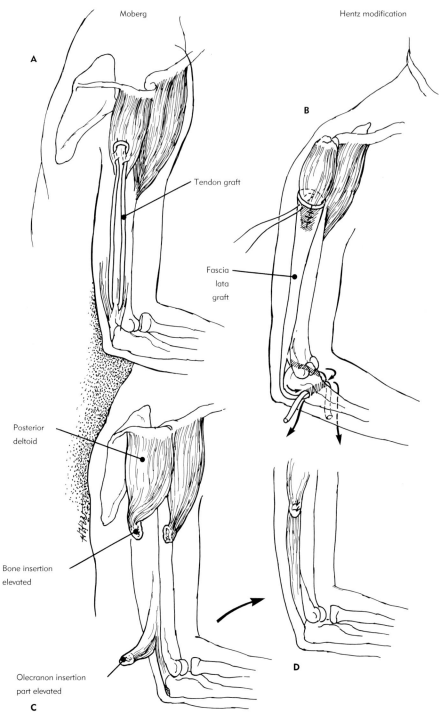

Figure 9.17 Methods to attach the deltoid to its intended site of action. (A) Moberg originally advocated using toe extensors.[1] Later (B) Hentz et al. described using fascia lata,[8] and still later (C, D) Mennon and Boonzaier[28] modified the technique of Castro-Serra and Lopez-Pita[27] by harvesting bone blocks from the humerus and olecranon and attaching the bone blocks together. (Modified with permission from Hentz and Chase 2001.)[29]

Commonly used donor muscles

Deltoid

The posterior portion of the deltoid muscle, as described by Merle D'Aubigne et al.,[24] is commonly used for rehabilitation of elbow extension. The posterior part of the muscle is dissected free from the humerus, elevated, and attached to the distal tendon of the triceps or into the olecranon. Harvesting the muscle is not easy, as there is no anatomical separation between the posterior, middle, and anterior portions of the deltoid muscle. Recommendations as to the quantity of muscle to be harvested vary according to different authors, with Moberg[1] using one-third and Hentz et al.[8] one-half of the muscle. Proximal separation of the muscle must stop at the point of penetration of the axillary nerve into the muscle. Distally, all its available tendinous portions must be harvested, so as to provide a strong hold for sutures. Some authors recommend including the periosteum in continuity with the tendon, and the fibrous origin of the brachialis muscle, if present.

The detached deltoid does not reach the tendon of the triceps and some interposition material is needed to bridge the obvious gap. In his initial description of the procedure, Moberg used toe extensors to the second, third, and fourth toes, which were inserted proximally in the deltoid tendon and distally in the triceps aponeurosis (Fig. 9.17A).[1] Hentz et al. suggests using the fascia lata (Fig. 9.17B) (see details in Chapter 10),[8] while Freehafer et al. prefer the tibialis anterior.[25]

Lamb favors use of the extensor carpi ulnaris, which does not require a second surgical field.[26] However, turning up the proximal part of the muscle may be difficult because of its bulk and, for the same reason, insertion of the muscle into the olecranon requires a large tunnel, which may weaken the bone.

Other authors, to avoid harvesting a distant tissue, have used a strip from the central part of the triceps tendon, detached distally and dissected proximally to join the terminal tendon of the deltoid. Castro-Sierra and Lopez-Pita, who described this technique, harvested the periosteal insertion of both muscles and sutured them together.[27] Mennen and Boonzaier made the suture stronger by harvesting the bony insertion of both tendons, and suturing them together with a wire (Figs 9.17C and 9.17D).[28] This technique allows a much earlier re-education, which the authors initiate at 1 week.

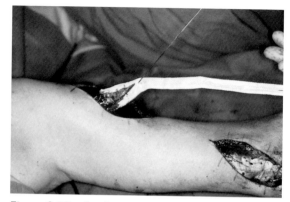

Figure 9.18 Synthetic material, alone or wrapped in autogenous tissue, has been used to connect deltoid muscle to the olecranon.

Finally, other authors have made use of artificial tendons, either surrounded with a strip of fascia lata, as described by Allieu,[30] or alone, as recommended by Tessier.[31] The latter, made of woven Dacron, is shaped as a funnel at its proximal end and divided into two strips at its distal end, which makes sutures to both tendons much easier (Fig. 9.18).

One of the frequent complications of this procedure is elongation of the interposed graft or of the sutured areas. To avoid this problem, postoperative re-education is different from that following other tendon transfers, with a very slowly progressive gain in ROM. Principles of re-education have been clearly elucidated by Moberg,[17] and are fully described in Chapter 9.

At higher levels of tetraplegia in which the pectoralis major is paralyzed, transfer of the deltoid may be less efficient because the stabilizing effect of the pectoralis major on the shoulder is lost. Buntine advocates advancing the clavicular origin of the deltoid muscle medially.[32] The medial third of the origin of the deltoid muscle is elevated with a large bony insertion, and transferred 3–4 cm (1–1.5 inches) medially on the clavicle (Fig. 9.19). This procedure restores some adduction and stabilizes the shoulder.

Biceps brachii

The biceps may also be used as a transfer to restore elbow extension. Residual elbow flexion is effected by the brachialis muscle, and assisted by the BR

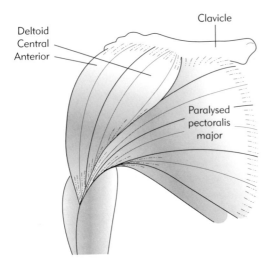

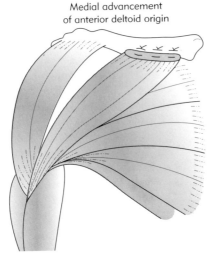

Figure 9.19 Medial advancement of the clavicular origin of the deltoid major muscle is advocated when the pectoralis major is paralyzed. (From Johnstone et al. 1988. With permission.)[42]

muscle if this is active. This procedure, initially performed by Leo Mayer (as cited by Zancolli[12]), was described by Friedenberg in 1954.[33] Its use in the tetraplegic population has been popularized by Zancolli,[34] who favors it over deltoid-to-triceps transfer because of its simplicity. This procedure can only be performed if there is an active supinator muscle (IC Group 2).

The biceps tendon is divided at its insertion on the radius and transferred posteriorly to the triceps. In the initial description of the procedure, the tendon was routed laterally, but some authors have experienced radial nerve compression and now favor a medial route (the procedure is described and illustrated in greater detail in Chapter 10).[35] Also, it was initially recommended that the biceps tendon be fixed distally to the olecranon, but this is often impossible to achieve because the tendon is too short. It can usually be fixed to the distal part of the triceps tendon. As there is no need for interposition grafts, postoperative re-education is much simpler and faster than with the deltoid muscle.

The biceps can also be transferred to restore pronation, while retaining its initial function as an elbow flexor.[15] This procedure is advocated for patients with no active pronation and a spontaneous tendency to permanent supination of the forearm, which is greatly impairing. This procedure requires a full passive range of pronation. If passive pronation is limited, the interosseous membrane must be freed during the same procedure. If there is a fixed attitude in supination, a pronation osteotomy is indicated instead. The biceps tendon is lengthened by longitudinal division of its tendon throughout its length. The distal strip, attached to the bicipital tuberosity of the radius, is rerouted around the radial neck and fixed to the proximal stump, attached to the muscle. Tension is obtained with the elbow flexed at 80° and the forearm pronated at 20°. The procedure is described and illustrated in Chapter 11.

Brachioradialis

The BR is available for transfer in IC Groups 1 and higher. Vulpius and Stoffel first described its transfer to augment wrist extension in 1920. Many authors have questioned its reliability as a donor, because the procedure is technically demanding (in 1990, Moberg stated 'This transfer requires perhaps the most delicate technique of all described procedures'[36]) and because it is more difficult to educate than are other transfers. On the other hand, except for the long antebrachial scar, its use causes no functional impairment in the tetraplegic patient, as the biceps and brachialis muscles are typically strong enough to preserve sufficient residual elbow flexion.

When considering transfer of this muscle, the presence or absence of active elbow extension is a significant factor. An active antagonist to elbow flexion makes the transferred BR a more reliable postoperative performer. In the absence of elbow extension, after transfer the BR continues to function as an elbow flexor. Occasionally, after transfer a flexion contracture of the elbow develops, and the BR becomes ineffective in its new task. If the triceps is inactive, a preliminary deltoid- or biceps-to-triceps transfer to restore active elbow extension should be considered strongly. Some authors advocate simultaneous BR and elbow extensor transfers.[37]

In tetraplegia, the BR may be used to restore or augment wrist extension (transfer to ECRB), finger extension (transfer to the EDC), thumb flexion (transfer to the FPL), thumb opposition, or finger flexion (transfer to FDP). Its use as a thumb abductor or extensor has been largely abandoned. Whatever its destination, the muscle is harvested in the same manner. Through a longitudinal incision, the distal tendon is divided from the radius as far distally as possible, leaving the periosteum undisturbed (so as to avoid local adhesions). Then the muscle is elevated from distal to proximal, during which two structures are at risk. These are the radial sensory nerve, which emerges dorsally from under the BR, 10 cm (4 inches) proximal to the wrist crease, and the radial vascular bundle, which follows the volar edge of the muscle throughout its length, and gives off several branches to the BR. The muscle must be dissected as far proximally as the elbow crease, so as to free it from its investing fascia. This part of the dissection is essential so as to obtain an adequate muscle excursion, which varies with the destination of the transfer. Freehafer found that the average total excursion (passive stretch plus active contraction) for the undissected muscle was 41 mm (1.6 inches) and for the dissected muscle 78 mm (3.05 inches). He recommended freeing the muscle to a level 2 cm (0.75 inches) distal to radial head. To restore wrist extension by transfer to the ECRB, Moberg advocates a minimum of 5 cm (2 inches) excursion, whereas for thumb flexion or adduction 3–4 cm (1.2–1.55 inches) of excursion is sufficient.[1] The vascular and nervous supplies of the BR are not at risk during this step, as they enter the muscle more proximally. These various transfers are illustrated in detail in later chapters.

If the BR is routed dorsally to the ECD or ECRB tendons, care must be taken not to compress the radial sensory branch. If the muscle is routed volarly to the thumb or the FDP, it must be passed deep to the radial vascular bundle.

When the BR is sutured to the recipient tendon, the position of the elbow must be considered to establish the appropriate tension. Also, the destination of the transfer influences the tension. For example, when the BR is transferred to the ECRB muscle, Zancolli advocates placing the elbow at 70° of flexion, and suturing the tendon in maximal extension of the wrist.[12] For a transfer to the FPL, the tension should be somewhat less.

Many surgeons believe that the BR is a 'dumb' muscle in that its postoperative re-education is frequently difficult. Most patients are relatively 'unaware' of the muscle ostensibly, since it normally plays such an accessory or subsidiary role. It is not natural to contract this muscle in isolation, a task that is almost impossible for the patient who cannot stabilize the elbow using the triceps muscle. The muscle seems to perform better in some roles than in others. Some authors have found it a more reliable performer after transfer to the ECRB to augment wrist extension than it is for providing independent thumb flexion after transfer to the FPL. The ability of the patient to trigger the muscle in isolation can be somewhat improved by such techniques as biofeedback. It has also been recommended to block the elbow in a splint at 90° flexion during therapy, to educate its new function.

Moberg[17] and others[8,10] noted that the power of the transferred BR muscle is greater in those patients who retained some triceps function. These observations led to several biomechanical studies, which have determined that the BR becomes a more effective wrist extensor following transfer if the patient can stabilize the elbow in space. Brys and Waters studied 15 patients who had undergone BR to FPL transfer.[37] Pinch strength was measured with the elbow free and with the elbow locked in 90° of flexion. Those patients who had 2 ft/lb or less of elbow extension torque had an average of 1.2 kg of pinch with the elbow free. With the elbow locked at 90°, pinch strength increased 153% to 3 lb. Patients having more than 2 ft/lb had an average of 4.1 lb of pinch with the elbow free, but no change with elbow immobilization.

Extensor carpi radialis longus

The ECRL muscle is one of the two radial wrist extensors that can be used as a transfer when both ECRL and ECRB are strong (IC Group 3 or higher).

One of these must be left in place to retain active wrist extension, and the choice is to leave the ECRB, as its moment arm for wrist extension is superior to that of the ECRL. The ECRB produces pure wrist extension, whereas ECRL also produces radial deviation. Postoperatively, strong full-wrist extension must be preserved to retain a good tenodesis effect, and to potentiate future transfers. This requires that the ECRB be at least MRC Grade 4. However, the relative contribution to the strength of wrist extension provided by either the ECRL or the ECRB cannot be easily tested preoperatively, since the patient cannot independently contract only one of these two muscles (see Chapter 6). Lamb reported residual weakness of wrist dorsiflexion in four out of 48 patients in whom the ECRL was used as a transfer.[38] To determine that the ECRB has sufficient strength in isolation to preserve strong postoperative wrist extension may require intraoperative testing, as suggested by Moberg, who insisted on many occasions that the ECRL should not be used if the ECRB is unable to support a 5 kg (11 lb) weight.[1,17] The testing procedure is described in Chapter 13. However, Moberg also states that it is more the rule than the exception for the ECRB to be MRC Grade 4 when ECRL is Grade 4 and above. If any doubt exists as to the strength of ECRB, then ECRL should not be used as a donor.

Harvesting the muscle is fairly straightforward. The tendon is exposed and divided distal to the dorsal retinaculum, which is left undisturbed. It is then retracted proximally, and dissected from distal to proximal. Its tendon lies radially to that of the ECRB, but its muscle belly lies superficially to the ECRB. To gain the maximal tendon excursion, the muscle must be dissected as far proximally as possible, up to its main neurovascular bundle.

In some cases a supernumerary radial wrist extensor muscle is found.[12] It can be a mere tendinous band, or a full intermediate radial muscle, with a separate muscle, as Wood described.[39] Leclercq's dissections of 104 cadaveric upper limbs showed that such an intermediate muscle was present in 25% cases, and was large enough to be used as a transfer in 15% cases.[14] These dissections also confirmed that when it has a separate belly, the muscle also has a separate motor nerve. It can therefore be transferred independently of the ECRL, during the same procedure, to restore a different function (usually, ECRL is used for finger flexion and the accessory muscle for thumb flexion). This intermediate muscle should always be checked for at the start of the procedure so as to be able to use it when present. It is assumed that its strength (MRC grade) is at the same level as that of the ECRL.

Pronator teres

The PT is a broad muscle with a short tendon. Its use as a transfer was popular among early authors, who felt it could partially retain its primary function, and therefore be used at little cost. In the main it was transferred to the FDP,[40] to the FCR,[20] and to the finger extensors or thumb abductors.[13] Today it is more often transferred to the FPL to restore thumb flexion, although it is still recommended by some authors for the FDP.[41]

As its tendon is short, it must somehow be extended to reach most recipient tendons. Although some authors have used a long periosteal strip in continuity with the tendon,[4] it seems safer strengthwise to use an intercalated tendon graft harvested from a locally paralyzed muscle.

Flexor carpi radialis

The FCR muscle should not be used as a transfer. When active, it stabilizes the wrist and contributes to the tenodesis effect by increasing passive extension of the fingers. It also enhances greatly any future tendon transfers to the finger flexors, and so brings greater power to the hand during grasp.

Other tendon transfers (e.g., extensor indicis, extensor digiti minimi, flexor, extensor carpi ulnaris) are utilized in lower levels of tetraplegia (IC Groups 8 and 9). These same muscles are transferred in distal median–ulnar palsies, and follow the same rules.

Fusions (arthrodeses)

A number of fusions or arthrodeses are performed in the tetraplegic hand, mainly for the joints of the thumb to make this multi-articular chain simpler and therefore more stable. Arthrodeses of the carpometacarpal, MP, and IP joints are carried out regularly, often at the same time as other procedures.

No techniques to effect fusion are specific to tetraplegic patients and many different techniques have been advocated, none of which seem better than another. However, some simple guidelines seem pertinent:

- Arthrodeses are usually performed along with other procedures that require long operative times (such as multiple tendon transfers), so the technique itself should not be too sophisticated or time consuming.
- Fixation of the arthrodesis should be sound, so as to allow mobilization of the part as early as 3–4 weeks postoperatively, when the plaster is removed and the tendon transfers allowed to move. Fusion healing should not delay the onset of therapy.
- Preferably fixation devices that need removal, such as Kirschner wires, should be avoided to reduce the number of operations.
- If Kirschner wires are used and are to be removed once fusion has occurred, the ends should be buried under the skin, rather than left protruding through the skin. Although removal is complicated by this step, it reduces the potential complications of pin-tract infections. Probably because tetraplegic patients bear weight even on the casted hand, they seem to have a higher incidence than ambulatory patients of problems associated with pins that protrude through the skin.

Very rarely is a wrist arthrodesis indicated. As mentioned above, usually every attempt is made to keep the wrist mobile to enhance the tenodesis effect, and thus favor the grasp and release scheme.

References

1. Moberg E. Surgical treatment for absent single-hand grip and elbow extension in quadriplegia. J Bone Joint Surg 1975; 57A(2):196–206.
2. Zancolli E. Structural and Dynamic Basis of Hand Surgery. Philadelphia: JB Lippincott, 1968.
3. Hentz VR, Hamlin C, Keoshian L. Surgical reconstruction in tetraplegia. In: Tubiana R, editor. Hand Clinics; Vol. 4. St Louis: CV Mosby, 1988:601–607.
4. House JH, Gwathmey FW, Lundsgaard DK. Restoration of strong grasp and lateral pinch in tetraplegia due to cervical spinal cord injury. J Hand Surg 1976; 1(2):152–159.
5. Allieu Y. Le membere superieur du tetraplegique. Conferences d'enseignment du GEM. Paris: L'expansion Scientifique, 1994: 1–17.
6. Bunnell S. Tendon transfers in the hand and forearm. In: American Academy of Orthopedic Surgery, Instructional Course Lectures. St Louis: CV Mosby, 1949:102–112.
7. Wilson J. Providing automatic grasp by flexor tenodesis. J Bone Joint Surg 1956; 38A:1019–1024.
8. Hentz V, Brown M, Keoshian L. Upper limb reconstruction in quadriplegia: functional assessment and proposed treatment modifications. J Hand Surg 1983; 8(2):119–131.
9. Zancolli E. Correccion de la 'garra' digital por paralisis intrinseca. La operacion del 'lazo'. Acta Ortop Latinoam 1974; 1:65–71.
10. Curtis RM. Tendon transfers in the patient with spinal cord injury. Orthop Clin North Am 1974; 5(2):415–423.
11. Bunnell S. Surgery of the Hand. Philadelphia: JB Lippincott, 1944.
12. Zancolli E. Structural and Dynamic Basis of Hand Surgery. 2nd edn. Philadelphia: JB Lippincott, 1979.
13. Moberg E. Upper limb surgical rehabilitation in tetraplegia. In: Evarts CM, ed. Surgery of the Musculoskeletal System, Vol. 1. New York: Churchill Livingstone, 1990:915–941.
14. Hentz V, House J, McDowell C, et al. Rehabilitation and surgical reconstruction of the upper limb in tetraplegia: an update. J Hand Surg, 1992; 17A:964–967.
15. Brummer H. The winch operation. In: McDowell C, Moberg E, eds. The Second International Conference on Surgical Rehabilitation in Tetraplegia, Giens, France: Journal of Hand Surgery, 1984:608–611.
16. House J. Two stage reconstruction of the tetraplegic hand. In: Strickland J, ed. Master Techniques in Orthopaedic Surgery. Philadelphia: Lippincott, 1998: 229–255.
17. Moberg E. The Upper Limb in Tetraplegia. A new approach to surgical rehabilitation. Stuttgart: George Thieme, 1978.
18. House JH, Shannon MA. Restoration of strong grasp and lateral pinch in tetraplegia: a comparison of two methods of thumb control in each patient. J Hand Surg 1985; 10A(1):22–29.
19. Riordan D. Tendon transplantation in median nerve and ulnar nerve paralysis. J Bone Joint Surg 1953; 35A(2):312–320.
20. Zancolli E. Surgery for the quadriplegic hand with active, strong wrist extension preserved. Clin Orthop Rel Res 1975; 112:101–113.
21. Mohammed KD, Rothwell A, Sinclair S, et al. Upper limb surgery for tetraplegia. J Bone Joint Surg 1992; 74B:873–879.
22. Pulvertaft G. Repair of tendon injuries in the hand. Ann Royal Coll Surg 1948; 3:14–24.

23. Ejeskar A. Elongation in profundus tendon repair. Scand J Plast Surg 1981; 15:61–65.

24. Merle D'Aubigne, Seddon H, Hendy A, et al. Tendon transfers. Proc Royal Soc Med 1949; 48:831–838.

25. Freehafer AA, Kelly CM, Peckham PH. Tendon transfer for the restoration of upper limb function after a cervical spinal cord injury. J Hand Surg 1984; 9A:887–893.

26. Lamb DW The current state of management of the upper limb in tetraplegia. Paraplegia 1992; 30:65–67.

27. Castro-Serra A, Lopez-Pita A. A new surgical technique to correct triceps paralysis. Hand. 1983; 15:42–46.

28. Mennen U, Boonzaier A. An improved technique of posterior deltoid to triceps transfer in tetraplegia. J Hand Surg 1991;16B:197–201.

29. Hentz V, Chase R. Hand Surgery: A Clinical Atlas. Philadelphia: WB Saunders, 2001.

30. Allieu Y. Fascia lata enveloped Dacron interposition graft in posterior deltoid to triceps transfer. In: the proceedings of the congress 'Les Journees de Propara a Montpellier' February 7, 8 1992; 55–82.

31 Tessier SC Personal communication.

32. Johnstone B, Buntine J, Sormann G, et al. Surgical rehabilitation of the upper limb in quadriplegia. Aust NZ J Surg 1987; 57:917–926.

33. Friedenberg Z. Transposition of the biceps brachii for triceps weakness. J Bone Joint Surg. 1954; 36A:656–658.

34. Zancolli E. Mid-cervical tetraplegia. In: Keith M, ed. Abstract of the Sixth International Conference: Surgical Rehabilitation of the Upper Limb in Tetraplegia. Cleveland: 1998: 56–61.

35. Ejeskar A. Upper limb surgical rehabilitation in high-level tetraplegia. In: Tubiana R, ed. Hand Clinics, Vol. 4, 1988:585–599.

36. Moberg E. Surgical rehabilitation of the upper limb in tetraplegia. Paraplegia 1990;28(5):330–334.

37. Brys D, Waters R. Effect of triceps function on the brachioradialis transfer in quadriplegia. J Hand Surg 1987; 12A:237–239.

38. Lamb D, Chan K. Surgical reconstruction of the upper limb in traumatic tetraplegia. J Bone Joint Surg 1983; 65B(3):291–298.

39. Wood TL. Les Anomalies Musculaires chez L'Homme Expliquees par L'anatomie Comparee, Leur Importance en Anthropologie. Paris: Mason and Cie, 1884.

40. Maury M, Guillaumat M, François N. Our experience of upper limb transfers in cases of tetraplegia. Paraplegia 1973; 11:245–251.

41. Gansel J, Waters R, Gelman H. Transfer of the pronator teres tendon to the tendons of the flexor digitorum profundus in tetraplegia. J Bone Joint Surg 1990; 72A:427–432.

42. Johnstone BR et al. A review of surgical rehabilitation of the upper limb in quadriplegia. Paraplegia 1988; 76: 317–339.

10

Surgical rehabilitation of active elbow extension

Introduction – the disability

Erik Moberg stressed the importance of restoring active elbow extension for the spinal cord injury patient in terms of locomotion, transfers, accurately positioning the arm in space, and improving the effect of more distal tendon transfers to restore hand function.[1] Dawn-Demagone et al. found that triceps strength was a good predictor of daily self-care abilities in tetraplegic patients.[2]

The wheelchair-bound individual depends upon good shoulder and elbow power and stabilization to push a wheelchair, transfer from bed to chair, and perform pressure releases to prevent pressure sores. Since the patient in a wheelchair must ambulate using the upper limbs for locomotion, the absence of a strong elbow extension means that power to propel the wheelchair is applied primarily through the shoulders. Without triceps function, the individual cannot 'push-through' with a full motion. This makes pushing a wheelchair less efficient and more energy consuming. In addition, individuals who do not have a triceps function cannot push their wheelchairs up any incline, which restricts their wheelchair 'environment' to level ground. Many tetraplegic patients who lack triceps function ultimately turn to the full-time use of a powered chair, in spite of the disadvantages of such chairs (i.e., cost, increased size and weight, and occasional mechanical failure).

For the tetraplegic patient, the lack of functional elbow extension results in a much-reduced functional environment. When seated in the wheelchair, the range of motion of his or her upper extremity determines the immediate 'world'. How far the patient can reach without having to move the wheelchair defines

the immediate environment. Without active elbow extension, the tetraplegic patient cannot reliably reach for overhead objects, such that even as simple a task as turning on a room light switch may be impossible. The ability to extend the hand away from the body in all planes by an additional 30 cm (12 inches) results in an additional 800% of space that the hand can reach. This is the difference between the arm that can versus the arm that cannot be fully extended at the elbow.

Without active elbow extension, the tetraplegic's hands frequently fall onto the face when the patient is lying supine. In addition, the patient must learn various adaptive maneuvers to lift his or her thighs and buttocks to relieve the effects of pressure. If the elbows have retained full passive extension, the tetraplegic may be able to lock them in full or slight hyperextension and, by leaning forward, perform effective pressure relief. This same ability allows these patients to assist their caregivers in safely performing transfers from bed to chair or from chair to toilet. If the trunk is unstable, however, patients may pitch forward.

Even a relatively small elbow extension torque, much less than that required to reach high overhead or to propel a manual chair up a gradient, and far less than that needed to self-transfer, is of major functional significance if controllable. A small extension torque may be the difference between a patient being able to direct the arm accurately to the target in a controlled and coordinated manner, versus having to launch the arm in the general direction of the target. If they have no triceps function, patients must depend solely on the braking function of their elbow flexors to control the trajectory and velocity of their arms in space. Restoring this critical element of control may be the most beneficial aspect of reconstruction of elbow extension.

Finally, Moberg stressed the beneficial effect of restoring elbow stability on the functional outcome of procedures that utilize either the brachioradialis (BR) or extensor carpi radialis longus for muscle–tendon transfers.[1] Brys and Waters found that pinch strength following BR to flexor pollicis longus transfer increased by 150% when the elbow could be stabilized.[3]

Today, two surgical procedures are advocated to restore active elbow extension. One is transfer of a strong portion of the deltoid muscle into the triceps, and the other commonly performed procedure is transfer of the biceps muscle into the triceps

Surgical techniques to restore active elbow extension

Deltoid-to-triceps transfer

In the USA, transfer of the posterior half of the deltoid into the triceps tendon or olecranon, as described by Moberg,[4] has been more frequently performed than the biceps-to-triceps transfer. One of us (VRH) prefers this procedure when the posterior deltoid is strong and the elbow has near normal passive extension.

Merle d'Aubigne recognized the synergism between the posterior part of the deltoid and the triceps muscles,[5,6] and suggested that the posterior half of the deltoid might substitute for the paralyzed triceps. Moberg[4] was the first to establish that this transfer could provide predictable elbow extension power in the tetraplegic patient.

Indications and contraindications
The procedure is potentially indicated in the tetraplegic patient who has maintained a good passive range of motion at the elbow, and who has sufficient strength in the posterior half of the deltoid. An initial concern was that transferring part of the tetraplegic patient's deltoid muscle might result in functional loss at the shoulder. Such has not been the case, although few studies have addressed this question with truly quantitative measurements. Logically, simply moving the insertion of the deltoid more distal on the humerus should not change its biomechanical properties relative to its function at the shoulder, save the potential for weakening this part of the muscle by surgical manipulation.

An absolute contraindication is inadequate strength of the deltoid muscle. A relative contraindication is a fixed elbow flexion contracture greater than 45°. Any significant flexion contracture should be treated first by progressive splinting, serial casting, or dynamic rubber-band stretching. If these conservative measures fail, surgical release prior to the deltoid-to-triceps transfer should be performed. Some authors caution against this procedure for patients with total paralysis of the pectoralis major muscle, since paralysis of the pectoralis, by robbing the posterior deltoid of its antagonist, reduces the ability of the patient to modulate the function of the posterior deltoid.[7] Other relative contraindications are associated with the particular rigorous time demands necessary for a good outcome following surgery, including up to 6 weeks in a cast and an equal number of weeks of progressive exercise. This rigorous rehabilitation schedule is a significant challenge even for the tetraplegic patient with strong assistive support from the family or attendants. Deltoid-to-triceps transfer surgery should be approached with caution if there are doubts about the patient's ability to participate fully in the vigorous and relatively complex rehabilitation process.

Some surgeons recommend simultaneous bilateral deltoid-to-triceps transfer.[8] As surgery on one arm renders the patient essentially totally dependent on others for most activities, they argue that patients who have both sides done simultaneously are only slightly more inconvenienced. As the time and cost savings are so much more substantial, these override the relatively short period of essential total dependence.

Preoperative assessment and patient preparation
Critical issues such as adequate attendant care and proper motivation are addressed in Chapter 8, and cannot be overstressed. Additional assessment includes a careful determination of the strength of the deltoid (see Chapter 6). It is important to assess the posterior part of the muscle and not simply test the patient's ability to abduct against resistance horizontally. We have seen instances in which shoulder abduction

were assessed to be Medical Research Council (MRC) Grade 4+, and yet little bulk remained in the posterior part of the deltoid. The ideal candidate possesses nearly MRC Grade 5 strength in this part of the deltoid. In such cases, it is almost impossible for the observer to push the arm forward into shoulder flexion using only his or her triceps muscle as the force of displacement. If the patient's arm can be easily pushed out of the extended position, the strength of the posterior part of the deltoid is probably insufficient to permit a predictable outcome after surgery. For some patients, a period of directed strengthening exercises might improve candidacy.

Moberg, in his 1978 monograph,[1] reports adding the anterior half of the deltoid to the transfer as a secondary procedure in an attempt to improve elbow extension power or salvage an initially suboptimal outcome. We have had similar experience in three patients and have not seen changes in postoperative

shoulder function following transfer of the entire deltoid muscle to the triceps insertion, at least as assessed by manual muscle testing. No patient complained about loss of preoperative shoulder function or strength.

In addition to deltoid strength, the active and passive range of elbow movement is assessed. Tetraplegic patients commonly exhibit some loss of passive elbow extension as a consequence of the unopposed pull of the biceps and other elbow flexors. The observer must distinguish whether the loss of extension range is a soft or firm one. If gravity alone is extending the elbow, the elbow may not fully straighten. To determine whether the loss is soft or firm, the observer must passively extend the elbow to measure the true level of contracture. If the elbow can be passively extended to within 30° of full extension, the patient is a potential candidate for deltoid-to-triceps transfer. The postoperative splint-

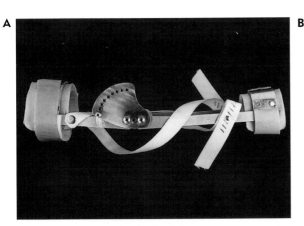

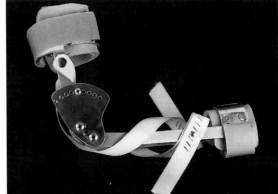

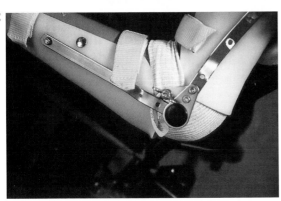

Figure 10.1 A special flexion-block orthosis is constructed from measurements of the patient's arm. The brace consists of three parts, humeral and forearm supports joined at a polyaxial center. A series of holes is drilled about the periphery of the polyaxial center piece and these holes are threaded to receive a simple screw. The screw-head creates a block against elbow flexion while allowing complete elbow extension. The brace is placed on the operated arm following removal of the postoperative cast and the screw is placed into the first hole. This allows only a small amount of elbow flexion. The screw is progressively moved farther around the axis of the device as time passes. The device is illustrated in its fully extended (A) and fully flexed (B) range. (C) A more sophisticated device.

ing regimen must be altered, but this amount of contracture can be stretched to nearly full extension in the postoperative period.

A fixed extension contracture greater than 30° should be corrected by therapy or may require a preliminary surgical release. Once nearly full passive extension has been achieved and the patient has regained strong elbow flexion, deltoid-to-triceps transfer can proceed. For such patients, especially if the elbow flexion contracture exceeds 45°, a biceps-to-triceps transfer may be preferred, as discussed later.

Occasionally, a patient presents with a significant spasticity in the biceps muscle. Such patients may benefit from constructing an antagonist to this spastic elbow flexor. In such cases, we have occasionally employed botulinum toxin placed into the spastic biceps muscle at the time of surgery.[9] The use of botulinum toxin in the tetraplegic patient is discussed more fully in Chapter 4.

Additional preoperative steps include measuring the patient's arm so that the postoperative exercise brace (*Fig. 10.1*) can be constructed or ordered so that it is available for placement when the patient's postsurgical cast is removed.

Fascia lata interposition

The fascia lata interposition (*Fig. 10.2*) is the authors' preferred surgical technique. The procedure is usually carried out under a general anesthetic or a supraclavicular brachial plexus block. Allieu pioneered performing this procedure under a cervical epidural anesthetic in the tetraplegic patient.[10–13]

The patient is positioned in a slightly lateral position, accomplished using a 'bean-bag' immobilizer or by elevating the hip and shoulder on the operated side with several towels or intravenous fluid bags. The anterior and lateral shoulder and the entire arm are draped free for exposure.

The surgical landmarks (*Fig. 10.3A*) at the level of the shoulder include the tip of the acromion superiorly, the interval between the posterior margin of the deltoid and the triceps muscle posteriorly, and the estimated point of insertion of the deltoid on the humerus. The landmark at the level of the elbow is the tip of the olecranon. The surgeon should keep in mind the neurovascular anatomy of the region, including the course of the axillary nerve, the circumflex humeral artery, and the radial nerve and its

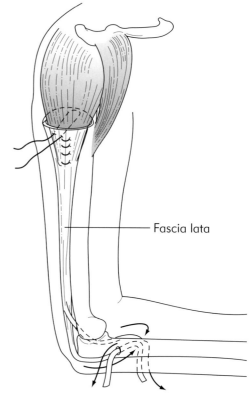

Fascia lata

Figure 10.2 Deltoid-to-triceps transfer using fascia lata to lengthen the deltoid.

relationship to the insertion of the deltoid (*Fig. 10.3B*).

The upper incision is centered half way between the mid-axial line of the humerus and the posterior margin of the deltoid (*Fig. 10.3A*). Since the skin in this area is very vascular, it is beneficial to infiltrate the proposed line of the incision with a solution of long-acting local anesthetic, such as bupivacaine containing epinephrine (adrenaline) at a concentration of 1:200,000, before the patient undergoes skin preparation and draping. This gives sufficient time for the epinephrine (adrenaline) to exert its vasoconstrictive benefits.

The skin incision is carried to the level of the muscle fascia and the skin and subcutaneous tissue are elevated anteriorly to just past the mid-axial line of the humerus. Posteriorly, the skin flap is elevated to the confluence of deltoid and the long head of the triceps (*Fig. 10.3C*). The plane between these two muscles is developed by sharp or finger dissection. The interval is relatively bloodless and easily dissected

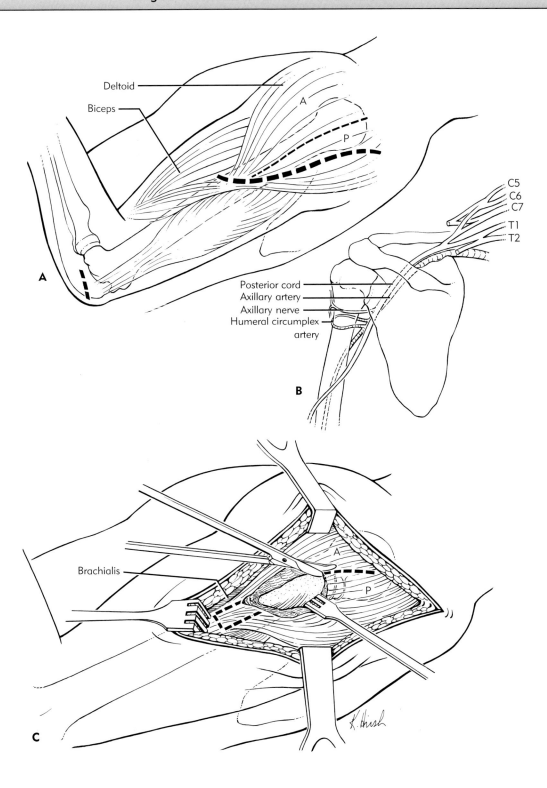

Figure 10.3 The deltoid-to-triceps surgical technique; see the text for details.

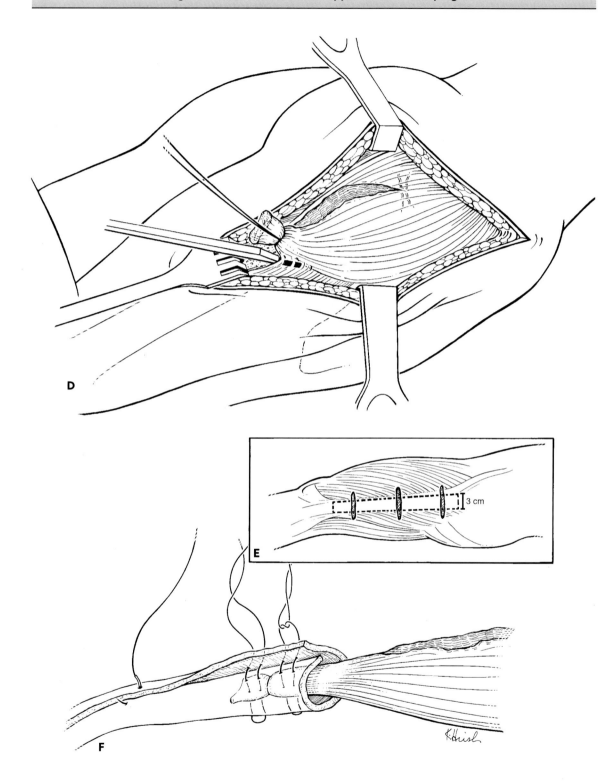

Figure 10.3 (continued)

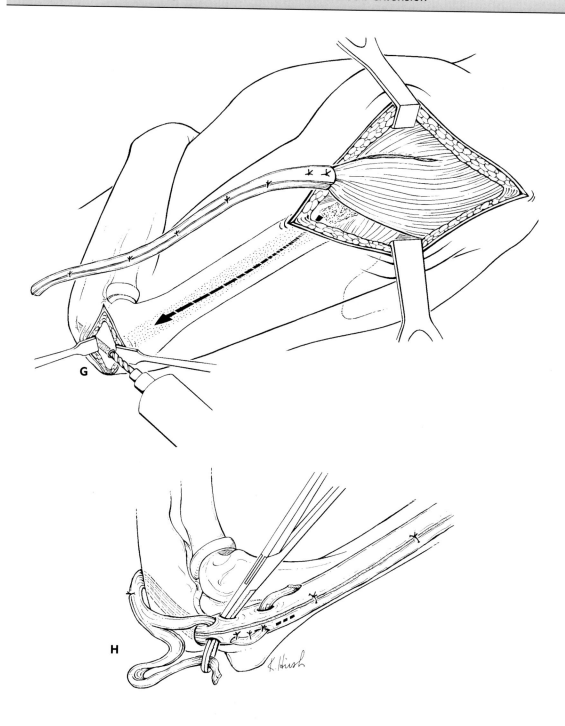

Figure 10.3 (continued)

so that a finger slips easily under the posterior half of the deltoid at about the mid-portion of this muscle. The lower retractor in *Figure 10.3C* is in this space. As the finger strikes the humerus, the fingertip can be insinuated upward through the fibers of the deltoid, separating anterior and posterior halves. The fibers of the deltoid are split in the direction of the muscle fascicles by inferior and superior sharp and blunt dissection.

It is helpful to detach the insertion of the posterior half of the muscle from its point of insertion onto the humerus. This is achieved by sharply incising a rectangle of periostium at the point of attachment and elevating the periostium and fibers of attachment off the humerus (*Fig. 10.3D*). Some surgeons include a small block of humerus at the point of muscle attachment. Care is taken to incorporate as much fascia and fibrous insertion as possible, including some of the fascial origin of the brachialis muscle. The radial nerve emerges from behind the humerus several centimeters distal to this point. Injury to this nerve has been reported as a rare but devastating complication of this procedure, so care must be exercised regarding the anatomic landmarks.

A suture is placed in the fibrous origin of the posterior half of the deltoid muscle (*Fig. 10.3D*) and the dissection is carried superiorly until the branches of the axillary nerve are visualized. These must not be injured and the superior dissection should stop at this point.

Several methods have been proposed to attach the posterior deltoid to the triceps or olecranon, including:

- autogenous tendons such as toe extensors (*Fig. 10.4A*),[4] tibialis anterior tendon,[14] or extensor carpi ulnaris;[15]
- strip of fascia lata (*Fig. 10.4B*);[16]
- turned up strip of the central part of the triceps tendon,[17] with synthetic reinforcement (see *Figs 10.4C, 10.4D,* and later);[18]
- bone-to-bone attachments;[19] or
- various synthetic materials.[10]

For many years, one of us (VRH) favored using a wide strip of the patient's own fascia lata, especially for the patient whose triceps tendon is relatively short or insubstantial. A second surgical team working simultaneously may obtain the fascia lata strip.

The fascia is harvested through several transverse incisions placed over the iliotibial band (*Fig. 10.3E*). The ideal width is about 2.5 cm (1 inch). The fascia lata is placed as a tube about the fibrous insertion of the deltoid using mattress sutures of nonabsorbable braided suture (*Fig. 10.3F*). This needs to be a secure attachment because it will be subject to some stress during surgical testing and in the healing period. The fascia is wrapped as a tube over its remaining length and will be tunneled subcutaneously to the distal incision to be made at the olecranon.

The tip of the olecranon is exposed just distal to the insertion of the triceps. The triceps tendon is split longitudinally to further expose the tip of the olecranon and a 5 mm drill bit is used to create an oblique tunnel through the olecranon (*Fig. 10.3G*). A Bunnell tendon-stripper is a useful instrument to 'polish' this channel so that the fascia lata tube can be passed smoothly in a proximal to distal direction (*Fig. 10.3H*). The fascia lata is passed into the distal exposure, separated into two tails, and the tails are passed through the bone channel and woven back on themselves.

The shoulder is abducted about 30° and the elbow is flexed about 30°. The two fascia lata tails are pulled to tense the transfer maximally and anchored to the fascia lata tube, again with nonabsorbable sutures. Once suturing is complete, the fascia lata tube should be under moderate but definite tension. A suction drain is placed in the upper wound and the incisions are closed using a layered closure with subcuticular absorbable sutures.

Deltoid-to-triceps transfer using the triceps tendon 'turn-up' technique

The technique attributed to Castro-Serra and Lopez-Pita (CSLP) is another option and is appropriate when the triceps tendon is long and broad.[17] A central triceps strip measuring 1.5 cm (0.5 inch) is harvested in continuity with a periosteal flap from the proximal ulna. The central strip of triceps tendon is dissected proximally until there is sufficient length to reach the deltoid insertion. The posterior deltoid is detached from the humerus along with a periosteal flap as described above (*Fig. 10.4C*). The two fresh periosteal flaps face each other when the triceps tendon is turned superiorly. The point of superior reflection of the central triceps is anchored to the adjacent triceps tendon on both sides, using heavy nonabsorbable

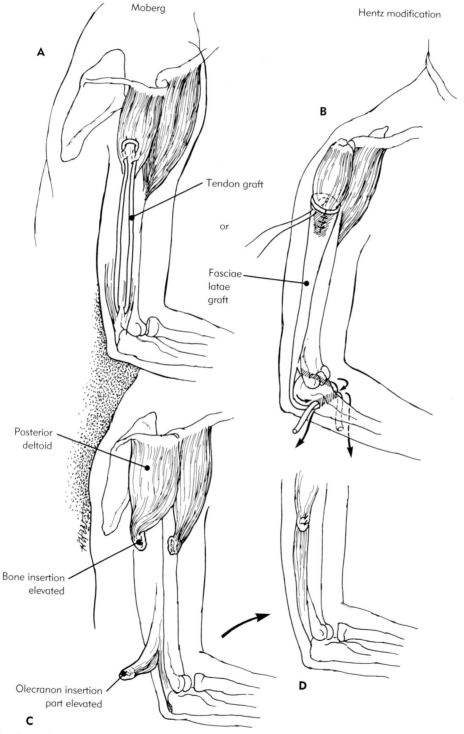

Figure 10.4 Several other methods can be used to attach the posterior half of the deltoid to the triceps tendon; see the text for details.

sutures. This prevents the turned-up strip of tendon from tearing more superiorly when tension is exerted on the transfer (*Fig. 10.4D*). The mass of reflection (i.e., the tendon reflected and all reinforcing material) is buried within the substance of the muscle itself with additional sutures. The periosteal faces of turned-up triceps and deltoid are fixed together with additional nonabsorbable sutures.

A modification of this technique described by Mennon utilizes a bone-to-bone juncture between a segment of the humerus with deltoid attachment and a segment of olecranon (*Figs 10.4C* and *10.4D*). The olecranon bone is harvested in continuity with a central strip of triceps tendon. This central strip with attached bone is split from the adjacent triceps tendon in a proximal direction and just enough to allow the tendon–bone end to be turned up to meet the deltoid–humeral bone segment. The two bone segments are wired or screwed together under appropriate tension.

Regardless of the technique chosen, the elbow is immobilized in full extension using a light plaster or fiberglass cylinder cast for 3.5 weeks (*Fig. 10.5*). A thin layer of moderate density foam (Rest-on Foam, 3-M Company) is used under the cast to protect insensate skin. This has an adhesive side that is applied directly to the skin of the patient, except where the surgical wounds are covered by dressings, such as about the elbow. Potential pressure points receive additional padding. Plaster or fiberglass placed over the foam wrap will also adhere to the foam material. This results in a very stable construct with little

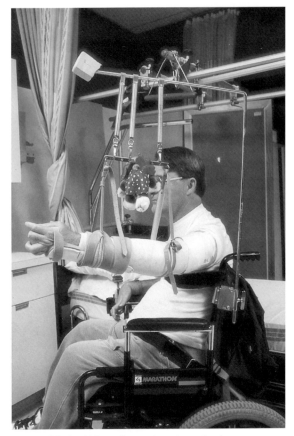

Figure 10.6 When the patient is up in the wheelchair, the operated arm is supported in a balanced overhead sling mounted on the chair.

tendency to slide up and down or twist about the patient's arm during the 3–4 weeks that the cylinder cast is worn. The shoulder is kept somewhat abducted and the patient and other caregivers are cautioned to not allow the shoulder to flop accidentally across the chest. The patient is encouraged to begin transferring into his or her wheelchair on the second postoperative day. Essentially, these patients are totally dependent for all transfer activity while their arm is in this cast. An overhead, chair-mounted sling is fitted to the wheelchair (*Fig 10.6*). This holds the arm elevated to a degree, which prevents distal edema and helps keep the arm somewhat abducted from the body, a position that relaxes the deltoid. The overhead frame is used whenever the patient is up in the wheelchair and until the cast is removed.

The suction drain is removed typically on the second postoperative day and the patient may be

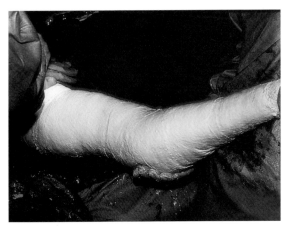

Figure 10.5 The arm is immobilized in a cylinder cast with the elbow held in about 15° of flexion.

discharged from hospital, either to home if sufficient attendant care is available or to an extended care facility.

The initial cast is left undisturbed for 3.5 weeks if the elbow had essentially normal passive extension preoperatively. If the elbow had a preoperative flexion contracture between 15 and 30°, the elbow is extended as much as possible at the time of surgery and held in that position in the cast. This cast is removed between 10 and 14 days postoperatively. Great care must be taken to keep the elbow extended during this maneuver. Typically, the elbow can be further extended at this time by slow stretch and the arm is again set in a cast, now typically in near full or even full extension.

Postoperative rehabilitation*

*See Appendix IV for a detailed postoperative rehabilitation regimen.

The cast is removed about 3.5 weeks following surgery, although other authors (including Moberg[20]) recommended periods of casting up to 6 weeks. Still others, using synthetic materials either in lieu of tendon or to reinforce autograft tissues, advise very short periods of cast immobilization, often only a few days, before beginning carefully directed exercises.[19] The patient begins active exercises in a protective polyaxial brace that limits the amount of flexion, but permits full extension (see *Fig. 10.1*). Measurements for the brace are made before surgery so that it is available at the time the patient is ready to be freed from the cylinder cast. The brace does not rigidly stabilize the elbow. Rather, about 30° of initial flexion is permitted by the brace, even with the elbow hinge 'locked' at maximum extension. We do not feel that this initial 30° of early movement constitutes a significant risk of overstretching the transfer. This active brace is worn essentially full time during the day.

Various exercise regimens are employed, including functional stimulation of the muscle beginning at about the sixth postoperative week.[21] Biofeedback may help assist the patient to trigger the muscle. Typically, the patient at first attempts to trigger the transfer while the arm is supported in a horizontal, gravity-eliminated position on a friction-free surface, such as a heavily powdered table or a specially designed ball-bearing rolling surface. As time passes, the patient attempts to trigger the transfer against

gravity, but without any additional resistance. Extension against resistance is avoided for the initial 8 weeks. The dynamic brace is removed for bathing, provided the arm is protected against accidental excessive flexion. At night, the patient dons a softer brace to maintain the elbow nearly fully extended. The degree of flexion allowed is gradually increased so that by the eighth postoperative week, the patient is allowed to fully flex the elbow. The dynamic brace can be abandoned at this time, but the patient has to wear the soft nighttime brace for at least 6 months following surgery. Also, the patient avoids transfer on the extended elbow for at least 10 weeks. Some months of cautious use are necessary to prevent overstretching of the transfer and many months pass before maximal strength is obtained (*Fig. 10.7*).

Biceps-to-triceps transfer

A second procedure, biceps-to-triceps transfer, has been advocated to improve elbow extension (*Fig. 10.8*).[22] The biceps tendon can be detached from its insertion on the greater tuberosity of the radius and the muscle–tendon unit routed either medially, as recommended by Kuz and House[23] and Revol,[24] or laterally[22,25] and the tendon attached to the triceps aponeurosis.

Indications, contraindications, and preoperative preparation

Many surgeons utilize biceps-to-triceps transfer as their primary means of helping the patient achieve improved elbow control. One of us (VRH) prefers to perform this transfer when there is a pre-existing fixed flexion contracture of the elbow greater than 30–45° (*Fig. 10.8A*). The greater the flexion contracture, the more likely is the recommendation for biceps-to-triceps transfer, since in such cases the biceps is usually a deforming force, both contributing to the flexion contracture at the elbow and keeping the forearm in a supinated posture. This deforming force must be treated either by tendon lengthening or tenotomy if increased passive elbow extension is to be regained. Rather than lengthen the biceps tendon, which always weakens this muscle, it is transferred at the time of contracture release. Transfer of an antagonist is frequently associated with postoperative difficulty in rehabilitating the transfer. However, by teaching the patient to conjointly supinate the

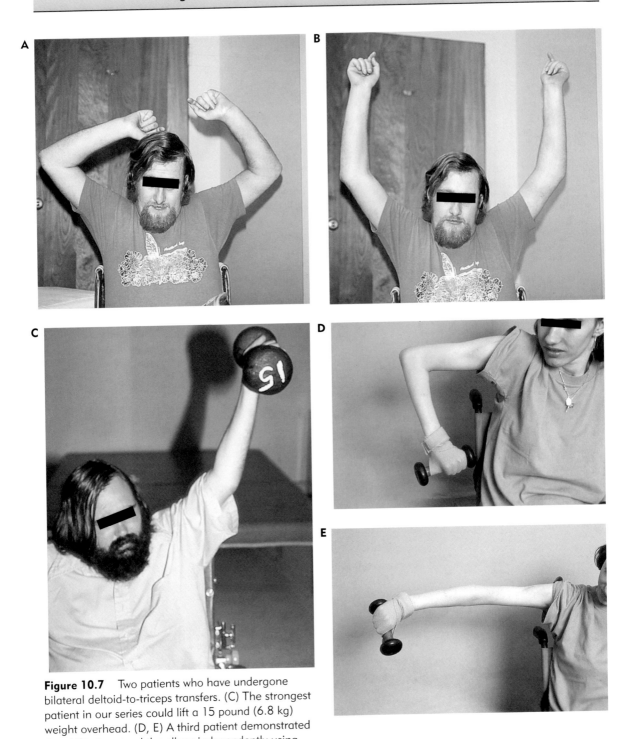

Figure 10.7 Two patients who have undergone bilateral deltoid-to-triceps transfers. (C) The strongest patient in our series could lift a 15 pound (6.8 kg) weight overhead. (D, E) A third patient demonstrated the ability to extend the elbow independently using the deltoid-to-triceps transfer.

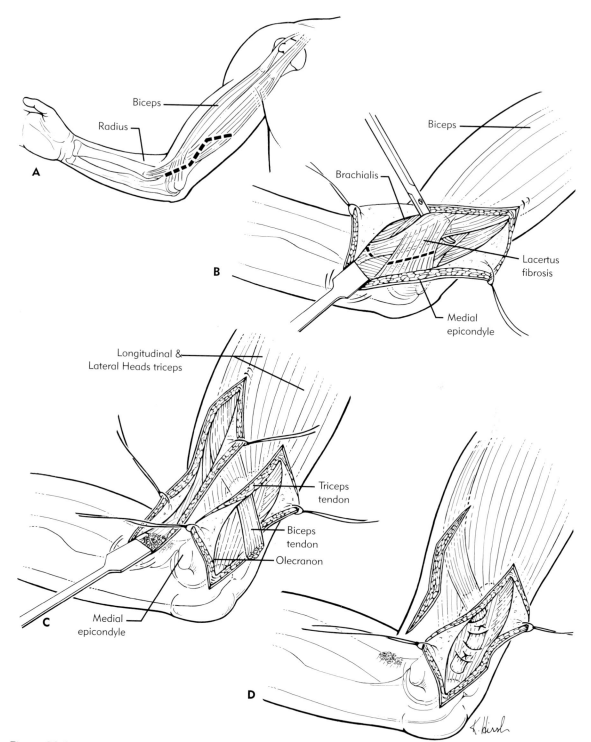

Figure 10.8 The surgical steps for the biceps-to-triceps transfer; see text for details.

forearm and extend the elbow, he or she can take advantage of the supinator function of the biceps in re-educating this transfer.

A potential contraindication to biceps-to-triceps transfer is the absence of any function in the remaining supinator muscle of the forearm. If the biceps is transferred, the patient will be unable to supinate actively the forearm. Some patients need to be able to supinate the forearm at least enough to direct an object, such as a fork or spoon held in the hand or mounted on an orthosis fitted to the hand, toward the mouth. If they cannot supinate the forearm, a fork held on the radial (normal) side of the hand cannot be brought easily toward the mouth, unless the patient elevates the arm at the shoulder or brings his or her mouth to the hand.

It is difficult to assess the function of the supinator preoperatively. It rarely functions in complete isolation from the biceps and no amount of elbow flexion totally eliminates the supinator effect of the biceps, although fully flexing the patient's elbow will weaken the biceps. We have always performed electromyographic analysis of the supinator in an attempt to determine whether the patient has retained some voluntary control over the supinator and could demonstrate a reasonable recruitment pattern. In one patient, we performed a preoperative local anesthetic block of the musculocutaneous nerve, temporarily paralyzing the biceps, to confirm supinator muscle activity.

Operative procedure

The procedure is typically performed under a general anesthetic, but it can be carried out under a supraclavicular brachial plexus blockade. A tourniquet cannot be accommodated.

The incisions that are employed depend in large measure on whether a wide exposure to the anterior aspect of the elbow joint is needed to allow adequate release of contracture (*Fig. 10.8A*). The distal extent of the incision should allow complete dissection of the tendon of the biceps, so that it can be detached as close as possible to its point of insertion on the bicipital tuberosity of the radius.

The incision is carried through the subcutaneous tissue, protecting the large tributaries of the basilic and cephalic veins. The soft tissues that overlie the lacertus fibrosus are elevated and the lacertus is either divided off the primary tendon or dissected distally as

far as possible to provide another point of fixation to the triceps (*Fig. 10.8B*).

The primary tendon of the biceps is dissected to its point of insertion on the radius. Flexion of the elbow and supination of the forearm assists in this exposure. The tendon is sectioned as far distally as possible (*Fig. 10.8B*). The biceps muscle is dissected proximally from within its dense investing fascia, and the dissection proceeds proximally until the cutaneous portion of the musculocutaneous nerve is identified as it courses between the overlying biceps and the deeper brachialis muscle (*Fig. 10.8C*). This nerve is protected while dissection of the biceps proceeds proximally, until the most distal motor branches arising from the musculocutaneous nerve are visualized.

Both medial and lateral routings of the transfer have been described. Since the ulnar nerve is typically nonfunctional in this population, we have preferred to route the biceps medially (*Fig. 10.8C*). It is necessary to dissect widely the arcade of Struthers and all other fascial communications about the medial intermuscular septum. However, we know of one case in which the medial route was used when a biceps-to-triceps transfer was carried out at the time of implantation of a functional neuromuscular system. After surgery, those ulnar nerve muscles that could be stimulated preoperatively could no longer be; ulnar nerve compression by the transfer was suspected and the transfer was subsequently routed laterally. There is reason to be concerned about compression of the radial nerve when the lateral route is chosen.

A second incision located posteromedially is made to expose the medial aspect of the triceps insertion. Through this incision, the medial border of the triceps is elevated and dissected to its insertion on the olecranon. The biceps muscle and tendon are passed from the anterior to the posterior incision through the widely dissected subcutaneous tunnel. The anterior incision may be closed at this point (*Fig. 10.8D*).

The biceps tendon typically just reaches the tip of the olecranon, but occasionally there is insufficient tendon length to permit a strong attachment into the olecranon. Instead, the tendon of the biceps is woven into the medial border of the triceps tendon and anchored in multiple locations with stout sutures. We have judged that the proper tension is achieved when the biceps is pulled distally enough to permit the end of the tendon to touch the olecranon with the elbow in about 20° of flexion. Bottero has recently described a technique to measure the length of the intramuscular portion of the biceps tendon, to aid in setting tension in transfer.[26] House recommends creating a bony tunnel in the tip of the olecranon and drilling several holes from the base of this tunnel out the cortex of the ulnar, several centimeters distal to the tip of the olecranon.[23] As much distal biceps tendon as possible should be introduced into this short tunnel by passing sutures woven into the distal biceps tendon into the tunnel and out through the predrilled holes. Tension on the suture ends brings the end of the biceps tendon snug against the bony tunnel. This is reinforced with additional sutures.

Once the tendon-to-tendon junctures have been made, the elbow is fully extended to relax the site of approximation. The posterior incision is closed and the arm is placed in a cylinder cast, as described above for the deltoid-to-triceps transfer.

The postoperative regimen is exactly like that described for the deltoid-to-triceps transfer, except that the patient learns to trigger the transfer by extending the arm at the shoulder while trying to supinate the forearm. A similar flexion arrest brace is worn, as described for deltoid-to-triceps transfer, and elbow flexion is gradually increased. Electrical stimulation and biofeedback therapy have been used on occasion with improved results (Fig. 10.9). Just as for the deltoid-to-triceps transfer, too rapid a remobilization of the transfer is an important concern.

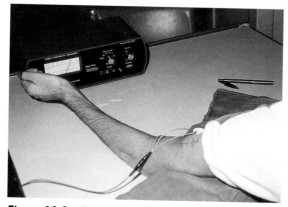

Figure 10.9   Electrical stimulation and biofeedback therapy to trigger the muscle after biceps-to-triceps transfer.

Other surgical procedures to restore elbow extension

Other procedures that might be considered for the tetraplegic patient include shifting the body of the BR muscle more posteriorly, though not the muscle origin, as described by Ober.[27] This removes the effect of the BR on elbow flexion and makes it more of an elbow extender. Ober reported the outcomes in five patients, all apparently successful. The muscle was easily educated. Typically, the posterior half of the muscle is used for the transfer. However, in the tetraplegic population, the BR is frequently the only available muscle for transfer and should be reserved to restore or strengthen more useful distal functions, such as thumb pinch or finger grasp. Most of the other procedures described to restore or strengthen elbow extension, such as transfer of the latissimus dorsi, are not applicable to the tetraplegic patient. The muscle is either too weak or its normal function too valuable to permit sacrifice.

Outcomes, complications, and their treatment in deltoid-to-triceps transfers

The authors' patients

Outcomes

In our experience the results of deltoid-to-triceps transfer have not been totally consistent. The great majority of patients can achieve full or near-full extension against partial gravity. In those patients who had a full passive range of motion preoperatively, almost all achieved full or near-full extension against partial gravity. However, only two-thirds were able to fully or near-fully extend (within 15°) the elbow in the completely overhead posture. Except for two patients, who were judged failures in spite of secondary procedures, all have gained the ability to better control the elbow. The majority of patients achieve more efficient transfers, pressure releases, and wheelchair mobility. Other functional gains include:

- ease of turning in bed;
- improved writing ability;
- improved ability to groom themselves;
- improved ability to feed themselves; and
- improved ability to drive an automobile.

We have not been able to correlate preoperative deltoid strength with the level of final elbow extension torque. Other authors have reported similar inconstant results, though failure of the procedure to provide any useful function is rare.

Complications and their treatment

Complications are rare provided the patient follows the exercise protocol and does not overstretch the transfer by too rapidly performing full elbow flexion. We have reviewed 45 deltoid-to-triceps transfers performed in 30 of our own patients. One patient experienced rupture of the CSLP tendon-to-tendon juncture on the second postoperative day when his arm was accidentally allowed to fall across his chest while still in the hospital. He reported sensing the juncture rupture and was returned to the operating room that day and the juncture re-established. His ultimate outcome was very acceptable. Two patients achieved very little useful function following their initial procedure. In both, the transfer was tightened at a second procedure, without much improvement.

If, at exploration, the transfer is found to be overstretched, the tendon must be shortened or tightened. Shortening involves resecting a portion of tendon and re-approximating the tendon ends. A better alternative involves osteotomizing the olecranon, in continuity with the triceps tendon, or a tendon graft attachment and re-attaching the olecranon more distally on the ulna. Firm attachment by a lag-screw technique allows earlier resumption of exercises than with a tendon-to-tendon re-approximation.

In the two patients with little improvement, the entire deltoid muscle was subsequently transferred without measurably changing the shoulder function, and one of the two patients improved significantly. Another patient reported the loss of a formerly good elbow extension gained by deltoid-to-triceps transfer. This patient was forced to lie in bed for many weeks as part of pressure sore management and apparently used his flexed elbow frequently to raise himself in bed. On re-exploration, we found evidence of loosening of the tendon-to-tendon juncture. The loose tendon was advanced more distal on the ulna and a very acceptable outcome obtained.

Outcome of other series of deltoid-to-triceps transfers

Moberg reported on his initial 16 deltoid-to-triceps patients, of whom 15 experienced significant functional improvement.[4] Two patients experienced overstretching of the transfer. A re-operation with tightening of the transfer in one resulted in satisfactory function. The other patient represents the only failure.

Bryan, working at the Mayo Clinic, Minnesota, USA, reported on seven patients who had bilateral transfers, several simultaneously.[8] The results were inconsistent, with some patients demonstrating great postoperative strength and others little strength.

Working initially in conjunction with Moberg at the Long Beach VA Spinal Unit, DeBenedetti reported the outcome of 20 transfers in 17 patients.[28] Prior to surgery, the average elbow extension strength was MRC Grade 0.5 (range, 0–2). Following surgery, elbow extensor power averaged MRC Grade 3.6 (2.5–4.5). Using a weight and pulley system, with the shoulder abducted about 45° and the elbow flexed to about 90°, the weight that could be lifted by their patients averaged 4.6 (1–9) pounds [2, (0.5–4) kg]. All 13 patients were satisfied with their results and 11 stated that they would have the procedure again.

Castro-Sierra and Lopez-Pita, working in Toledo, Spain, reported the outcomes of 10 elbows in seven patients utilizing their novel method of tendon attachment (described above).[17] The elbow is immobilized for 21 days and protected during progressive exercises of flexion to 30°, and then flexion to 60° for an additional 2 weeks only. They state that tendon part does not measure more than 10 cm (8 inches) and thus is a relatively short graft, so less likely to elongate. They report that all patients had a satisfactory outcome.

Raczka *et al.* reported the outcomes of a series of 23 transfers in 22 patients operated on at the Rancho Loa Amigos Center, California.[29] Their evaluation included preoperative assessments of motion, strength, and activities of daily living (ADLs), including transfers, hygiene, self-grooming, driving, turning in bed, writing, and use of wheelchair. The subjective assessment included the patient's opinion of the types of functional improvements obtained relative to the above ADLs, and the overall gain or loss in independence. The average follow-up time was 49 months (7–79).

Of these patients, 15 said they had gained functional improvement, and 13 gained increased independence. Frequently mentioned improvements included stability of the arm (15), reaching overhead objects (15), turning in bed (10), and functional improvement in hygiene. Also, 12 patients said that they were able to relieve pressure more easily and that writing speed and clarity had improved, and 50% said their driving ability was better. Six patients were not able to drive before surgery, but were able to do so after. One patient went to a manual chair exclusively. One patient said he was worse because of decreased supination, perhaps secondary to prolonged casting.

A few patients were now able to transfer from a bed to a chair using a sliding board; most others said they could, but that it was too difficult and time consuming so they used a lift. Those that did gain had bilateral transfer.

On objective testing, nine patients had MRC Grade 4 to 4+ postoperatively (seven were MRC Grade 0 prior to surgery), four patients had MRC Grade 3+, and three had only MRC Grade 2+ postoperatively, but these patients experienced good functional improvement.

Initial failures occurred in three patients. One was revised, but the results are unknown. At surgery it was noted that the original graft had failed in its midsubstance. In a second patient, the anterior deltoid was transferred with a gain to MRC Grade 2+.

Allieu et al. from the Propara Center in Montpellier, France, reported the results of their initial 21 cases.[10] They used fascia lata reinforced with Dacron sutures to join the deltoid to the triceps, followed by a 3 week period of immobilization. The excursion and power of the transfer was less than expected, but subjectively the results were considered by the patients to be satisfactory in spite of an inability to actively fully extend elbow.

Lacey and his medical and engineering colleagues from Case Western Reserve University, Cleveland, USA, reported the first biomechanical analysis of this transfer.[14] A 5 kg (11 pound) pull was used to stretch the muscle into its full passive length. Then, using intraoperative electrical stimulation as described by Freehafer et al.,[30] they determined the excursion of posterior deltoid to be 7.31 cm (2.88 inches). A surprisingly flat, active length–tension curve was obtained.

The tibialis anterior tendon was used as the interpositional graft and the elbow immobilized in 30° of flexion for 4 weeks. No special flexion block brace was used and the patients were permitted as much active flexion as they could tolerate. No resistance exercises were permitted for the first 8 weeks. A night resting splint was used for 3 months. Postoperatively, using a specially designed device and with the shoulder abducted 90° and forward flexed to 45°, the elbow extension torque averaged 3.57 N-m (2.63 ft-lb) with a deviation range of 5.69 to 2.06 N-m (4.2 to 1.52 ft-lb). The maximum strength occurred when the elbow was between 30° and 90° of elbow flexion. Lacey et al. noted a large effective range for the deltoid. Clinical results were judged to be excellent in 10 patients with 16 transfers.[14] The average MRC Grade was 3 with a range of 2–4. They measured 3 cm (1.2 inches) of excursion of the tendon graft to achieve full motion of the elbow, substantially less than that measured for the posterior deltoid. They recommend that tension be adjusted by putting in the distal site first, flexing the elbow to 90°, abducting the shoulder to 30°, and then performing the proximal juncture while the deltoid is pulled to its normal insertion length. Lacey et al. believe that this positioning maximizes the force production in the most useful elbow range.[14]

A later biomechanical study looked at the length tension relationship of the posterior deltoid-to-triceps transfer and compared it to the normal triceps.[31] Using force transducers, Rabischong et al. found that the maximum torque was in 130° of elbow flexion, and that the normal triceps produced an average of 27 N-m (19.91 ft-lb) while deltoid-to-triceps transfer, measured in eight tetraplegic patients, produced 7.8 N-m (5.75 ft-lb).[31] They concluded that the initial tension set by the surgeon is the most significant variable and also difficult to control without some type of device dedicated to attaining nominal length–tension relationships

In 1988, Ejeskär updated results of the reconstructions of elbow extension from Gothenburg, Sweden (some of the reported patients were the original patients operated on by Moberg).[32] Between 1970 and 1983, 40 elbows in 32 patients had surgery, 30 by Moberg's method and 10 by the CSLP method. Eight patients of the 30 who were treated with the Moberg method had full extension against gravity; only one of the 10 treated with the CSLP method achieved this. Extension against gravity was measured with the shoulder elevated fully and the elbow extended against the weight of forearm. Thirteen of the 30 Moberg-methods patients and seven of the 10 CSLP-method patients had a greater than 60° extension lag with the arm overhead, but could still control the elbow. However, there was little improvement in transfers in these 20 patients (i.e., half the total series). Ejeskär advocated placing steel sutures on either side of the tendon junctures to enable the estimation of tendon elongation in the postoperative period.[32]

Mennen described a modification of the CSLP technique and reported on his results in 35 procedures performed since 1983.[19] His patients achieved, on average, the strongest level of elbow extension torque reported so far. In this method, bone blocks are harvested at the deltoid and triceps insertions, connected to a 10 mm strip of triceps aponeurosis; the bone blocks subsequently are wired together. A saw is used to cut a 10×30 mm bone block from the humerus at the point of deltoid attachment. A bone block of similar size is taken slightly medial to the center of triceps insertion. Special 'U' stitches are placed into the corners of the triceps, plus an additional attachment of reflected tendon to the remaining tendon. The gap in the tendon is closed. A splint is used for only 1 week, during which time the patient does isometric exercises. Elbow flexion is increased over the next 6 weeks, avoiding resistance except that of gravity. If, preoperatively, the forearm is contracted into supination, simultaneous biceps 'Z' lengthening and rerouting is carried out. The elbow is held in 45° of flexion, with Kirschner-wire pinning of the pronated forearm for 6 weeks while elbow flexion exercises continue.

Mennen do not state the average length of follow-up.[19] Manual muscle testing was performed. Seven patients achieved MRC Grade 5 strength, another 25 achieved MRC Grade 4, and three achieved Grade 3 strength. Postoperative strength seemed less critical than better balance. Three patients were able to perform self-transfers. One patient required re-exploration and was found to have developed a boutonnière deformity of the remaining triceps insertion. This was repaired with a good result. One patient suffered a fractured humerus.

The authors concluded that the main reconstructive goal is stabilization of the forearm for better distal reconstruction and/or function, to reach out and pick-up objects, and to provide a wider range of manipulation. Synchrony, balance, and control lead to better patient motivation. The ability to institute early motion impressed the staff.[19]

Outcomes of biceps-to-triceps transfer

The results of biceps-to-triceps transfers in our patients have not been as impressive as those of deltoid-to-triceps transfers. This is most likely a consequence of patient selection. All biceps-to-triceps cases performed by one of us (VRH) were for patients with significant fixed preoperative elbow flexion contracture, usually exceeding 45°. Most patients required some form of anterior capsular release and some intramuscular tendon lengthening of the contracted brachialis muscle.

The typical postoperative patient cannot actively extend through a large range against the force of gravity. However, these patients do appreciate a gain in the ability to position the arm more accurately in space. The removal of a deforming supinator force and the strengthening of the antagonist decreases the chances of recurrence of the elbow contracture.

Two patients developed extension contractures following anterior release of their preoperative elbow flexion contracture and simultaneous biceps-to-triceps transfer. Both responded well to a limited posterior capsulotomy.

Zancolli of Buenos Aries, Argentina, reported on six cases of biceps-to-triceps transfer using the lateral route of transfer.[33] He favored this procedure over the deltoid-to-triceps method in those patients with residual wrist extension, because he felt that the supinator functioned reliably in these patients. Extension power measured 0.25–0.9 kg (0.6–2.0 pounds) and he reported no loss of flexor power. In a later report of 13 patients,[25] Zancolli stated that 80% of the patients experienced a good to excellent result. There were no poor results. Loss of elbow flexion strength averaged 24%, but no functional complaints were associated with this loss.

In 1988, Ejeskär updated the results for this operation in Gothenburg.[34] Although his evaluation of their patients who had undergone biceps-to-triceps transfer by lateral routing was still preliminary, he reported that in five patients, two had full extension against gravity, 1 lacked 80° to full extension and 2 had no active extension. He mentioned reduction in elbow flexion strength as a disadvantage and reported one patient who had a prolonged radial nerve palsy. Ejeskär tested for supinator function by palpating the muscle belly while resisting supination. Ejeskär's specific indication for the procedure is a contracted elbow along with a supination deformity of the forearm. He rationalizes that even if no active extension is gained, the patient achieves better passive elbow extension and better forearm pronation, which is necessary to use a surgically constructed one-hand grip. Ejeskär recommends biceps-to-triceps transfer if the strength of elbow extension is not important and some elbow flexion contracture is present. He recommends deltoid-to-triceps transfer if there is a fear of losing elbow flexion strength and strong elbow extension is the primary goal.

Moberg[35] updated his results in 1989, reporting on 10 patients. He stated that most had good results, especially those with pre-existing elbow flexion contractures. He noted a few cases where the insertion had lengthened.

Kuz and House from the University of Minnesota reported their results in four biceps-to-triceps transfers performed in three patients.[23] They used a medial route for their transfers. All had preoperative supination function and none had an elbow flexion contracture beyond 15°. All the patients achieved at least MRC Grade 4 elbow extension strength, with little extension lag, and all were highly satisfied with their outcomes. None reported the loss of any preoperative function. They mentioned functional improvements in many or all of the activities made easier by restoring elbow extension, such as driving, eating, transfers, etc.

Revol reported the experience of his colleagues from Hôpital Saint-Louis in Paris, France. The study comprised 13 elbows in eight patients.[24] The biceps was routed medially, and mean follow-up was 18 months after surgery. The authors measured elbow extension torque, although they do not describe the methodology; the mean postoperative torque was 3.7 N-m (2.73 ft-lb). They measured elbow flexion torque preoperatively and postoperatively and found that flexion torque decreased by a mean of 47% following transfer. However, no patient complained about this loss of flexion power and no ADLs were impaired. No complications were encountered.

Long-term outcomes (10-year follow-up)

To provide some current perspective to this issue, we located and personally examined 45 patients who had been operated at least 10 years prior to evaluation. We analyzed these patients according to the proposed major preoperative goals.

A primary goal was restoration of elbow extensor stabilization and active elbow extension. Two surgical procedures were employed, with relatively specific indications for each. Most commonly (and exclusively until 1985), transfer of the posterior deltoid to the triceps, as popularized by Moberg, was performed. Beginning in 1985, for patients who presented with a preoperative elbow contracture greater than 30°, contracture release was combined with medial routing of the biceps to the triceps as popularized by Zancolli.

We examined 21 patients who had undergone elbow extensor reconstruction more than 10 years previously. In the 15 patients who had posterior deltoid-to-triceps transfer, 10 were bilateral transfers. All 15 had required a motorized wheelchair as their primary means of movement before surgery. 10 years following surgery, nine now used a push chair as their standard chair and four others used a push chair at least some of the time. Three patients who had undergone bilateral posterior deltoid-to-triceps transfer had been able to self-transfer in the early postoperative period. All three continued to be able to perform this monumental, for a tetraplegic, task. In the posterior deltoid-to-triceps group, four patients had required a preliminary release of elbow flexion contracture. One of the four examined 10 years postsurgery had developed a recurrence of contracture greater than 30°.

In the six patients who had biceps-to-triceps transfer (all needed contracture release), two could use a push chair, but not exclusively so. None developed a recurrence of elbow contracture.

Conclusion

Reconstruction of elbow extension is the single most satisfying reconstruction for our patients. Even though the overall time for rehabilitation can be relatively lengthy, the functional gain is substantial, predictable, and easily appreciated by the patient. Furthermore, the risks to residual preoperative function are practically nil. It represents an important addition to our reconstructive surgical armamentarium.

References

1. Moberg E. The Upper Limb in Tetraplegia. A new approach to surgical rehabilitation. Stuttgart: George Thieme, 1978.
2. Dawn-Demagone B, Ross D, Zafonte D. Triceps strength as a predictor of daily self-care in quadriplegics. J Am Paraplegia Soc 1991; 14:66–72.
3. Brys D, Waters R. Effect of triceps function on the brachioradialis transfer in quadriplegia. J Hand Surg 1987; 12A:237–242.
4. Moberg E. Surgical treatment for absent single-hand grip and elbow extension in quadriplegia. J Bone Joint Surg 1975; 57A(2):196–206.
5. Merle d'Aubigne, Seddon H, Hendy A, et al. Tendon transfers. Proc Royal Soc Med 1949; 48:831–837.
6. Merle d'Aubigne' M, Benassy J, Ramadir J. Chirurgie orthope'dique des paralysies. Paris: Masson, 1956.
7. Revol M. Biceps versus deltoid transfer for elbow extension in tetraplegia. In: Keith M, ed. Abstracts from the Sixth International Conference: Surgical Rehabilitation of the Upper Limb in Tetraplegia. Cleveland, 1998:25.
8. Bryan R. The Moberg deltoid–triceps replacement and key-pinch operations in quadriplegia: preliminary experience. Hand 1977; 9(3):207–214.
9. Cromwell SJ, Paquette V. The effect of botulinum toxin A on the function of a person with poststroke quadriplegia. Physical Ther 1996; 76:395–402.
10. Allieu Y, Tessier J, Triki F, et al. Réanimation de l'extension du coude chez le tétraplégique par transplantation du deltoide postérieur. Rev Chir Orthop 1985; 71:195–200.
11. Allieu Y, Benichou M, Tessier J, et al. La réanimation du membre supérieur du tétreplégique par transferts tendineux. Chirurgie 1986; 112:736–743.
12. Allieu Y. Fascia lata enveloped Dacron interposition graft in posterior deltoid to triceps transfer. In: 1986:
13. Deschodt J, Mailhe D, Lubrano J, et al. Anesthesie selective sensitive par péridurale cervicale dans la chirurgie et la rééducation de la main. Ann Chir Main 1988; 7:217–221.
14. Lacey SH, Wilber RG, Peckham P, et al. The posterior deltoid to triceps transfer: a clinical and biomechanical assessment. J Hand Surg 1986; 11A:542–547.
15. Lamb DW. Upper limb surgery in tetraplegia. Br J Hand Surg 1989; 14B(2):143–144.
16. Hentz V, Brown M, Keoshian L. Upper limb reconstruction in quadriplegia: functional assessment and proposed treatment modifications. J Hand Surg 1983; 8(2):119–131.
17. Castro-Serra A, Lopez-Pita A. A new surgical technique to correct triceps paralysis. Hand 1983; 15:42–46.
18. Johnstone B, Buntine J, Sormann G, et al. Surgical rehabilitation of the upper limb in quadriplegia. Aust NZ J Surg 1987; 57:917–926.
19. Mennen U, Boonzaier A. An improved technique of posterior deltoid to triceps transfer in tetraplegia. J Hand Surg 1991; 16B:197–201.
20. Moberg E. Upper limb surgical rehabilitation in tetraplegia. In: Evarts CM, ed. Surgery of the Musculoskeletal System, Vol. 1. New York: Churchill Livingstone, 1990:915–941.
21. Bajd T, Kralji A, Turk R, et al. Use of functional electrical stimulation in the rehabilitation of patients with incomplete spinal cord injuries. J Biomed Eng 1989; 11:96–102.
22. Friedenberg Z. Transposition of the biceps brachii for triceps weakness. J Bone Joint Surg 1954; 36A:656–660.
23. Kuz M, House J. Biceps to triceps transfer in tetraplegic patients: report of the medial routing technique and follow-up of three cases. J Hand Surg 1999; 24A:161–172.
24. Revol M. Biceps to triceps transfer in tetraplegia. The medial route. J Hand Surg (Br) 1999; 24(2):235–237.
25. Zancolli E, Zancolli E. Tetraplegies traumatiques. In: Tubiana R, ed. Traite' de Chirurgie de la Main. Paris: Masson, 1991.
26. Bottero J. Anatomical study of the distal tendon of the brachial biceps muscle. Application to biceps–triceps transfer in tetraplegic patients. Ann Chir Plast Esthet 1999; 44(5):541–544.
27. Ober F, Barr J. Brachioradialis muscle transposition for triceps weakness. Surg Gynecol Obstet 1938; 67:105–111.
28. DeBenedetti M. Restoration of elbow extension power in the tetraplegic patient using the Moberg technique. J Hand Surg 1979; 4:86–89.
29. Raczka R, Braun R, Waters R. Posterior deltoid-to-triceps transfer in quadriplegia. Clin Orthop 1984; 187:163–167.
30. Freehafer AA, Peckham PH, Keith MW. Determination of muscle–tendon unit properties during tendon transfer. J Hand Surg 1979; 4:331–339.
31. Rabischong E, Benoit P, Benichou M, et al. Length–tension relationship of the posterior deltoid to triceps transfer in C6 tetraplegic patients. Paraplegia 1993; 31:33–39.

32. Ejeskär A, Dahllöf A. Results of reconstructive surgery in the upper limb of tetraplegic patients. Paraplegia 1988; 26:204–208.

33. Zancolli E. Structural and Dynamic Basis of Hand Surgery. 2nd edn. Philadelphia: JB Lippincott, 1979.

34. Ejeskär A. Upper limb surgical rehabilitation in high-level tetraplegia. In: Tubiana R, ed. Hand Clinics, Vol. 4. Philadelphia: WB Saunders, 1988:585–599.

35. Moberg E. The present state of surgical rehabilitation in tetraplegia. Third International Congress of the International Federation of Societies for Surgery of the Hand, Tokyo, Japan. J Hand Surg 1989: 14:354–355.

11

Surgical rehabilitation for the very weakest (International Classification Group 0) patients

Introduction

Patients whose injuries result in no useful muscle strength (less than MRC Grade 3) distal to the elbow have limited potential for improvement of the upper limb function by surgery. While they may retain some shoulder and elbow strength, most must depend on various orthoses to enhance hand function. Some of these patients might benefit from functional neuromuscular stimulation described in Chapter 17. Nearly all are candidates for improved elbow control procedures, such as deltoid to triceps or biceps to triceps, described in Chapter 10.

The limited strength in the muscles about the shoulder girdle means it is difficult to propel manual chairs and to perform pressure relief maneuvers. Thus these patients are prone to the development of pressure sores, a risk that may limit the amount of time many of them are able to spend sitting in their wheelchairs. Limitations in the control of shoulder muscles may make it difficult or impossible for these patients to operate standard electric wheelchair controls. Some patients will require a mouth control device to maneuver their wheelchair.[1]

Patients within this International Classification (IC) Group 0 are dependent on others for the majority of their activities of daily living (ADLs). Their level of relative independence depends in large part on their ability to position their forearms in pronation, which enables them to have at least one hand and wrist fitted with a static orthosis to hold adaptive aids, such as a fork or spoon. Unfortunately, patients with high-level injuries find it difficult to control the posture of their upper limbs. Several pathologic positional states are seen:

- If the deltoid muscles are innervated, but other shoulder stabilizers such as the pectoralis major muscle remain paralyzed, the arm tends to be held in abduction, a position that accentuates elbow flexion. If the biceps muscle is at all spastic, these patients quickly develop flexion contractures of their elbows. The absence of adequate proprioceptive impulses from the arms and hands means that the patient is essentially unaware of the status or position of his or her arms and hands, and cannot easily alter an inappropriate position.

- If the biceps or brachialis muscle is at all spastic, it tends to keep the elbow somewhat flexed and the forearm supinated. At the onset, the forearm is held in a supinated posture, but can be passively pronated. Persistence of this supinated posture leads to a fixed supination contracture of the forearm (*Fig. 11.1A*). With the forearm held supinated, the hands are turned palm upward. This is a disabling state because any orthosis that might be prescribed to stabilize the wrist, such as a long opponens splint, cannot be fitted with an eating utensil in the usual way. If the utensil is attached in the normal manner onto the radial side of the orthosis, the patient cannot move it far enough to reach the plate to acquire food. With the utensil attached to the ulnar side of the orthosis, the patient may be able to put it into the food, or spear food from the plate. However, he or she cannot

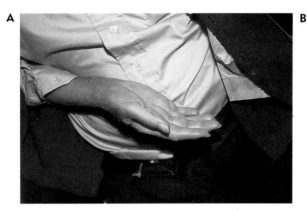

Figure 11.1 The unopposed action of a spastic biceps has led to loss of even passive forearm pronation. (A) The patient's hand remains in a dysfunctional supinated posture, so the patient must place his adaptive spoon on the ulnar side of the universal cuff. (B) While he can place the spoon into his food in this position, he cannot easily and accurately direct the spoon to his mouth.

further supinate the arm to guide the end of the utensil toward his or her mouth (*Fig. 11.1B*). The patient whose forearms remain in a supinated posture is then dependent on others for all aspects of feeding and almost all aspects of self-care.

Functional rehabilitation

Splinting

The majority of patients injured at this high level must depend on various devices to enhance their upper limb function, and for most only static orthoses are appropriate. In many patients, an attendant must apply even the simplest device. Few patients are able to self-don and -doff their orthotic device.

Orthoses for the shoulder
The very weakest patients in this group benefit from the use of a mobile arm support (MAS). Most are

variations of a ball-bearing platform for increased arm mobility used to treat quadriplegic and hemiplegic patients (*Fig. 11.2*).

Orthoses for the elbow and forearm
Several splints to improve function in the arm that is held flexed at the elbow and supinated at the forearm have been developed. Abrahams *et al.* described a functional splint for the C5 tetraplegic arm designed to overcome the problem of the flexed and supinated arm by providing active extension and pronation of the forearm.[2] The elbow piece has an adjustable coiled spring that keeps the elbow extended and the patient can flex the elbow against the resistance of the spring. The forearm piece swivels by means of a force couple to push the forearm into pronation as the elbow is flexed.[2]

Two pronation splints designed for tight biceps and lack of active pronation have been described that can substitute for the more cumbersome mobile arm support.[3] These splints use a lever that pushes the

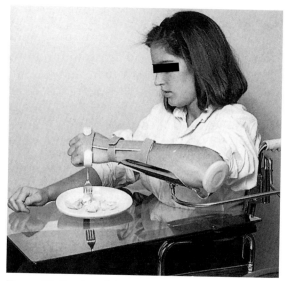

Figure 11.2 A mobile arm support may provide some additional upper limb function for the patient with poor shoulder and elbow control.

forearm into pronation as the elbow is flexed. They are simple and inexpensive to construct.

Orthoses for the wrist and hand

The most commonly prescribed static orthosis for this group of patients is termed a 'long opponens' splint (*Fig. 11.3*). It is designed to stabilize the wrist in a somewhat neutral posture. Various fasteners are used to affix the device to the forearm of the patient,

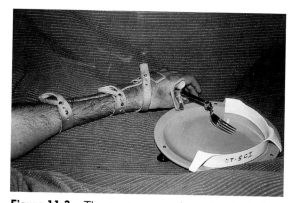

Figure 11.3 The most commonly used orthosis for the IC Group 0 patient. The long-opponens splint stabilizes the wrist and prevents undue tightening of the finger and thumb flexors.

including Velcro straps or an inelastic strip of cloth or leather into which are cut several slots. The slots are pulled over a rivet-like stanchion at the proper tension. Some patients are able to doff and don this splint, and may be able to take advantage of a plastic or metal ring attached to the end of the straps. They can be taught to hook the thumb or another finger of the opposite hand through the ring and pull the strap to the correct location and affect fastening. Other patients use their teeth as another grasping device to perform the same maneuver.

Once the splint is securely fastened to the patient's arm, various terminal devices can be placed into specially constructed adapters built into the long opponens splint. The device may be nothing more elaborate than a slot into which an eating utensil is placed, usually by the attendant. It seems advisable to position the utensil in different planes relative to the palm to encourage different shoulder movements.[4] For example, placing the utensil perpendicular to the palm encourages flexion and adduction, while placement parallel to the palm encourages abduction and internal rotation and supination of the forearm. It is desirable to provide sophisticated splints early to encourage function and acceptance of the device. Use of the splint encourages mobilization and strengthening of the extremity. Other devices useful for attaching specialized end pieces include a coiled spring into which a typing stick can be wedged. Similarly, a toothbrush or a writing implement can be positioned in such a spring.

A few patients with good bilateral shoulder control are able to take advantage of a modification of the wrist extension–finger flexion orthosis introduced in Chapter 4. As they lack wrist control, the device cannot be powered similarly to the more commonly prescribed brace. These patients need a way to lock the device in either the open or closed position. Locked open, the stabilized thumb ray and index and middle finger combination is ready to receive an object. The patient must first maneuver the opened first web space around the object to be obtained. Then, using the opposite hand as a brace, the patient pushes the splinted wrist into extension, which causes the index and middle fingers to approach the stabilized thumb ray. This requires some skill to avoid forcing the object to be grasped out of the closing terminal device. The patient must keep pushing the wrist into extension until sufficient closing force is achieved. A ratchet mechanism is used to fix the grasp at the desired tension and this tension is maintained until released. The patient is able to release tension in the grip by again using his or her opposite hand or mouth to push a lever that unlatches the ratchet mechanism. Again, using the opposite hand, the grasp is opened by pushing the wrist of the splinted hand into wrist flexion. This is a rather complex set of maneuvers and studies indicate that very few patients continue to use such complex devices for any lengthy period. Some studies indicate that more than 50% of patients with electric grasp devices or ratchet splints that require mouth control discard them within 1 year.[5] Other studies indicate that only 36% of patients prescribed these devices still used the device 2 years after discharge.[6]

Surgical indications in the IC Group 0 patient

Few patients with high-level injuries benefit significantly from functional surgery, but occasionally, surgery is indicated in these patients. Commonly this is to correct a postural imbalance of one or both upper limbs, such as to release a contracted elbow, simplify the use of orthotic devices, or (rarely) add a level of functionality that did not exist prior to surgery. Five circumstances and associated surgical solutions stand out:

- the abducted shoulder;
- flexion contracture of the elbow;
- supinated but not contracted forearm;
- fixed supination contracture – osteotomy of the radius versus release of contracture; and
- unstable or contracted wrist – wrist fusion.

The abducted shoulder

The pectoralis major muscle is one of the principal antagonists of the deltoid muscle. When the deltoid is strong and unopposed, the shoulder assumes an abducted posture; this may be improved by medial transfer of the anterior portion of the deltoid, as described by Johnstone *et al.*[7] The origin of the anterior part of the deltoid is elevated off the acromion and reinserted more medially into the clavicle. The arm is protected against shoulder abduction for several weeks, after which range of motion exercises are begun. In their series Johnstone *et al.* reported

that, following surgery, patients were better able to move their hands toward their faces for feeding and smoking.[7] They also demonstrated better control of their wheelchair. See Figure 9.19 page 92.

Flexion contracture of the elbow

This problem of the contracted elbow and its solutions are addressed in detail in Chapter 10.

The supinated but not contracted forearm

Often associated with a flexed and contracted elbow are a forearm and hand held in supination by the unopposed action of the innervated and perhaps spastic biceps muscle. In the absence of any activity of the pronator teres muscle, the patient's hand remains in a supinated posture, whether contracture exists or not. The dysutility of this posture is discussed above. Initially, it is possible for the therapist or physician to passively rotate the affected forearm into the pronated position. As time goes by, unless extraordinary attention to passive exercises is provided, the forearm becomes contracted in supination and the hand cannot even be passively pronated.

The management of the supinated forearm is determined by whether or not the forearm can be passively pronated. If this can be done, muscle rebalancing by biceps rerouting is possible. If the forearm cannot be passively pronated, an osteotomy may be indicated.

Rerouting the biceps

Eduardo Zancolli of Buenos Aries, Argentina, is credited with describing this surgical technique.[8] The complexity of the procedure is determined by whether or not an associated flexion contracture of the elbow must be addressed simultaneously. The indications for this approach include:

- presence of a functioning supinator muscle; and
- nearly full passive pronation of the forearm.

It is essentially impossible to perform preoperative manual muscle testing of the supinator since the biceps, a strong supinator, cannot be willed quiet by the patient and always contribute to supination. An electromyograph (EMG) may help to assess whether innervation of the supinator muscle has been retained. Occasionally, it may be necessary to anesthetize the musculocutaneous nerve to assess the strength of the supinator muscle.

Several different incisions might be considered. An above-elbow incision only may be preferred or one that crosses the elbow flexion crease (*Fig. 11.4*). The biceps tendon and its associated lacertus fibrosis or aponeurosis is dissected from the surrounding tissues. The lacertus portion is left attached to the proper

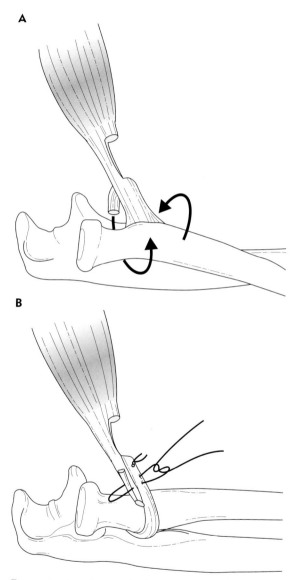

A

B

Figure 11.4 The surgical technique to restore some forearm pronation. (A) The biceps tendon is detached from the tuberosity of the radius and the tendon is rerouted about the radius so that (B) contraction of the biceps now causes pronation of the forearm. (Adapted from Zancolli, 1975.[9])

tendon and its attachments into the forearm fascia are divided. The primary tendon of the biceps is split longitudinally into two segments and the attachment of one-half of the tendon is divided at its point of attachment into the tuberosity of the radius. The other half of the tendon is sectioned near the muscle–tendon junction. This length of tendon, still attached to the tuberosity, is passed from the medial side of the forearm around the neck of the radius to the lateral side of the forearm, so that a pull on this now rerouted tendon causes the forearm to pronate. To achieve this the strip of biceps tendon is passed counterclockwise (from the perspective of the surgeon) for the left arm and clockwise for the right arm. The rerouted tendon half is then strongly anchored to the remaining proximal half of the biceps tendon to re-establish muscle–tendon continuity. This juncture is reinforced with the lacertus part of the tendon. Proper tension at the repair site is judged by fully pronating the forearm, with the elbow in 45° of flexion, and suturing the transfer under strong tension. After tendon repair, the elbow is flexed to about 75°, which relaxes the tendon juncture. After wound closure, the elbow is placed in a cast with about 75° of flexion and near-full forearm pronation. After 4–5 weeks, the cast is removed and the elbow and forearm are fitted with a splint that maintains the forearm pronated and the elbow flexed. Gradually, increasing periods of time are spent performing directed exercises out of the brace.

The fixed supination contracture – osteotomy of the radius versus release of contracture

If the forearm cannot be pronated passively, the less complicated biceps rerouting procedure will fail. One solution to a forearm fixed in supination, despite vigorous therapy, is the aggressive surgical release of contracted periarticular and interosseous soft tissues, followed by aggressive therapy. If passive pronation is restored, it may be possible to perform biceps rerouting, as described above, at a later operative procedure. Alternatively, the biceps could be rerouted at the time of soft-tissue release. However, early aggressive passive motion is vital to a good outcome and biceps rerouting precludes early aggressive range of motion exercises.

A simpler, more reliable, alternative involves performing a rotational osteotomy of the radius. The goal is to pronate the wrist and hand relative to the pathologically supinated proximal radius. This procedure does not alter the arc of rotatory motion; it simply shifts the preoperative arc toward pronation. If the patient is able to abduct the shoulder, even a small movement toward pronation may allow better function, since shoulder abduction is the principal substitutional movement used by these patients to assist pronation of the hand.

A period of preoperative and intensive passive pronational stretching is usually indicated before the required amount of rotation can be determined. Once improvement has reached a plateau, the amount of pronational rotation that can be achieved by surgery depends in large part on the severity of the preoperative supination contracture. Usually, between 45° and 60° of radial rotation can be obtained easily with an osteotomy performed through the middle third of the radius. This is a favored site because an osteotomy at this level allows the thickest parts of the contracted interosseous membrane to be released. If much more pronational rotation is required, for example, when the forearm is solidly fixed in full supination, osteotomy of both radius and ulna may be necessary.

Surgical technique

The desired degree of rotation must be determined preoperatively. The middle third of the radius is approached through an interval developed between the radial wrist extensors and the brachioradialis muscle. The attachment of the pronator teres is preserved. The attachments of the stabilizing band of the interosseous membrane are detached from the radius distal to the point of proposed osteotomy. Rigid fixation of the rotated radius is achieved with compression-plating techniques. It is useful to pre-drill the distal half of the radius prior to making the osteotomy, since this half becomes more unstable than the proximal half following osteotomy. The plate can be swung aside to complete the osteotomy. The circumference of the radius can be estimated from a preoperative radiograph, and this value used to determine the desired amount of rotation. For example, if 60° of rotation is desired, the distal radius must be rotated one-sixth (60°/360°) of the circumference of the radius. Just prior to completing the osteotomy, the radius is scored longitudinally across the proposed osteotomy site to create a reference line so that the rotational movement can be judged. Sturdy bone clamps are placed on either side of the osteotomy site,

the osteotomy is completed, and the radius is rotated the desired distance, as judged by the reference lines. The pre-positioned plate is fixed to the distal radius and another bone clamp used to compress the proximal half of the plate to the proximal radius. Standard compression techniques are used to provide rigid fixation at the osteotomy site. Rigid fixation enables this technique to be combined with biceps rerouting, since exercises can begin as soon as tendon healing is achieved.

Osteotomy of radius and ulna

If the supination contracture is severe, an osteotomy of both bones of the forearm may be necessary. The ulna is first osteotomized somewhat more proximally than the radius to minimize the possibility that a radioulnar synostosis will develop.

Coulet and Allieu from Montpellier, France, reviewed their experience with 18 supination contractures in 15 patients.[10] Biceps rerouting gave the best forearm motion, but then only deltoid-to-triceps transfer could achieve elbow extension. Elbow extension strength was weaker than in those patients who underwent forearm osteotomy and biceps-to-triceps transfer. These authors prefer to perform a forearm osteotomy, conserving the biceps for transfer to the triceps.

The unstable or contracted wrist—wrist fusion

The occasional IC Group 0 patient may benefit from fusion of the wrist. These patients are typically totally dependent on others in all transfer activities and a surgically stiffened wrist does not interfere with their transfers. The IC Group 0 patient is unable to control the posture of the wrist and must depend upon an external device if wrist stabilization is necessary for improved hand function. Typically, stabilization is achieved by means of a long orthosis, either a long opponens splint or a wrist 'cock-up' splint (*Fig. 11.3*). Self-application of either splint is a challenge. Internalizing the long brace by a formal wrist fusion may allow the patient to use a much simpler device, one that might be self-donned and -doffed, such as a universal cuff that can hold adaptive devices (*Fig. 11.5*).

The other indication for fusion of the wrist is the patient who has developed a fixed contracture of the wrist (*Fig. 11.6*). In this group of patients, the wrist may have become contracted in either excessive extension or flexion, or excessive radial deviation.

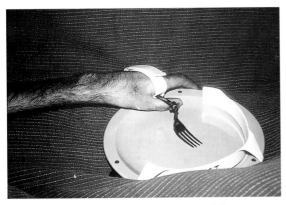

Figure 11.5 Fusion of the wrist allowed this patient to use a much simpler and more easily donned 'short-opponens' splint, fitted with slots for attachment of ADL aids.

Both these extremes may interfere with ADLs, and such positions of the wrist make fitting an orthosis difficult.

Wrist fusion can be accomplished by one of many well-described surgical techniques. The goal is stabilization in a nearly neutral position. A simple technique that works well in this group of 'low-demand' patients involves obliteration of the radiocarpal and intercarpal joint spaces and stabilization with a large diameter Steinmann pin placed down the shaft of the third metacarpal and into the distal radius. The distal end of the pin is countersunk well into the metacarpal. More complicated fixations with plates

and screws are unnecessary. The wrist is immobilized within a short-arm cast for 4–6 weeks and then protected within a removable orthosis for several more weeks.

If the wrist is contracted into a flexed or extended posture, it may be necessary to excise the proximal row of carpal bones or shorten the radius as part of the fusion procedure to overcome the contracture. The postoperative care is as described above.

Active grasp for the IC Group 0 patient – the Brummer winch operation

Brummer[11] proposed a clever surgical procedure that has the potential to provide a weak, but perhaps useful, key pinch for this very disadvantaged population. The procedure couples the active forearm supination vector of the innervated biceps with the automatic flexion of the thumb to provide a key pinch between the pulp of the thumb and the side of the index finger. The requirements include a near normal passive range of motion of the elbow and forearm, and good biceps strength. The fingers and thumb must be flexible. The wrist must be in a useful position (not contracted in excessive flexion or extension) and stabilized either by a splint (commonly) or by wrist fusion.

The operative procedure (*Fig. 11.7*) is carried out by first stabilizing the interphalangeal joint of the thumb in slight flexion with a Steinmann pin. Next, the flexor pollicis longus is divided at its muscle–

A
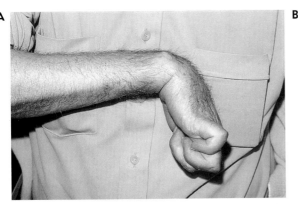

B
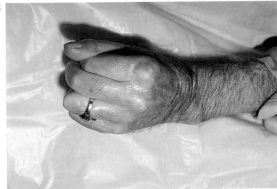

Figure 11.6 (A) One indication for wrist fusion is the weak patient who has developed a severe flexion (or extension) contracture of the wrist. Fusion may need to be combined with excision of the proximal carpal row to overcome the more severely contracted wrist. (B) The repositioned wrist allows the patient to use standard orthoses, such as a short-opponens splint.

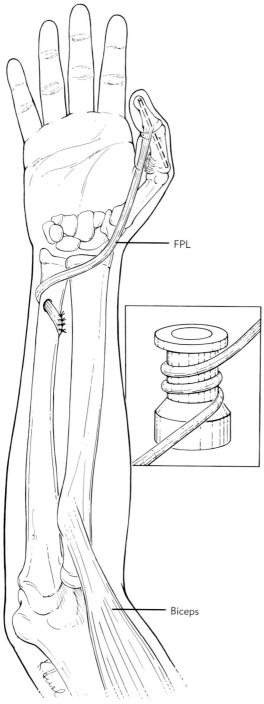

tendon juncture. The tendon of the flexor pollicis longus is passed ulnarward (deep to the remaining flexor tendons, median and ulnar nerves, and ulnar artery) and is firmly anchored into the ulna using a bone anchor or similar technique. The tension on the flexor pollicis longus tendon is adjusted so that, with the forearm in full pronation, the thumb tip just touches the side of the flexed index finger in the position of a lateral or key pinch. As the forearm is supinated, the thumb tip begins to apply greater and greater pressure against the side of the index finger. Active supination leads to passive thumb flexion by this tenodesis effect. It may be necessary to prevent excessive flexion of the thumb at the metacarpophalangeal joint with one of the procedures described for Moberg's key pinch operation in Chapter 12.

After wound closure, a long arm cast is placed to maintain the forearm in full pronation for about 4 weeks. The cast is removed and exercises begun. The patient is taught how to grasp objects by pronating his or her arm and sliding the thumb and index around the object. The patient is next taught to contract the biceps and, as the forearm begins to supinate under the influence of the biceps, the thumb is forced against the side of the index finger, and the object stabilized. If more power is needed, the patient further supinates the forearm.

Few of these procedures seem to have been carried out, judging by the paucity of follow-up studies.[12] The grasp achieved is challenging to control and its value must necessarily be limited. Our personal experience is small, but two of three patients benefited.

Functional neuromuscular stimulation

Patients injured at such high cervical cord levels have few splinting and surgical options, as described above. It was for this group of patients that investigators studied and developed methods of functional neuromuscular stimulation. The indications and current technology are discussed in detail in Chapter 17.

Figure 11.7 The Brummer winch operation, for which a supple forearm is a prerequisite; see the text for details.

References

1. Blaine H, Nelson E. Mouthstick for quadriplegic patients. J Prosthet Dent 1973; 29:317–322.

2. Abrahams D, Shrosbree R, Key A. A functional splint for the C5 tetraplegic arm. Paraplegia 1980; 17:198–203.

3. Hage G. Brief or new: Two pronation splints. Am J Occup Ther 1985; 39(4):265–267.

4. Kester N, Lehnis H. A combined ADL-long opponens orthosis. Arch Phys Med Rehabil 1969; 50(4):219–222.

5. Garber SL, Gregorio T. Upper extremity assistive devices: assessment of use by spinal cord-injured patients with quadriplegia. Am J Occup Ther 1990; 44:126–131.

6. Ditunno JF, Stover S, Freed M, et al. Motor recovery of the upper extremities in traumatic quadriplegia: a multicenter study. Arch Phys Med Rehabil 1992; 73:431–436.

7. Johnstone B, Buntine J, Sormann G, et al. Surgical rehabilitation of the upper limb in quadriplegia. Aust NZ J Surg 1987; 57:917–926.

8. Zancolli E. Structural and Dynamic Basis of Hand Surgery. 2nd edn. Philadelphia: JB Lippincott, 1979.

9. Zancolli E. Surgery for the quadriplegic hand with active, strong wrist extension preserved. Clin Orthop Rel Res 1975; 112:101–113.

10. Coulet B, Chamas M, Allieu Y. Supination contracture of the forearm in tetraplegics: Etiology and surgical treatment. In: Keith M, ed. Abstracts of the Sixth International Conference: Surgical Rehabilitation of the Upper Limb in Tetraplegia. Cleveland, 1998:23.

11. Brummer H. The winch operation. In: McDowell C, Moberg E, eds. The Second International Conference on Surgical Rehabilitation in Tetraplegia, Giens, France. J Hand Surg 1984:608–611.

12. Ejeskär A. Upper limb surgical rehabilitation in high-level tetraplegia. In: Tubiana R, ed. Hand Clinics, Vol. 4. Philadelphia: WB Saunders, 1988:585–599.

12

Surgical rehabilitation of key pinch by tenodesis (International Classification Groups 1 and 2)

Introduction

The International Classification (IC) Group 1 and 2 patient has relatively normal function in the deltoid and biceps and/or brachialis muscle groups. By definition, the IC Group 1 patient has one MRC Grade 4 forearm muscle, typically the brachioradialis (BR), and the IC Group 2 patient an additional MRC Grade 4 muscle, typically the extensor carpi radialis longus (ECRL). In these patients, most of the distal functioning muscles that remain are innervated by elements of the C5 and the C6 cervical spinal levels. In the American Spinal Injury Association (ASIA) system, the lowest muscle of at least MRC Grade 3 defines the motor level, provided that the key muscles above that level are judged to be normal. Therefore, IC Groups 1 and 2 patients are classified by the ASIA system as either C5 or C6 level tetraplegic patients.

The IC Group 1 or 2 patients represent a relatively large proportion of the overall tetraplegic population. In Moberg's series of 321 arms,[1] 54% were classified as IC Group 0 or 1 and 31% as IC Group 2 patients. From Zancolli's series of 100 patients, 26% were classified as IC Group 0 or 1 and 43% as IC Group 2 patients.[2] Of 122 patients examined at the Palo Alto Veterans Affairs Spinal Cord Injury Center, 20 were determined to be IC Group 0 or 1 while 48 were IC Group 2 patients.[3] These statistics represent a period of time before seatbelt and shoulder restraint systems became mandatory in most industrialized countries, so current statistics may provide different proportions. Nonetheless, this group, characterized by absent or weakly functioning wrist extension, still constitutes a significant percentage of tetraplegic patients.

Goals

IC Group 1

For the IC Group 1 patient the principal functional goal is active wrist extension. If this critically important function can be achieved, the hand becomes a far more useful tool. Absent or barely anti-gravity wrist extension (MRC Grade 2+ or 3−) renders the hand essentially incapable of performing any but the simplest single-handed activities of gripping, sensory functions, or human contact. Aside from the two latter functions, touching the environment and human contact, the isolated hand serves primarily as a weight used to stabilize, balance, or push light objects. Some IC Group 1 patients may have weak active wrist extension (below MRC Grade 3 or 3+). These patients may be able to extend their wrist against gravity and demonstrate a rudimentary tenodesis grip, but with the existing natural tenodesis effect of the paralyzed finger and thumb flexors, they can exert only the most minimal force [probably less than 50 g (1.8 oz) of pressure] between the digits and thumb. However, active wrist extension powerful enough to overcome gravity (MRC Grade 3) and still do some work (MRC Grade 4 or 5) allows the patient to use passive finger flexor forces to lift and manipulate very light objects with a tenodesis grip. Restoring wrist extensor strength may enable the IC Group 1 patient to be fitted with a dynamic orthosis such as a wrist-driven, flexor-hinge splint (WDFH, as described in Chapter 4). Finally, restoring adequate wrist extension power may make it possible for the IC Group 1 patient to have the strength of the grasp between thumb and fingers surgically enhanced by a tenodesis of the flexor pollicis longus (FPL) to the radius.

IC Group 2

For the weaker IC Group 2 patient, defined as having barely MRC Grade 4 wrist extensor strength, the principal reconstructive goals are to augment the power of active wrist extension surgically, and at the same time surgically enhance a tenodesis grip between thumb and digits. For the fortunate IC Group 2 patient who has retained or spontaneously recovered strong active wrist extension, the reconstructive options include a surgically created pinch activated by wrist extension (tenodesis) or by tendon transfer. These procedures are discussed in detail in the following sections.

Restoring or strengthening wrist extension by brachioradialis to wrist extensor muscle–tendon transfer

In IC Group 1 or 2 patients, the BR muscle, an accessory elbow flexor innervated by both C5 and C6 segments, is the only available transferable muscle. Transfer of the BR into the tendon of the extensor carpi radialis brevis (ECRB) can augment wrist extensor strength.[4] The ECRB tendon attaches to the base of the third metacarpal, and so the ECRB is a more efficient wrist extensor than its adjacent ECRL muscle, the tendon of which attaches to the radial side of the second metacarpal. The ECRB tendon is chosen as the transfer target because it functions more purely as a wrist extensor, unlike the ECRL, which both extends and radially deviates the wrist.[5,6]

Prerequisites, indications, and preoperative assessment

A general discussion of surgical prerequisites and indications is given in Chapter 8. The specific pre-

requisites for constructing or strengthening wrist extension in the IC Group 1 or 2 tetraplegic patient include:

- adequately strong BR;
- functional range of passive wrist extension and flexion;
- shoulder control to assist forearm pronation; and
- elbow stabilization.

An adequately strong brachioradialis

Determining whether the BR has sufficient power to be transferred successfully is discussed in Chapter 6. A muscle that is deemed too weak at the initial examination may respond to a course of directed exercises designed to isolate, as much as possible, the muscle's action. A period of many months of both isometric and isotonic conditioning may yield a muscle that can be transferred with the expectation of a functionally useful outcome. This is more often the case for a patient examined relatively soon after injury than for one examined many years following injury. If the patient has been using only a power driven wheelchair, a switch to the frequent use of a manual push-chair may also significantly strengthen the BR muscle.

A functional range of passive wrist extension and flexion

Since the goal of the procedure is to construct an active, useful wrist extension, a reciprocal passive wrist flexion must also be present for the patient to benefit most from a natural tenodesis grasp, a grasp achieved with the aid of a dynamic orthosis, or a surgically constructed grip. In the simplest concept, wrist extension tightens whatever grip exists and wrist flexion loosens the grip, which allows either opening of the grasp or release of whatever object is in the grasp. In the IC Group 1 or 2 tetraplegic patient, wrist flexion depends upon gravity. Since the ECRL muscle crosses the elbow, a contracted ECRL (a common finding in IC Group 1 and 2 patients) may allow gravity to flex the wrist only when the elbow is in the flexed position. However, when the elbow is extended, as in reaching out to acquire an object, the ECRL tightens and the wrist may no longer respond to the flexor forces of gravity. This makes it difficult for the patient to open the tenodesis grip to grasp an object located any distance away from his or her body.

Since flexion of the wrist is of significant functional importance in opening the hand, a wrist that is contracted in extension must first be rehabilitated through exercise and splinting so that some wrist flexion via gravity is possible. Chapters 4 and 11 discuss the management of the contracted upper limb.

Shoulder control to assist forearm pronation

Only when the forearm is pronated can gravity cause the wrist to flex. In the IC Group 1 or 2 tetraplegic patient, the normal muscles that pronate the forearm, the pronator teres and pronator quadratus, are paralyzed. Thus the biceps, a strong supinator and the supinator muscles, are unopposed. When the patient flexes the elbow, the forearm has a tendency to supinate. These patients quickly learn to abduct the shoulder to effect forearm pronation. In addition, if the forearm is in a position of supination, contraction of the BR muscle tends to return the forearm to the neutral position. A fixed supination contracture is a strong contraindication to the construction of a wrist extension, and must be treated by exercise, splinting, or surgery before proceeding.

Elbow stabilization

If no active elbow extension is present, because the BR crosses the elbow joint after the transfer some of its excursion and power may be wasted in flexing the elbow rather than in extending the wrist. It is difficult for many patients to isolate the BR without co-contracting the biceps muscle. For this reason, the BR has gained, not unjustly, the reputation of being a poorly educable or 'dumb' muscle.[7] A prerequisite for the optimum function after BR transfer is active elbow extension. For this reason, it is preferable first to reconstruct active elbow extension if no triceps function remains, as discussed in Chapter 10. Some authors report combined deltoid-to-triceps and BR-to-ECRB transfers,[8] but others prefer to perform the elbow stabilization procedure as a preliminary step.[7,9,10] The latter authors believe that the simultaneous rehabilitation of these two transfers is difficult for the patient and that the outcome of each part, elbow stabilization and wrist extension, is compromised somewhat by combining the two procedures.

Once adequate BR power, passive wrist motion, and the ability to pronate the forearm have been established absolutely, the patient is assessed from the point of view of motivation, general good health, adequate physical and psychological support from other care-givers, and so on. These vital issues are discussed in more detail in Chapter 8.

In addition, the surgeon must make a decision regarding whether or not the elbow should be immobilized within the postoperative cast. We have not routinely immobilized the elbow after this procedure and have experienced two early ruptures of the tendon-to-tendon juncture in more than 100 BR transfers performed over the past 25 years. Other authors advise immobilization of the elbow.[4,9,11] If the elbow is to be left free (and even if included within the cast) the patient must be instructed carefully in how to avoid any inadvertent strong contraction of the BR during the postoperative period. Family members and the patient's attendant must be cautioned against allowing the patient to pull up with the operated arm, as stress of this type may elongate or even rupture the tendon-to-tendon repair. The consequence is either a less than optimal result or complete failure.

On the day of surgery, care is taken with the standard preoperative issues, such as bladder drainage, preoperative antibiotics, correct positioning on the operative table, adequate padding of any pressure points, etc. Many of these details are discussed in Chapter 8. Regional anesthesia is preferred. Allieu and colleagues have published their novel method of cervical epidural anesthesia, which both allows the patient to maintain some motor control and provides adequate pain control to carry out the procedure.[12]

Surgical technique

The BR arises proximal to the elbow on its lateral aspect and has a tendon of insertion at the level of the radial styloid distally. However, its effective insertion is over a long length of the distal radius secondary to the dense investing fascia around the tendon. Essentially, no tendon glides past the mid-forearm. Therefore, though it is possible to detach the tendon of insertion through a small incision, to obtain the most effective potential excursion of the muscle it is better to perform a wide dissection of the distal muscle and tendon from its insertion at the radial styloid up to the very proximal forearm level.[13]

Under tourniquet control a zigzag or curvilinear incision over the course of the BR is drawn from near the radial styloid to the junction of the proximal and middle one-third of the forearm (*Fig. 12.1A*). Beginning distally, the incision is carried down through the subcutaneous tissues and the dorsal sensory branch of the radial nerve is identified and protected. Locating this nerve also guides the approach to the BR tendon since the radial nerve comes from beneath the BR muscle and swings around its tendon. With the nerve protected, the dense investing fascia on either side of the tendon is sharply incised. The tendon insertion is elevated and detached close to the radial styloid (*Figs 12.1A* and *12.1B*). A small hemostat is used to grasp the tendon end and, with traction, additional fibrous attachments to the radius are identified and divided. As dissection proceeds proximally, the dorsal sensory branch of the radial nerve becomes prominent as does the radial artery and its accompanying veins. As the muscle belly is reached, small arteries and veins from the radial artery should be ligated or cauterized.

To test the effect of the dissection, pull the undissected (but cut) tendon end distally and measure how much distal stretch can be achieved (*Fig. 12.1D*). After dissection repeat this test and an additional 2–3 cm of distal stretch should be gained (*Fig. 12.1E*).

Just adjacent to the BR are the paired radial wrist extensor tendons, the tendons of the ECRL and ECRB. The ECRB is identified and its investing fascia cleared for a short distance. Traction on the ECRB causes wrist extension, whereas traction on the ERCL causes both extension and radial deviation of the hand. A heavy Keith needle is placed through the tendon close to the muscle–tendon junction of the ECRB. A heavy suture looped around this tendon allows the surgeon to apply proximal traction as part of adjusting the tension of the tendon juncture (*Figs 12.1B* and *12.1C*).

The tendon of the BR is passed superficially over the tendon of the ECRL and woven back and forth several times through the substance of the tendon of the ECRB (*Figs 12.1F* and *12.1G*). By grasping the very distal end of the BR tendon with a clamp and pulling distally, the length and tension of this muscle can be adjusted. At the same time, the needle and suture anchors through the ECRB are pulled proximally to lift the wrist into the neutral position. The tension on the BR should be adjusted to re-establish the normal resting length of the muscle. Freehafer

et al. described a method to quantify this value using specially designed force sensors.[13] A more practical way to estimate the appropriate tension is to stretch the muscle passively to its maximum length and place a mark on the BR tendon at its most proximal intersection with ECRB tendon. Next, relax all the tension and mark this 'zero-tension' site of BR relative to ECRB. The tension on the BR is adjusted so that the first proximal intersection between BR and ECRB is mid-way between the maximum and no-tension marks. Multiple sutures of braided nonabsorbable material are used to anchor the BR tendon at the several points where it is woven through the tendon of the ECRB. In adjusting the tension, it is important to place the elbow in some flexion while tension is set at the junction. Moberg recommended that the elbow be set at about 40° of flexion,[15] and we follow this guideline so that the transfer does not lose significant power as the elbow is flexed.

In the IC Group 1 patient, the wrist extensors may be absent or very weak. If so, Moberg recommends resecting an 8–10 cm (3.2–3.9 inch) segment of tendon and muscle proximal to the point at which the BR is woven into the tendon of the ECRB.[1] His assertion is that the lack of any pull from the ECRB results in postoperative adhesions that form about the ECRB tendon just proximal to the BR–ECRB junction and prevent tendon gliding and restrict the excursion of the transfer. If preoperative wrist extension is at the MRC Grade 3 level, this resection is not necessary. We have not followed this recommendation.

If BR to ECRB transfer is performed in isolation, the wounds are irrigated and the skin closed. The wrist is splinted in near full extension to relax the tendon-to-tendon juncture and this position is maintained for approximately 4 weeks.

Postoperative management

Following a 3–4 week period of healing, rehabilitation is begun, although Zancolli describes how his patients actively contracted the BR within their long arm cast soon after surgery.[2] If the elbow is unsplinted, this muscle is exercised to some degree each time the patient actively flexes the elbow.

The cast is removed at the fourth week, the surgical incision sites are inspected, and a removable orthosis is fitted. This can be custom-made by the hand therapist, or an off-the-shelf commercial ortho-

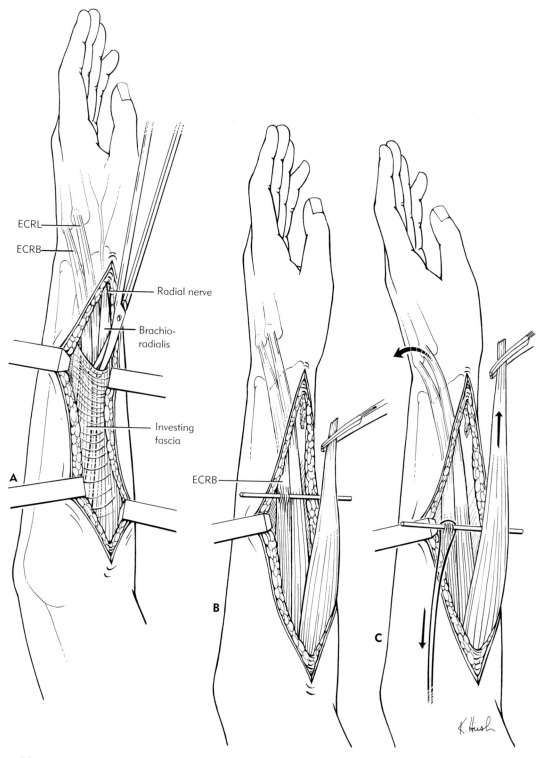

Figure 12.1(A, B, C) The operative steps of brachioradialis to extensor carpi radialis brevis (ECRB) transfer; see text for details. (Reproduced with permission from Hentz and Chase in press.)[14]

D

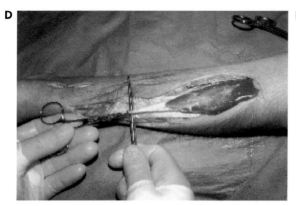

E

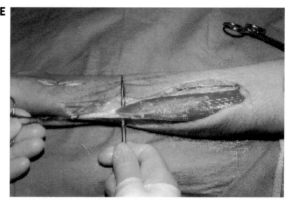

Figure 12.1(D, E) *(continued)*

sis, suitably fitted, serves equally well. The orthosis is designed to maintain the wrist in some extension to further protect the tendon-to-tendon juncture. The orthosis is removed, initially and preferably under the supervision of the therapist, and the patient and attendant are instructed in the exercise protocols. The orthosis is replaced between exercise sessions, and is best worn at night for many additional weeks.

If the elbow was immobilized as part of the initial casting, the aim of the initial exercises is to regain the preoperative elbow range of movement. All exercises are primarily active exercises, with the possible exception of elbow extension if active elbow extension is not present or was not restored at the same time as the BR to wrist extensor transfer. Until about postoperative week six, the patient utilizes the orthosis except when exercising. At about postoperative week six, the orthosis is removed during much of the day and the patient begins to strengthen the transferred muscle by actively contracting the BR against no resistance.

As the BR muscle can be notoriously difficult to re-educate, adjuncts to the exercises may be useful, including biofeedback devices. The goal is to assist the patient in contracting the BR muscle. Electrical stimulation of the transferred muscle may also help the patient to 'find' the muscle. Keith *et al.* percutaneously insert fine wire electrodes into the muscle either at the time of surgery or after removal of the postoperative immobilization.[16] With these electrodes, the muscle can be progressively contracted more strongly. This exercise may help to reduce adhesions, help the muscle to regain strength,

and assist the patient in acquiring the proper proprioceptive information needed to re-educate this transfer.

If the patient had any preoperative active wrist extension, exercises usually progress more easily. The patient begins to learn how to better use either the normal tenodesis effect of the finger flexors and extensors or, if a surgical tenodesis has been performed, begins to learn how to use this efficiently. This is discussed in more detail below.

The transfer is protected against resistance for an additional 3–4 weeks, depending on whether or not this procedure was combined with additional procedures such as a key grip procedure or reconstruction of elbow extension by deltoid- or biceps-to-triceps transfer. Therapy protocols applicable to each of these procedures are discussed in the appropriate chapter.

Outcomes of brachioradialis to wrist extensor transfer

At our two centers we have transferred the BR to the ECRB to augment wrist extension 26 times in 16 limbs. The literature contains little information about the outcome of this now commonly performed procedure, except in the context of the key grip procedure described below. Freehafer reported results in six patients,[4] four of whom were able to grasp effectively postoperatively and three could use a WDFHS. Two others had improved posture. Freehafer mentioned that a flexor tenodesis may be possible, but no patient had this.

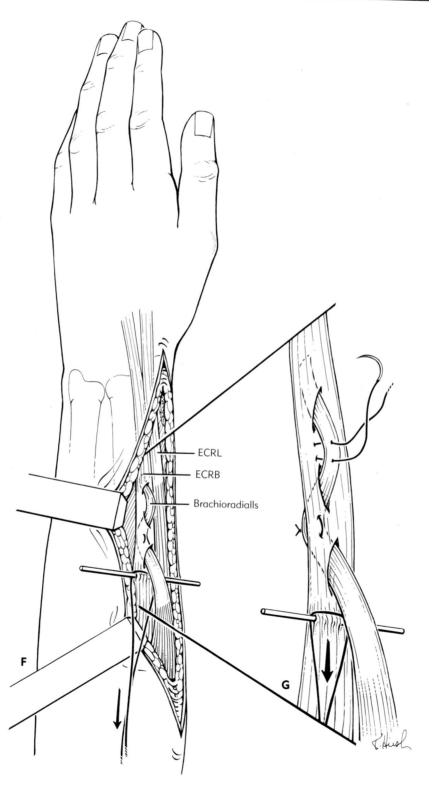

ECRL

ECRB

Brachioradialls

F

G

Figure 12.1(F, G)   (*continued*)

Johnson *et al.* performed a BR transfer for wrist extension in 16 tetraplegic patients who had neurological function at the fifth cervical level;[9] of these, nine were studied. At surgery, tension of the transfer was adjusted to hold the wrist neutral with the elbow flexed at 90°. The limb, including the elbow, was placed in a cast for 3 weeks. Five patients had key grip constructed by FPL tenodesis, and biofeedback and electrical stimulation were used to teach BR contraction without flexing the elbow.

All the patients could use a WDFHS orthosis postoperatively. The average active wrist extension was 39° and passive flexion averaged 34°. Seven patients had functional improvement, and two had questionable improvement. All the patients said that the operation was successful. Johnson *et al.* do not recommend concomitant FPL tenodesis and BR transfer, because the wrist cannot be fully extended postoperatively if FPL tenodesis is performed.[9]

Other procedures to restore wrist extension

McDowell described another tendon transfer to augment wrist extension in the tetraplegic patient. He extended the biceps with a tendon graft to restore wrist extension.[17] These patients needed weights as an antagonist to elbow flexion. Today, this could be accomplished with a deltoid-to-triceps transfer.

Reconstruction of key pinch by flexor pollicis longus tenodesis

If patients in the IC Group 1 achieve MRC Grade 3+ or greater wrist extension by BR-to-ECRB transfer, they become candidates for the creation of a lateral or key pinch as described by Moberg.[1,15] This is also true for the weaker IC Group 2 patient. Erik Moberg is credited with demonstrating that this is a reliable and attainable function and that the procedure has a predictable outcome if several tenets are kept in mind. Conceptually, this is a very simple operative procedure that provides a key pinch between the pulp of the thumb and the radial side of the index finger and, importantly, is essentially totally reversible should the patient decide that he or she was more functional before surgery. This is an important consideration for a patient with a weak wrist extension many years after his injury.

The key pinch is an automatic pinch in that the tendon of the thumb flexor, the FPL, is anchored to

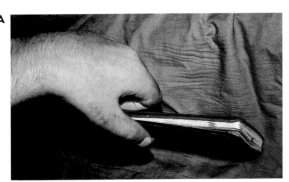

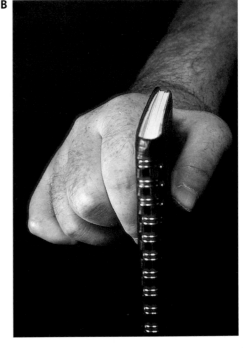

Figure 12.2 Key or lateral pinch following Moberg's key pinch procedure. (A) The patient flexes the wrist to loosen the tension on the FPL and to open the grip. The fingers must be rolled somewhat into flexion to provide a platform against which the thumb presses (B) as the wrist is extended.

the palmar surface of the radius under such a tension that, with wrist extension, the thumb tip is pulled against the side of the index finger (*Fig. 12.2*). The other fingers are usually left supple and, unless these digits automatically flex as the wrist extends, the patient must learn to roll them into some flexion to provide a platform against which the thumb can act by the tenodesis effect. Gravity is needed to flex the wrist, relaxing the FPL tenodesis and allowing opening of the grip. This implies that preoperatively the wrist must have a good passive range of motion and that the patient will be sitting much of the time so that gravity can affect opening of the grip.

Key pinch was achieved in Moberg's original design (*Fig. 12.3*) by tenodesis of the tendon of the FPL to the radius. In addition, Moberg recommended the interphalangeal (IP) joint of the thumb be stabilized with a large Steinman pin, designed to be left permanently in place. Several additional steps were suggested, depending on the preoperative assessment of the patient's thumb, particularly the stability and passive range of motion of the thumb metacarpophalangeal (MP) joint. The goal of the procedure was to transfer the force of wrist extension into a force that flexed and slightly adducted the thumb ray toward the side of the index finger. The key pinch is most successful when neither the IP nor the MP joints of the thumb flexes excessively. Indeed, the pinch function is best when most of the active motion takes place at the thumb's carpometacarpal (CMC) joint.

Prerequisites, indication, and preoperative assessment

Since the original description in 1975, Moberg's procedure has been modified (*Fig. 12.4*) by other authors to address several shortcomings of the original design seen in occasional patients, although the prerequisites for the procedure remain much as they were when Moberg first introduced the concept.[15,18] These include:

- stability in a wheelchair, that is the ability to sit for extended periods in a wheelchair;
- sufficient control of the elbow;
- ability to pronate the forearm so that gravity can effect wrist flexion;
- useful power in the extensors of the wrist or provision to restore useful antigravity or better wrist extension;
- sufficient passive flexion of the wrist aided by gravity when the patient pronates the forearm;
- at least one thumb joint (usually the CMC joint) with essentially normal passive range or motion;
- ability to position the index and preferably the middle fingers so that they serve as a platform against which the thumb can push during key pinch.

The primary contraindication to this procedure is absence of these requirements. A number of secondary relative contraindications must be considered,

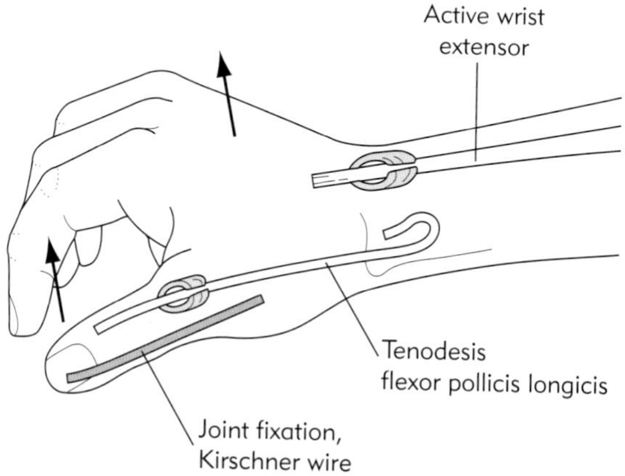

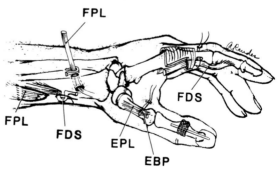

Figure 12.3 Moberg's original procedure; see the text for details. (Modified with permission from Moberg 1978.)[1]

Active wrist extensor

Tenodesis flexor pollicis longicis

Joint fixation, Kirschner wire

Figure 12.4 One of several modifications of Moberg's original procedure. The FPL tendon is passed through the radius, the flexor digitorum superficiales (FDS) to the index and middle digits are tightened to assist these fingers to become reliable platforms, and the A1 and proximal A2 pulleys are resected to increase the FDS moment at the MP joint.

however. Most involve the manner in which the patient uses the limb to be considered for surgery preoperatively. These include the methods used to propel a wheelchair, perform pressure relief actions, and carry out other activities that put stress against the thumb, such as transfer from bed to chair or chair to toilet, etc. These are discussed in greater detail in Chapters 4 and 6. Since the success of this procedure depends on the long-term stability of the FPL tenodesis, all activities that might disrupt or excessively elongate the tenodesis must be considered during the preoperative assessment. Failure to address these issues is a principal reason why earlier surgical procedures designed to restore hand function in the tetraplegic patient were judged unsuccessful.

The manner in which the surgical candidate pushes on the extended thumb is most critical. Many tetraplegic patients are taught to relieve pressure or to perform transfers by locking their elbows in full extension and then leaning forward on their fully extended wrists and hyperextended fingers and thumbs (*Fig. 12.5*). This hand and wrist position is

useful as it helps prevent the patient who lacks the muscles necessary to stabilize the trunk from falling forward. However, as discussed above, with time such stresses overstretch the collateral ligaments of the thumb, especially at its CMC joint, and the collateral ligaments of the MP joints of the fingers. Such positioning clearly leads to elongation of any passive reconstructive procedures such as tenodeses. The same deleterious forces work against the hand's anatomy if the patient propels the wheelchair using the extended thumb against 'quad-knobs' or the chair's wheel rims.

Prospective surgical candidates who perform transfer or pressure relief activities in this manner, either by education or by force of habit, must be re-educated in the preoperative period. They must be taught and allowed to practice safer methods of transfer and pressure relief, as illustrated in Chapter 4. Only when they have clearly mastered these safer techniques are they appropriate surgical candidates.

Additional relative contraindications include pathologic extensor postures of the index finger (*Fig. 12.6*). This reflexive posture makes it very

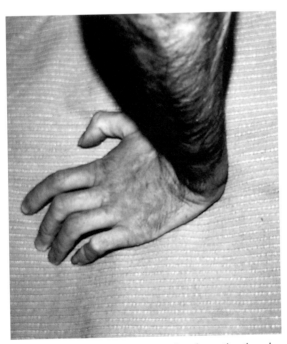

Figure 12.5 Transfer postures that force the thumb into extension stretch out the tenodesis over time. Unless this patient learns a more protective method of transfer, his key grip will deteriorate.

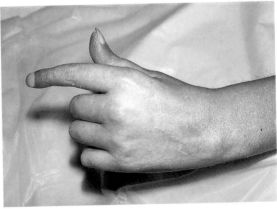

Figure 12.6 This spastic index extensor muscle must be treated if this patient is to become a good candidate for a key-pinch procedure. Surgical treatment might include detaching one of the two index finger extensors from the extensor aponeurosis, passing this tendon volar to the intermetacarpal ligament between index and middle fingers, and re-attaching this tendon into the tendon of the extensor mechanism over the proximal phalanx (see *Fig. 9.3*). This maneuver creates a mild flexion posture at the index finger MP joint. The index finger then becomes a better platform for thumb pinch.

difficult for the patient to position the index finger to provide a useful platform against which the thumb can work during key pinch. Such an abnormal posture must be addressed at the time of the key-pinch procedure by surgical re-balancing (see Chapter 9 for a tenodesis procedure that addresses this problem).

Finally, surgery for the patient many years after his or her injury who has a marginally strong BR should be approached with great caution. These patients will not achieve strong wrist extension and therefore will not reap the benefit of restoration of a strong key pinch. Typically, they have developed many adaptive or trick maneuvers or utilize unusual finger postures to perform their activities of daily living (ADLs). If they must 'unlearn' these trick maneuvers to profit from the surgical creation of a key-pinch, they may be disappointed in the result, especially if achieving even a weak grasp requires a great deal of retraining in how they use their hands.

Wrist extension at the MRC Grade 3+ level is required if the key grip created is to be at all useful. The more powerful the wrist extensors, the more powerful is the key pinch that will be achieved after surgery. The most common indication is a patient who requires transfer of the BR to augment wrist extensor strength. If the wrist extensors function pre-operatively at the MRC Grade 2+ or greater level, the BR is transferred into the tendon of the ECRB (as described above) and the FPL is fixed to the radius.

If the IC Group 2 patient already possesses MRC Grade 4+ wrist extension, the BR transfer to the ECRB may not be necessary. If the BR is not needed to augment wrist extension power, the patient and the hand should be assessed carefully in terms of utilizing the BR for another potentially beneficial function, which might include:

- Transfer to the FPL (discussed in greater detail later in this chapter). Moberg observed that the average power after BR-to-FPL transfer was less than that obtained by FPL tenodesis. We studied a number of our own patients who were at least 10 years post surgery and found the same.
- Transfer to the flexor carpi radialis (FCR) to aid in wrist flexion. The patient would be less dependent on wrist position and gravity to flex the wrist and open the key grip.
- Transfer to the abductor or extensor pollicis longus (EPL) or to the extensor pollicis brevis (EPB) for

thumb abduction. This procedure is designed to provide active opening for the first web space in preparation for a key pinch. Moberg reported less than optimal results with this procedure, perhaps because it is difficult to isolate this muscle in functional activities. Patients seem to compensate well for the lack of active first-web opening. They quickly learn to push the first web around the object to be grasped, although this usually requires that lighter objects be stabilized with the other hand so that the grasping hand does not push the object away. Bryan advised putting the BR into the EPB and abductor pollicis longus to give the best separation.[19]

- Transfer to the extensor carpi ulnaris to assist in pronation of the forearm. The patient would not need to rely only on shoulder movement to pronate the forearm.

Our preferred surgical technique

Provided that wrist extension power is adequate, the key steps of the procedure have evolved to include:

- stabilization of the IP joint of the thumb, by pin fixation of the IP joint, fusion of this joint, or a tenodesis of the joint effected by splitting the FPL insertion and transferring half the tendon dorsally, where it is attached to the tendon of insertion of the EPL;
- fixation of the tendon of the FPL to the radius at the correct tension;
- stabilization of the thumb's MP joint against excessive flexion (necessary if this joint can be passively flexed more than 45°), or against excessive extension (necessary if the joint passively hyperextends beyond 10°).

It is preferable to carry out the procedure under a regional arm block. Depending on the status of the MP joint, either four or five small incisions are planned in addition to the incision on the radial aspect of the forearm for transfer of the BR to the radial wrist extensor, if this is to be done (*Fig. 12.1A*). If this transfer is indicated, it is performed as the initial operative step.

The next step is stabilization of the IP joint of the thumb. Moberg originally described stabilization of the IP joint of the thumb with the insertion of a heavy

Steinman pin of 3 mm diameter (3/16ths of an inch). He initially used a smooth pin, but because of a high incidence of pin migration he evolved toward using a threaded Steinman pin that had a slot cut into one end so that the pin could be fully buried within the bone. Hiersch described how to construct a slotted screw that is threaded, and found that a 3.2 mm pin was sufficient to not break.[20]

We experienced similar complications of pin migration and, because no patient had ever requested reversal of the procedure, turned to formal fusion of the IP joint. More recently, we have adopted the procedure described by Mohammed *et al.*, termed the split FPL transfer.[21] This has proved a reliable alternative that preserves some active and even greater passive IP joint movement. It involves splitting the terminal several centimeters of the FPL, detaching the radial half of the FPL from the distal phalanx, and then re-attaching it to the tendon of the EPL just proximal to the IP joint.

Split flexor pollicis longus to extensor pollicis longus interphalangeal stabilization

For the optimum result, the critical pulleys, including the oblique pulley of the flexor sheath of the thumb, must be preserved (*Fig. 12.7A*). The procedure may be carried out using the incisions outlined in *Figure 12.7B*, or using just one incision along the radial mid-axis of the thumb (see *Fig. 12.8A*).

The zig-zag incision is made and the dissection commences by locating the neurovascular bundle on the radial side of the digit. The neurovascular bundle is included within the skin flap to protect it (*Fig. 12.7C*). Frequently, a small annular ligament or pulley is located at the level of the joint, and can be incised to visualize the FPL tendon.

A blunt probe can be used to find the small midline split in the tendon's structure. This split is lengthened both distally and proximally. When the distal dissection reaches the insertion of the tendon, the radial half of the split FPL tendon is divided at its bony insertion. The tendon end is delivered into the wound and, by pulling distally on the tendon, some additional as yet unsplit FPL is visualized. The proximal split is extended. Finally, a small window into the flexor sheath is created just proximal to the oblique pulley and the radial half of the tendon is brought through this window (*Fig. 12.7D*).

If a second incision is used, it is located on the mid-dorsum of the thumb, over the course of the EPL. The radial half of the FPL is tunneled under the intervening skin, deep to the radial digital nerve, and brought out at the dorsal incision (*Fig. 12.7D*).

The tendon slip is passed under the tendon of the EPL and then brought back over onto itself (*Fig. 12.7E*). Conversely, it can be passed through the substance of the EPL and then woven into itself. The thumb IP joint is temporarily stabilized in slight flexion with a 0.035 Kirschner wire placed across the joint (*Fig. 12.7E*). The transferred slip of tendon is pulled distally until a noticeable slackening of the remaining tendon half is noted, whereupon it is relaxed slightly to give equal tension on the slip of transferred tendon and on the original remaining half of the tendon (*Fig. 12.7F*). Pinning the IP joint before a final adjustment of the tension makes this step much more practical and more easily accomplished. The transferred half of the tendon is sutured to itself and to the EPL with absorbable 4–0 sutures. Conversely, a suture of clear monofilament nylon may be used. It is best to avoid the use of nonabsorbable dyed sutures, because the dorsal skin is so thin that the suture material or the knot of the suture shows through the skin.

Flexor pollicis longus tenodesis

The tendon of the FPL is to be anchored to the distal radius, and a number of variations in the routing of the FPL have been described. Moberg's original procedure left the FPL within its natural bursa, although he recommended releasing the A1 pulley under the thumb's MP joint to increase the moment of this tendon. He and Brand later modified the technique to include withdrawal of the FPL tendon from its bursa after dividing the muscle–tendon juncture in the forearm, and routing it across the palm deep to the finger flexors before passing it into the forearm via Guyon's canal. Moberg's original method is technically easier but Brand's modification provides, according to his biomechanical analysis, a more favorable FPL flexor moment. We continue to utilize both routes of FPL transfer and frequently test each method to determine which route seems to provide a more stable thumb posture in the key pinch position when the FPL is placed under tension.

The Moberg–Brand FPL tenodesis procedure requires three incisions (*Fig. 12.8A*). The first is

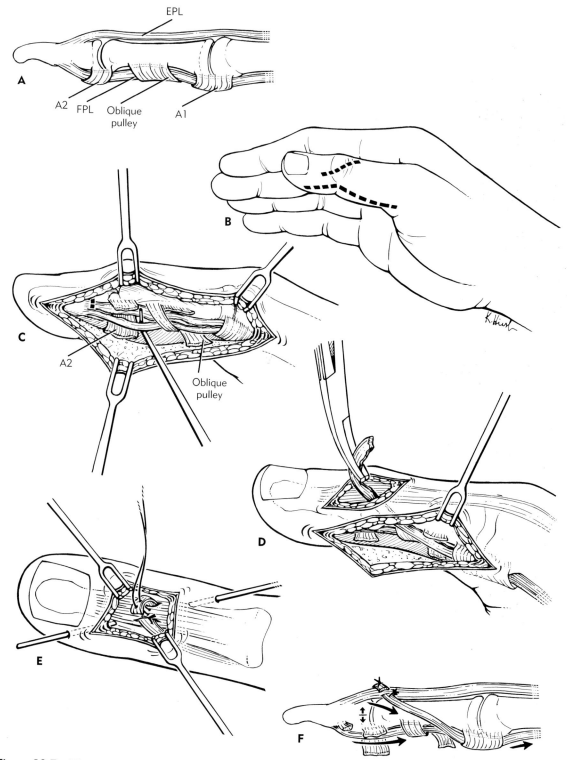

Figure 12.7 The operative steps of the New Zealand split FPL tenodesis; see the text for details. (Reproduced with permission from Hentz and Chase in press.)[14]

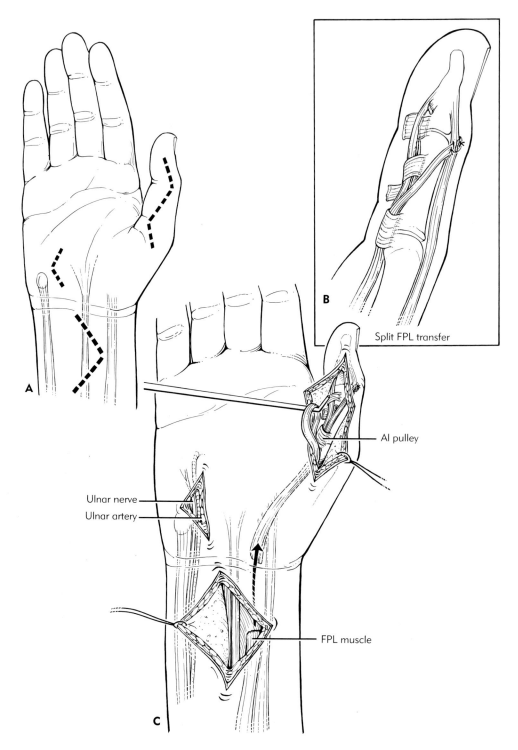

B

Split FPL transfer

AI pulley

Ulnar nerve

Ulnar artery

FPL muscle

A

C

Figure 12.8(A, B, C) The operative steps to achieve a reliable key grip; see the text for details. (Reproduced with permission from Hentz and Chase in press.)[14]

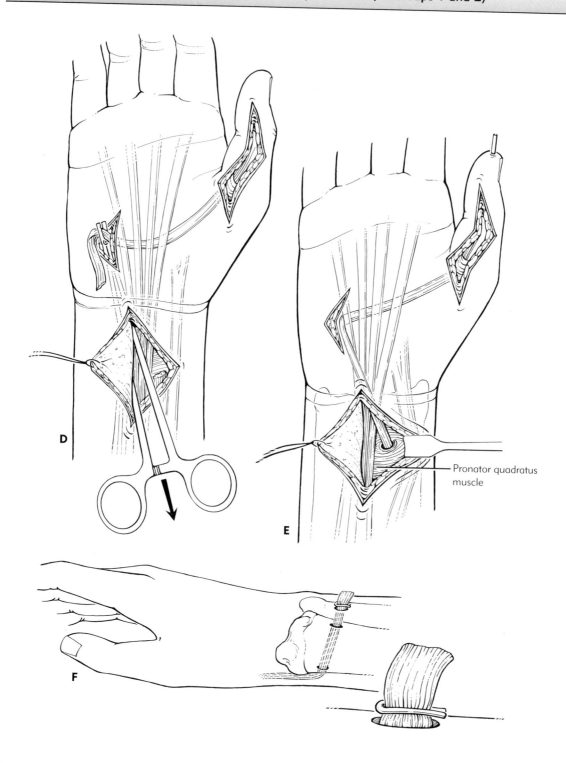

Pronator quadratus
muscle

Figure 12.8(D, E, F)   (continued)

designed along the radial aspect of the thumb and exposes the flexor sheath of the thumb from the IP joint to the level of the A1 pulley at the MP joint. The second incision is made in the palm at the level of the hook of the hamate. Access is gained to Guyon's canal through this incision. The third incision is located on the volar side of the distal forearm. The landmarks to determine the location of this incision are the FCR and the palmaris longus (PL) tendons. The fourth small incision is made last and is located on the dorsum of the distal aspect of the forearm (*Fig. 12.8F*).

After the FPL–EPL transfer has been performed, the FPL tendon is identified just proximal to the A1 pulley of the thumb. This pulley should be preserved, especially if the thumb MP joint can be passively flexed more than 30° on preoperative testing. A small probe is placed under the FPL tendon just proximal to the A1 pulley (*Fig. 12.8C*).

The volar forearm incision is made and the interval between the FCR and the PL tendons dissected. Just deep to this interval is the muscle–tendon junction of the FPL (*Fig. 12.8C*). The tendon is identified and the muscle fibers are dissected sharply from the tendon as far proximal as possible. After the final few muscle fibers have been divided, tension on the probe under the FPL at the MP joint level allows delivery of the FPL tendon into the thumb incision (*Fig. 12.8C*). The tendon is wrapped in a moistened sponge and protected from drying by frequent applications of sterile physiological solution.

The third (palmar) incision is made and the dissection is carried down through the hypothenar fat and the palmaris brevis muscle until the ulnar neurovascular bundle is located. The ulnar neurovascular bundle is retracted ulnarward to expose the flexor tendons to the little and ring fingers. A curved tendon-passing forceps is used to make a tunnel deep to the these flexors and then deep (dorsal) to the adjacent flexor tendons and neurovascular structures to the ring, middle, and index fingers. The tip of the curved tendon-passing forceps is next directed toward the thumb incision. The tendon of the FPL is grasped in the jaws of the tendon-passing forceps and delivered into the hypothenar incision (*Figs 12.8D and 12.9*).

The same tendon-passing forceps is introduced into the volar forearm incision and, staying deep (dorsal) to the flexor tendons and the median nerve,

the forceps is gently guided across the wrist crease in an ulnar direction, to exit at the hypothenar incision (*Fig. 12.8E*). The tendon of the FPL is grasped and withdrawn into the forearm incision.

The final part of this procedure involves firm fixation of the FPL tendon to the radius at the appropriate tension. This step can be simplified by first dissecting the pronator quadratus off a small window of volar radius. The ulnar aspect of the radius is exposed so that the hole to be drilled through the radius does not interfere with the radial wrist extensor tendons. A 3–4 mm drill point is used to drill a hole from volar to dorsal through the radius. The site at which the drill point exits the dorsal aspect of the radius is the location for the final incision (*Fig. 12.8F*). A loop of 30 gauge (3–0) monofilament wire is passed through the drill hole in a dorsal-to-palmar direction and the tendon of the FPL placed in the loop and drawn through the radius and into the small dorsal incision.

Moberg's original method of attaching the FPL to the ulnar edge of the volar surface of the radius can also be chosen (*Fig. 12.10*). In this case, two appropriately sized holes are drilled immediately adjacent to one another through the cortex of the volar surface of the radius. The intervening cancellous medullary bone is removed so that a monofilament wire loop can be passed into the distal hole and out of the proximal hole. The wire loop is used to guide the free end of the FPL tendon into the proximal hole and out of the distal hole. Only after all the other procedures have been accomplished and all the wounds closed (save the volar wrist incision) is the tension of the FPL tenodesis adjusted so that the thumb just contacts the

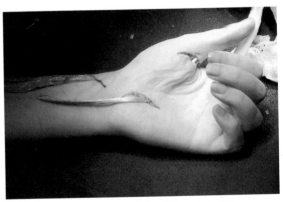

Figure 12.9 The path of the FPL; see text for details.

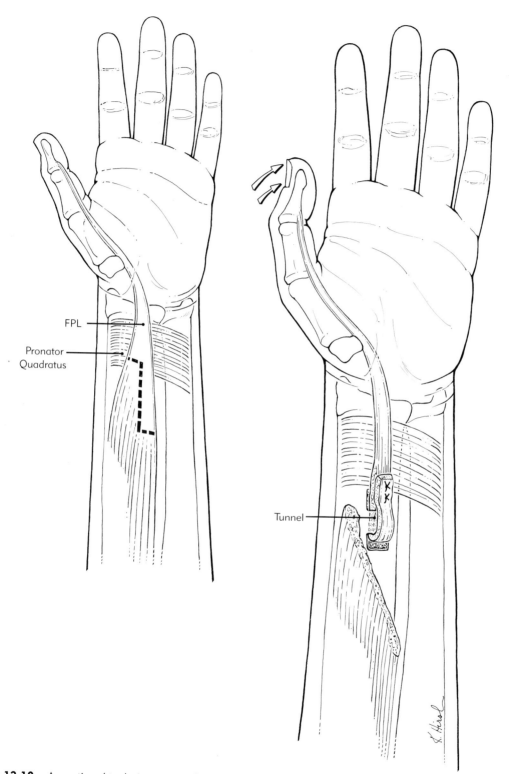

FPL

Pronator
Quadratus

Tunnel

Figure 12.10 An optional technique to anchor the tendon of the FPL to the volar surface of the radius; see the text for details.

side of the index finger with the wrist in the neutral position.

If the volar-to-dorsal, trans-radial FPL passage is selected, then all the skin incisions are closed with absorbable skin sutures or subcuticularly placed sutures. The tendon of the FPL that exits the skin on the dorsum of the forearm is grasped firmly in a large clamp. By pulling on the tendon, the tension can be adjusted according to the surgeon's preference. The proximal end of the FPL tendon is pulled so that the pulp of the thumb contacts the radial side of the index finger when the wrist is in the neutral position. When the wrist is flexed, the tension of the FPL is relaxed and the thumb ray extends in response to the dorsal tenodesis and/or viscoelastic forces. As the wrist is brought from the flexed to the neutral position, the thumb contacts the index finger. As the wrist is further extended, the thumb exerts greater and greater force against the side of the index finger.

Once the FPL tendon is positioned satisfactorily, a large vascular clip is fixed across the tendon at the level of the skin and one or two final skin sutures are placed to close the small dorsal wound (see *Fig. 12.8F*).

The position of postoperative immobilization depends on whether or not the BR was transferred as part of this procedure. If this transfer was performed, the wrist is immobilized in the neutral position and the thumb is flexed at the CMC joint to relax FPL tension. If this transfer was unnecessary, the wrist may be immobilized in 15–20° of flexion, again to relax tension at the FPL tenodesis site.

Additional technical variations

In his 1978 monograph, Moberg described several additional variations to his basic key-pinch procedure, either performed in conjunction with FPL tenodesis or frequently as a secondary procedure.[1] We have found indications for most of these.

Stabilization of the excessively flexible thumb metacarpophalangeal joint

If the MP joint of the thumb can be passively flexed beyond 45° an additional step is required. Through a small incision over the dorsum of the MP joint of the thumb, the tendons of the EPB and EPL are anchored to the thumb metacarpal using a Mitek suture anchor (*Fig. 12.11*). This extensor tenodesis checkreins the

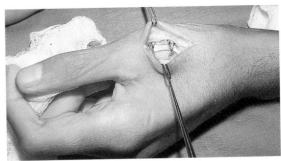

Figure 12.11 Preoperative measurement of the thumb's MP joint indicated the need to stabilize it at the time of FPL tenodesis. Otherwise, this joint will flex as the wrist is extended and the thumb tip may not contact the lateral aspect of the index finger. Stabilization is effected by anchoring the tendons of the EPB and EPL to the distal aspect of the metacarpal.

thumb MP joint against excessive flexion during key pinch (see *Fig. 12.4*).

The hyperextensible thumb metacarpophalangeal joint

If the MP joint of the thumb is excessively hyperextensible, strong consideration should be given to fusing it in slight flexion. Capsulodesis to stabilize against hyperextension rarely succeeds in the long term if the joint is very unstable into hyperextension.

Lack of wrist extensor power – division of the extensor retinaculum of the wrist

Division of the extensor retinaculum of the wrist permits bowstringing of the active wrist extensor carpi radialis tendon and increases the moment or torque of the wrist extensor. However, it reduces the amplitude of motion obtained. The risk of excessive displacement of the ECRL tendon may lead to subsequent radial subluxation and reduction of function.

Inadequate first-web opening – dorsal tenodesis of the extensor pollicis brevis or longus to the radius

This is usually performed as a secondary procedure for patients who experience great difficulty in curling the hand around objects. Inadequate tone in the paralyzed extensors may not allow sufficient extensor tenodesis and opening of the first web when the wrist is flexed. Dorsal tenodesis of the EPB or EPL to the radius may be a useful procedure when the ligaments of the thumb CMC joint have been so stretched that the thumb misses the side of the index finger in a key grip. Several technical variations of this procedure are discussed in Chapters 9 and 13.

Dysfunctional spasticity of various muscles – selective denervation of spastic and irreversibly contracted muscles

On several occasions we have had to perform selective division of the motor branch of the ulnar nerve in patients whose spasticity of the adductor pollicis made it impossible for them to open the first web space.

Difficulty in learning how to position the index finger in preparation for key pinch – Zancolli lasso procedure

The Zancolli lasso procedure includes steps to create more flexion at the MP joint of the index finger using a modification of the Zancolli 'lasso' procedure depicted in *Figure 12.4*. The A1 and the proximal one-third of A2 pulley of the index and middle finger are opened and the superficial flexor tendons of these digits tightened via the forearm incision. In this way, the platform against which the thumb can work is in a better position.

The excessively extended or spastically extended index finger can be treated as Hamlin suggested by redirecting the extensor indicis tendon to the volar side of the MP joint, as discussed in Chapter 9 (*Fig. 9.3*). This routing provides a MP flexor vector that reduces or eliminates the extended posture and assists in flexing the index finger in preparation for key pinch.

Postoperative management and rehabilitation*

*See Appendix V for a detailed postoperative rehabilitation regimen.

The thumb ray and wrist are immobilized in a cast for 4 weeks. The Kirschner wire placed to protect the split FPL interphalangeal tenodesis is usually left in place for a further 1–2 weeks and then removed. A small taped-on aluminum splint is substituted, which is removed frequently during the day and gentle pinching exercises begun. The joint is supported against significant stress for a total of 8 weeks.

During the following week, the patient is told to try and grip lightly with his or her hand. The initial exercises aim to restore wrist extension range and strength, which will have been compromised by the period of immobilization. The patient is encouraged to lift both arms over his or her head many times a day to pump out the edema. During the first week out of plaster the key grip action is demonstrated to the patient, who should not be trained yet but should be acquainted with how the grip feels.

At the end of the fifth week after surgery active training with therapist supervision can start, preferably twice each day. The patient is encouraged to practice the same grips on his or her own between the sessions. The goal of therapy is to provide the patient with a variety of activities in which he or she can utilize the key grip pinch, such as playing chess, handling pegs, picking up a small booklet, and moving small wooden cubes, a matchbox, etc. Generally, early pinch efforts may be somewhat ineffective, especially if the tenodesis is initially tight. Some gripping between the thumb and middle finger may usefully provide a small amount of resistance. By the sixth week, the patient may allow more resistance against the index finger. The patient is taught how to roll the index and middle fingers around an object so that grasp occurs:

- at the distal IP joint level (most unstable, but useful for grasping small objects);
- at the middle phalanx or proximal IP (PIP) joint level (more stable); and
- at the level of the proximal phalanx (most stable as the collateral ligaments of the MP joint tighten and the ulnar fingers help support the index and middle fingers).

Moberg has identified some regularly encountered difficulties in the training sessions. The potential problems and Moberg's novel solutions are taken from his monograph with the kind permission of the publisher (*Fig. 12.12*).[1]

Thumb does not meet the side of the index finger

The thumb may be too far into the palm and so does not meet the side of the index finger. This problem is temporarily counteracted by the pull of one small rubber-band acting as a thumb abductor. With the

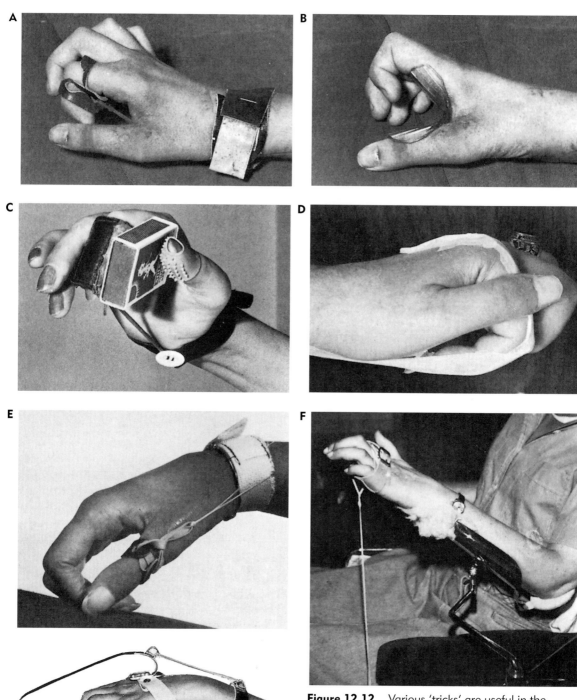

Figure 12.12 Various 'tricks' are useful in the postoperative period to assist the patient in learning how to use the new function; see the text for details. (Reproduced with permission from Moberg, 1978.)[1]

thumb out just a little bit the oblique inner surface of the thumb pulp faces in the correct direction to approach the object (*Fig. 12.12A*). The problem that the index and middle fingers are not flexed enough to meet the thumb is also temporarily relieved by a pull with the rubber-band, or the index may be fixed with a tape (*Fig. 12.12C*) or by other straps (*Fig. 12.12D*). The proximal end of this rubber-band or tape is anchored to the wrist. Very soon the patient is taught to 'roll up the fingers' against the surface (e.g., a table) the object is placed on (*Fig. 12.12E*). These patients have an amazing ability to adapt themselves to the rolling up function. If the tenodesis effect of the fingers is too great, the thumb strikes the index finger too far proximally for optimum function. Dynamic rubber-band extension splinting may help to overcome too tight a flexor tenodesis (*Fig. 12.12G*).

Insufficient passive abduction range of thumb

The passive abduction range of the thumb may not initially be sufficient, even in maximum flexion of the wrist. A rubber-tube or plastic-tube splint, cut as shown in *Fig. 12.12B*, can improve this. In a combined action with the wrist extensors, this splint will, of course, help increase the range of motion of the wrist, which will have stiffened to some extent during the necessary rest in plaster.

Temporary lack of mobility of the wrist

The temporary lack of mobility of the wrist must be treated. It is important to retrain the immobilized wrist muscles and commence new training of the transferred musculotendinous system. This should be performed actively using another strap, which can be fixed to the wheelchair (*Fig. 12.12F*), and permits almost isometric training of the BR and isotonic exercise with the radial wrist extensors. The forearm should be positioned in slight pronation. The skin also improves as a result of this edema-reducing pumping action.

Reduced hand friction

Friction in these hands is reduced considerably, even though innervation of the sudomotor function may be retained. With the limited power available, friction here is of paramount importance. The lack of friction

is another of the many reasons why the three-pulp pinch should be avoided in tetraplegia, as the gripping areas are too small. Friction can be supplied by using bank note counters (*Fig. 12.12C*), carborundum tape-on pens, forks and other utensils, or other means to make the surface rough, either temporarily during training or permanently. This training and the accompanying encouragement soon enables the patient to continue alone. The patient is shown the different gripping possibilities and makes a personal choice between them, or perhaps find another new way to achieve the desired activities. A mutual search develops between the patient and the occupational therapist to seek ways to perform the ADLs. Every patient and every hand is different and apparently small details can greatly enhance function. Strength of the wrist extensors, and thus pinch strength, may continue to improve over a period of years after surgery as a consequence of use. Again, it must be stressed that it is almost impossible to train a patient adequately if, for some reason, he or she is bedridden. All that can be done under such circumstances is to prevent loss until the patient is no longer bedridden.

The thumb is further protected against stress for several additional weeks while wrist flexion and extension exercises are carried out. Only very light pinching activities are allowed until the eighth postoperative week.

Illustrative patient

A 30-year-old man suffered a C5–C6 injury in a diving accident 2 years prior to being evaluated. His injury had left him with strong elbow flexion and essentially a normal range of elbow motion. The hand therapists assessed wrist extension strength at Grade 4–. He was stable in his wheelchair, and was able to sit for many hours. In the chair, he was able to position his elbow and shoulder so that gravity, assisted by the action of the BR, would pronate his forearm. With the forearm pronated, the wrist would flex to about 45° under the influence of gravity. With his wrist flexed, his thumb extended enough to provide a decent opening between thumb and index finger (*Fig. 12.13A*). It was felt that this position would allow him to curl his thumb and index finger around reasonably sized objects to grasp them. He had good attendant care and would be able to cope with a 4–6 week period of greater dependence associated with having one arm in a cast.

A

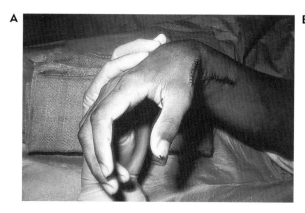

B

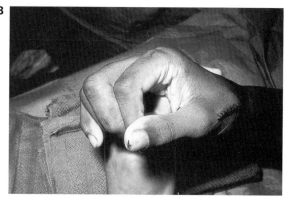

C

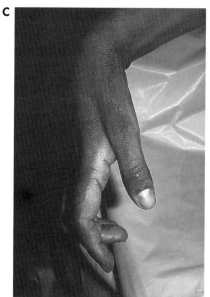

D

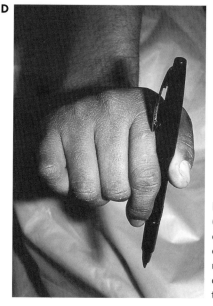

Figure 12.13   The (A) pre-, (B) intra-, and (C, D) post-operative opening and closing of the key pinch, in response to active extension and gravity-assisted flexion of the wrist.

The procedure described above was carried out and the posture of his thumb and fingers at the completion of surgery is shown in *Figure 12.13B*. After a period of rehabilitation, the patient was able to grasp and release objects of various sizes readily (*Figs 12.13C* and *12.13D*). The reconstruction of a key pinch allowed him to perform many activities in a more time-efficient manner. He related how prior to surgery it took him about 1 hour to dress himself. After surgery this time diminished to about 15 minutes.

Common complications and how to deal with them

Complications specific to the three procedures described above (transfer of the BR to the wrist extensor, the Moberg FPL tenodesis for key pinch, and the split FPL interphalangeal tenodesis) include those related to errors of omission and errors of commission.

Complications of BR transfer include accidental rupture of the transfer. The patient may report feeling or even hearing the juncture rupture. In our experience, this occurs as a result of the individual being pulled from a supine to a sitting position by someone tugging on the operated arm with the operated elbow semi-flexed and in an isotonic state of contraction. Immediate re-exploration has resulted in a good outcome.

Complications associated with the split FPL interphalangeal tenodesis are essentially nonexistent. Our experience is that little active flexion remains after

A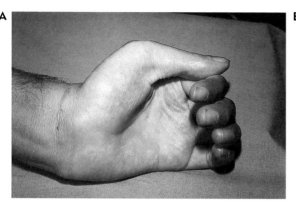

B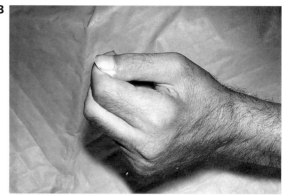

Figure 12.14 (A) If the force of pinch is strong, that is the wrist extensor power is great, in the context of a hyperflexible MP joint, the FPL will progressively bowstring at the MP joint. This increase in the moment of the FPL at the MP joint causes the joint to assume an excessively flexed posture. This may result in the tip of the thumb not contacting the side of the index finger as the patient tries to pinch. Occasionally, when the FPL tendon is left in its normal course, with a strong pinch the thumb tends to supinate as it presses against the index finger during pinch. In this case, (B) the side of the thumb becomes the contact surface rather than the broad pulp surface of the thumb. This is a less stable construct for function.

this procedure, as anticipated from the design of the procedure.

Our analysis of complications and less than ideal outcomes after FPL tenodesis led to the variations in the current technique compared to Moberg's original design. Until his death in 1993, Moberg himself constantly modified his own procedure according to outcome. We have learned the following from our favorable, but especially our less than favorable, experiences:

When wrist extension is MRC Grade 4+, the key pinch is strong. If the thumb's MP joint exhibits preoperative passive flexion greater than 30°, then the A1 pulley of the thumb should not be sectioned. Doing so invariably leads to increased MP joint flexion as time goes by (*Fig. 12.14A*). The FPL tendon bowstrings in an increasingly excessive manner. This enlarging flexion moment leads to even more MP joint flexion. Eventually, this results in a functional shortening of the thumb sufficient to preclude the thumb tip from easily contacting the radial side of the index finger. The thumb tip misses the index finger as the wrist is extended and the pinch becomes tenuous or is totally lost.

If the standard Moberg 'in-situ' FPL tenodesis is performed when the CMC joint of the thumb is unstable, secondary to laxity of the intrinsic ligaments, a forceful key pinch may result in the thumb supinating at the CMC joint (*Fig. 12.14B*). The result

is that the ulnar side of the thumb becomes the contact surface rather than the broad pulp surface of the thumb desired. The more the wrist is extended, the more unstable the pinch becomes. In these cases, the tendon of the FPL should be withdrawn from its normal course through an incision at the flexor crease of the thumb, preserving the A1 pulley. It should then be redirected, as recommended by Brand and Moberg (see *Fig. 12.8D*), across the palm deep to the flexor tendons and neurovascular bundles to emerge at the distal edge of Guyon's canal. It is wise to experiment with several different transfer routes, including ones that mimic those recommended by Royle[22] and Thompson[23] for their modifications of the opponens transfer. The goal is a route of transfer that effects as little rotational vector as possible when the FPL tendon is placed under tension, as occurs during wrist extension as part of the key grip.

Salvage procedures for suboptimal outcomes

The most commonly required secondary procedures are discussed above, and include procedures to ameliorate the consequences of an inability to open the first web space adequately and procedures to stabilize the MP joint that flexes excessively during key pinch.

Additional procedures that we have employed to try to improve function include MP joint fusion when the joint demonstrates flexion greater than 45°. Early in our experience we secondarily fused the thumb's IP joint when it became excessively flexed following pin migration and removal.

Several patients developed over time a tendency for the extensors of the index finger to become more and more spastic in the postoperative period (see *Fig. 12.6*). The consequence of this extended index finger posture is the loss of a suitable platform for the thumb. Hamlin's solution to this problem, volarly rerouting the extensor indicis tendon, is discussed in Chapter 9 (*Fig. 9.3*).

Perhaps the most common complication occurs gradually. The FPL tenodesis may stretch as time passes. If the laxity becomes significant, the force of pinch deteriorates. The wrist cannot be extended enough to create a force between the thumb and index finger. In such cases, it is possible to tighten the original tenodesis. This can be accomplished by exposing the distal insertion of the FPL, disinserting the tendon, advancing the tendon an appropriate distance, and re-anchoring the tendon to the distal phalanx at its new tension. The thumb and wrist should be immobilized so that tension on the point of reinsertion is minimized and the immobilization should be maintained for 4 weeks.

If the split FPL interphalangeal stabilization procedure was performed at the time of the initial key pinch surgery, this distal readjustment is not convenient. In such cases, the FPL tendon should be isolated at the site of tenodesis to the radius and tightened at this level, either by suturing a tuck in the tendon or reinserting the tendon of the FPL into the radius at the new tension. The thumb and wrist must be immobilized for 4 weeks and then protected against forceful resistance for an additional 4–6 weeks.

Outcomes

We have performed this procedure on over 50 hands and the results are very satisfying.[18] We measured the gain in pinch strength and it was typically proportional to the strength of the wrist extensor power, but somewhat dependent on the stability of the thumb and finger joints.

In an effort to assess the outcomes in our own patients, 23 patients at least 1 year post-surgery were evaluated to compare postoperative functional capabilities to the preoperative levels. Five patients (about 20% of the study group) with five operated limbs (15%) were dissatisfied with their hand function. However, only one patient believed his function had suffered from having undergone surgery and no patient asked that the procedure be reversed. Our analysis showed several factors to be important contributions to overall dissatisfaction. On preoperative assessment, these patients either possessed the fewest functional resources (those who required BR transfer to bring wrist extension to MRC Grade 4 level), or exhibited the longest intervals between injury and surgery (up to 15 years in one case). For these patients the insidious postoperative development of contractures, spasticity, and dystrophic-like pain severely limited function.

Seven patients (35%) with 10 operated limbs (30%) were moderately satisfied with their hand function. On analysis, these patients had stronger preoperative wrist extensions than those with poor results (averaging MRC Grade 4). Three patients had wrist strength augmented by BR transfer. All had increased their strength of wrist extension by half a grade or more postoperatively. For most, this increase helped in transfers using overhead frames.

Factors detrimental to function in these patient's hands included postoperative flexor instability of the thumb MP joint and poor index and long finger position when attempting key pinch. Two patients had procedures to further stabilize the MP joint against excessive flexion during key pinch. This succeeded in improving the position of the thumb relative to the other digits during pinch. Two patients had successful postoperative revisions to tighten the FPL tenodesis.

Eleven patients (45%) with 18 limbs (55%) were very pleased, especially at the greater ease with which they could perform functional activities related to self-care, communication, and mobility. Three patients required revision, either to tighten the FPL tenodesis, further stabilize the MP joint, or replace extruded IP joint pins. Five patients chose reconstruction of active elbow extension in eight limbs. Postoperatively, all could extend against gravity, some with great force. They were all very pleased with the result of their elbow extension procedures.

These patients as a group had the strongest pre-operative wrist extensors, although three required BR augmentation. Many had a normal natural flexor tenodesis when they extended their wrist preoperatively, although without any strength in this flexor tenodesis. This natural tenodesis effectively aided placing the index and long fingers in the correct position relative to the thumb, which obviated the need to learn to roll the fingers around the object to be grasped by pushing them against a platform .

Dissatisfaction related to:

- stretching of the FPL tenodesis with weakening of pinch (this usually occurred early in the postoperative course);
- thumb MP joint instability (occurring both early and late);
- breakage of the pin fixing the thumb IP joint (also occurring early or late); or
- difficulties in learning to position the fingers prior to pinch in those patients who lacked natural flexor tenodesis.

Interestingly, strength of pinch averaged only 2 lb (0.9 kg) greater in those patients judged to have a 'good' result as compared to those judged to have a 'fair' result. Very little difference was observed on functional testing, which again demonstrates the difficulty in objectively assessing results.

Long-term outcomes

We recently studied seven International Classification Group 1 or 2 patients whose surgical procedures had occurred more than 10 years previously to determine the durability of their FPL tenodesis procedures. Five had maintained pinch strength essentially equivalent to that demonstrated 6–12 months after surgery. The other two patients had a 30% reduction in power compared to 1 year postoperatively. Overall pinch strength in this group was 25 N.

Outcomes from other published series

Moberg reported his initial results after operating on 40 hands in 33 patients.[15] The average follow-up was 2 years. No significant deterioration had occurred over that time. All but two were significantly improved. In three patients the wire used to stabilize the IP joint

of the thumb migrated and had to be removed. The FPL tenodesis needed readjustment in a 'few cases'

Smith described the outcome in 29 key-grip procedures carried out at Rancho Los Amigos in California, USA, and Warm Springs Institute in Arkansas, USA.[24] Six pin complications occurred in the first 13 cases, in which a smooth pin was used. A slotted-threaded pin that could be fully buried within the bone of the distal phalanx using a screwdriver was developed and this eliminated pin migration. The surgical recommendation included tensioning the FPL tenodesis so that the thumb was firmly against the index finger with the wrist in neutral. Two of the 14 dorsal EPL–EPB tenodeses stretched out. These had been anchored to the periostium of the metacarpal with sutures that passed through holes drilled into the bone. Based on this experience, Smith recommended a looped tenodesis. Four patients had BR-to-ECRB transfer performed, but in two patients this transfer did not result in improved wrist extensor strength. Six of 29 patients required revision.

Reiser and Waters examined 10 patients at an average of 7.4 years after surgery.[25] They saw progressive flexion of the thumb's MP joint associated with excessive bowstringing of the FPL, probably associated with A1 pulley release. In these patients, the average MP joint flexion was 61°. The most effective pinch involved objects 2.5 cm wide. As a result of loosening of the pinch, patients had to extend their wrist more and more to achieve a pinch. The authors believe that the FPL did not stretch, but rather that the loosening occurred as a result of MP joint flexion. In their experience, if the patient needed to roll the fingers in preparation for gripping, functional pinch was only possible on a flat surface.

Subjectively, all the patients felt that their power had decreased; four said their pinch was still adequate and six said their pinch was now inadequate. Patients indicated that the procedure raised their independence level, improved their mental attitude, and overall was worthwhile. Eight patients had discarded their orthosis. No patient with a key grip had catheter independence.

The investigators also noted differences in functional levels if fingers had lost passive tenodesis and did not flex somewhat when the wrist was extended. They recommend tightening the finger flexors if passive tenodesis flexion is inadequate. They recommend a BR-to-ECRB transfer before key grip, because two patients who had this procedure failed to regain good wrist extensor strength.

Colyer reviewed eight patients who had 10 key grips constructed by Moberg's method.[26] The Jebsen test was used to assess six of the patients. The average improvement in the Jebsen score was 31%. Few new functions were gained. The most significant improvement was in terms of speed and ease of performing pre-existing functions. Three patients were able to self-catheterize, which made them totally independent. The investigators also experienced difficulties with the IP wire and recommend fusion. Key pinch strength averaged 0.9 kg (2 lb) postoperatively. No correlation was found between strength and score on the Jebsen functional test. No thumb was sufficiently stiff at the IP joint after the wire came out; all needed fusion.

Ejeskar reported results following reconstruction procedures in 50 hands in 40 patients.[27] Pinch strength was 0–3.5 kg (0–7.7 lb) with an average of 0.7 kg (1.54 lb). Ejeskar found that the position of thumb and fingers during the grip was more important than the ultimate strength. The FPL had been routed primarily by the transpalmar route. Ejeskar felt that this led to a weaker grip and did not necessarily eliminate the need for tenodesis of the thumb extensors to stabilize the MP joint against excessive flexion. Flexion at the thumb's MP joint of more than 30° caused the thumb's CMC joint to rotate, which reduced the tension of the FPL tenodesis. Flexion at the MP joint of the index finger greater than 60° gave a poorer function as it caused the thumb to be too long. Therefore, in postoperative splinting the MP joints should not be splinted in more than 45–50° of flexion.

Mohammed et al. reported their results with the Moberg key pinch procedure.[21] Key pinch in 52/68 cases averaged 2.1 kg (4.6 lb).

Reconstructive choices for the stronger International Classification Group 2 Patient

The IC Group 2 patient possesses wrist extension of at least MRC Grade 4 level. Our convention has been to grade the patient with a clearly MRC Grade 5 wrist extension as IC Group 3, that is they possess MRC Grade 4 ECRL and ECRB. If adequate wrist extensor

strength exists preoperatively, the patient is potentially a candidate for either a Moberg key pinch procedure, effected by FPL tenodesis, or an active pinch, effected by transfer of the BR to the FPL. Various authors have different recommendations, based on their own experience. For example, Waters et al. measures wrist extensor torque and makes a decision based on this.[11] He now recommends BR-to-FPL transfer if wrist extensor torque is greater than 10 ft-lbs (13.6 N-m). He correlates this to a good contraction of the muscle against moderate resistance and occasionally measures the torque under local anesthetic at the time of operation. If less than 10 ft-lbs (13.6 N-m), he transfers the BR to ECRB and performs a tenodesis of the FPL (Moberg procedure). Other authors who generally favor an active pinch using the BR as the motor for the patient with good preoperative wrist extension include Lamb[28] and House et al.[29] In contrast, Ejeskar recommends FPL tenodesis in the IC Group 2 patient.[30]

One of us (VRH) initially preferred FPL tenodesis for all IC Group 2 patients, as discussed above. More recently, BR-to-FPL transfer, along with thumb CMC stabilization, became the preferred recommendation for the patient with MRC Grade 4+ preoperative wrist extension. This is despite our observations that in patients with similar powers of wrist extension, pinch force is, on average, greater in those patients who have had tenodesis compared to those who have undergone BR-to-FPL transfer. In contrast, in House et al.'s series of 21 hands in 18 patients after BR-to-FPL transfer, pinch strength exceeded that observed in his Moberg FPL tenodesis patients.[29]

Active key pinch by brachioradialis to flexor pollicis longus transfer

The goal of this procedure is a strong key pinch between the pulp of the thumb and radial side of the semi-flexed index finger, not associated with an obligatory wrist extension. The patient should then be able to effect a pinch in many wrist positions, but will reflexively extend the wrist to augment the power of pinch. The corollary goal is the ability to open the pinch by allowing gravity to flex the wrist and release the tension of the transfer. These two primary goals are best accomplished by:

- prepositioning the thumb ray through an appropriately directed fusion at the CMC joint of the thumb, necessary because the number of active muscles is insufficient to control the normally complex movements of the thumb's CMC joint;
- stabilizing the IP joint of the thumb to avoid troublesome and potentially dysfunctional hyperflexion at the IP joint after transfer (Froment's sign);
- tenodesis of the EPL so that the MP and IP joints of the thumb extend as the wrist is flexed, which opens the grip; and
- powering the paralyzed by BR-to-FPL transfer.

The minimum prerequisites for this procedure include strong (at least MRC grade 4+) wrist extension, a transferable BR, a passively flexible wrist, at least 45° of gravity assisted wrist flexion, and a supple thumb MP joint.

Operative procedure

The operative steps are carried out via one longer and three or four smaller incisions, as illustrated in *Figure 12.15*. First, the FPL-to-EPL IP joint stabilization procedure is completed, as illustrated in *Figure 12.9*. Next, the CMC joint is exposed through an incision made along the juncture of the glaborous and hair-bearing skin over the palmar–radial aspect of the thumb's thenar eminence. The thenar muscles are reflected off the capsule of the CMC joint and the capsule opened. The adjacent joint surfaces are prepared for fusion by sharp excision of all the cartilage and by perforating the dense subchondral bone in several areas on the metacarpal base and face of the trapezium. Bone is removed with a small osteotome, curette, or powered burr, equally from both sides of the joint. This maintains the relative contours of the metacarpal base and trapezium and good bone-to-bone contact between the two surfaces.

Choosing the position for carpometacarpal fusion

The preoperative digital flexor tenodesis pattern and the passive range of motion at the thumb's MP joint mainly determine the angles of palmar and radial abduction for CMC fusion. The goal is to have the pulp of the thumb contact the radial side of the index finger over the middle phalanx as the wrist is extended. Opening of the grip is effected by wrist flexion and occurs almost exclusively at the MP joint. The ideal candidate has a well-preserved digital flexor tenodesis pattern and passive MP flexion that exceeds the range of CMC extension. For such a patient, the thumb ray should be positioned in only about 20° of palmar abduction and in almost maximum radial abduction. A thumb ray fixed by CMC fusion in a larger palmar abduction will interfere with transfers and pressure relief efforts and will be subject to great stress when the patient performs these maneuvers. If the patient demonstrates very poor finger flexion as the wrist is extended, the CMC joint should be fused in a slightly less palmarly abducted posture. If the range of passive MP flexion is small, the CMC joint should be fused in less than the maximal radial abduction. If too radially abducted, the patient with a poorly flexible MP joint will not be able to effect firm contact between the pulp of the thumb and the index finger.

The CMC joint is temporarily pinned with a 2 mm Kirschner wire to test the preoperative hypothesis. If the position seems ideal, the joint is further stabilized. A small four-corner plate (*Fig. 12.15D*) provides sufficiently rigid bone-to-bone contact. Bone staples also provide excellent immobilization at the fusion site.

Tenodesis of the extensor pollicis longus to the dorsal surface of the radius

The third step involves creating a firm tenodesis of the EPL to the dorsal surface of the radius. Since the CMC joint is now fused, no particular EPL rerouting is needed. Through a transverse incision made just proximal to Lister's tubercle, the tendon of the EPL is located and divided at its muscle–tendon junction. The end of the tendon is brought over the extensor retinaculum, and passed under the EPL tendon just distal to the retinaculum. The wrist is flexed to 45° and the EPL is tensioned so that the thumb extends maximally. Several nonabsorbable sutures are used to anchor the EPL to itself and to the dense extensor retinaculum. The wrist is then passively flexed and extended and the thumb's motion observed. The thumb should reach maximum extension as the wrist reaches 45° of flexion, but the pulp of the thumb should contact the radial side of the index finger as the wrist is extended to reach the neutral position.

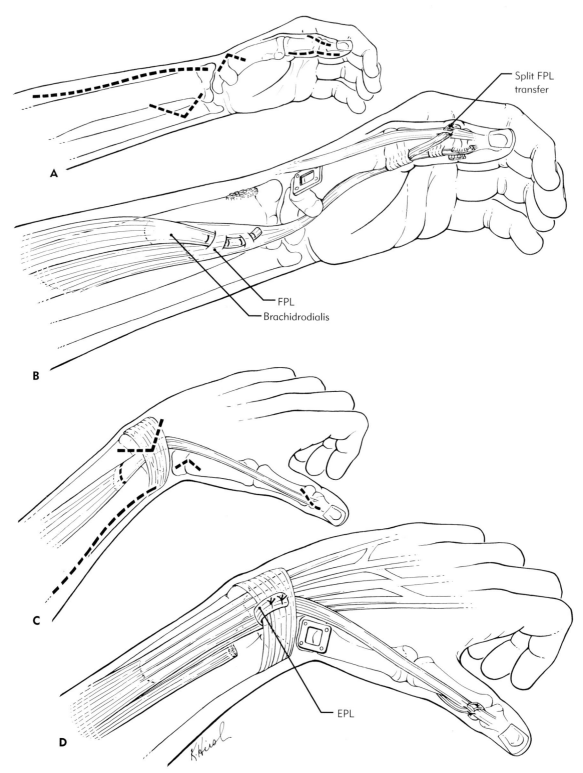

Split FPL
transfer

FPL

Brachidrodialis

EPL

Figure 12.15 The operative steps for providing an active key pinch by BR-to-FPL transfer; see the text for details.

Brachioradialis to flexor pollicis longus transfer

The final procedure involves BR-to-FPL transfer. The BR is exposed via a long serpentine incision, as illustrated in *Figure 12.15*, and is dissected as described above. The FPL is identified in the volar forearm, either through the same incision as used to dissect the BR or through a separate volar incision. The FPL is divided at its muscle–tendon junction and the two tendons are directed in as straight a line as possible toward one another. The ends of both tendons are passed through one another several times, interweaving them. The ideal tension for the transfer is established as described for the BR-to-ECRB transfer. The juncture is created with the elbow in 40° of flexion, the wrist in a neutral position, and the index finger held flexed at the MP and PIP joints. The BR is pulled distally to a point midway between the tensions of maximum passive stretch and full relaxation (zero), and the FPL tendon is pulled proximally so that the pulp of the thumb just touches the radial side of the index finger. The assistant maintains this posture of both tendons while the surgeon joins together the two tendons with three or four non-absorbable sutures. Once this tendon-to-tendon juncture is secure, the tension of the FPL transfer and the EPL tenodesis is tested by gently moving the wrist between 45° of flexion and 45° of extension. It is important that after BR transfer the thumb continues to fully extend at the MP joint with wrist flexion. The wounds are closed and the limb solidly immobilized in a below-elbow cast that maintains the wrist in a neutral position, and the thumb MP joint in some flexion. We typically place the thumb in contact with the flexed index finger.

Postoperative management

The immobilization is continued for 4 weeks and, on removal, a plastic splint is constructed to keep the thumb and wrist in the initial position of postoperative immobilization. The splint is removed for exercises and the initial exercises aim to regain the preoperative range of wrist movement. At the beginning of the fifth postoperative week, the patient is

A
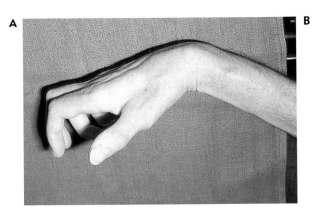

B
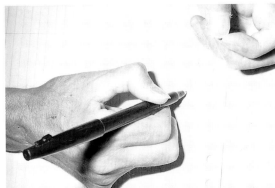

C
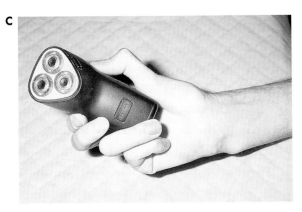

Figure 12.16 The ability to open the hand (A) and grasp objects of various sizes (B and C) is shown in this patient after EPL tenodesis, thumb CMC fusion, and BR-to-FPL transfer.

encouraged to start to practice grasping small, light objects; for these exercises, the therapist constructs a small hand-based splint to protect the CMC fusion. These exercises progress until the beginning of the eighth week when greater resistance is permitted. The splint is discontinued during the daytime, but is worn at night for an additional 4 weeks. The same weight-bearing precautions apply as for the FPL tenodesis procedure, with no transfers out of the splint until after the eighth postoperative week. The fused thumb CMC joint requires that the patient's transfer mechanics be closely monitored by the therapist.

Figure 12.16 demonstrates the postoperative result of this procedure in an IC Group 2–3 patient. The hyperextension of the thumb's MP joint became advantageous in assisting him to grasp objects.

Complications and salvage procedures

Radiographic evidence of less than a solid bone union at the fusion site is common, yet none of our patients have complained of postoperative discomfort in spite of apparent pseudoarthrosis. We cannot readily determine with clinical testing if the joint is solidly fused or not, since (rather quickly) the scaphotrapezial joint acquires useful compensatory movements, which probably provide some protective effect to the CMC joint. We have not had to re-operate on the CMC joint in any patient.

Prior to routinely adopting the FPL-to-EPL interphalangeal stabilization procedure, the IP joint was left unaltered during BR-to-FPL transfer. We accepted some hyperflexion at the IP joint as a necessary side effect of the procedure. In two patients this became so excessive that functional pinch was lost and we performed a secondary IP joint fusion. This solved the problem of hyperflexion, but resulted in a very stiff thumb ray that interfered with transfers and pushing a manual wheelchair.

Rupture of the BR-to-FPL transfer occurred in one extremely heavy patient, probably during the period of initial immobilization. We believe this problem potentially exists whether or not the elbow is included in the postoperative cast.

Long-term outcomes

Six of our IC Group 2 or possibly 3 patients who had transfer of BR to FPL to restore dynamic voluntary key pinch more than 10 years prior were evaluated and all six had maintained useful power (averaged 20 N). It has been difficult to determine through clinical examination when pinch function is primarily a consequence of an enhanced tenodesis effect brought about by wrist extension and when it functions as a dynamic transfer. In many patients, the BR muscle only visibly contracts when the patient attempts a maximal or near maximal effort. Using electromyographic analysis, Waters *et al.* determined that the BR, once transferred to FPL can function as a primary thumb flexor.[10]

Thumb IP joint instability seems to have played a major role in the diminished power seen in several of the BR–FPL patients. We now routinely employ the split FPL attachment described by Mohammed *et al.* to provide thumb IP stabilization and avoid IP joint fusion.[21]

Other reported series

House *et al.* reported their results using a procedure similar to that described above.[29] Average pinch was 3.3 kg (7.3 lb). House *et al.* also noted no difference between patients with solid fusion and stable fibrous nonunions.

Waters reported results in a series of 17 hands in 15 patients who had BR-to-FPL transfers. Of these hands, 16 had thumb IP fixation, and 11 had extensor tenodesis over the thumb dorsum. Pinch strength averaged 8.6 kg (18.9 lb) with wrist extension at 30°. Waters correlated the strength of wrist extension to pinch power and found that the ratio of wrist extension torque to pinch pressure was 5.3 to 1. Of the 15 patients, 13 said they were improved by surgery.

Summary

We have benefited from an initial large experience with the straightforward and predictable FPL tenodesis procedure and, after gaining experience, have continually modified it with the goal of customizing the procedure to each particular patient. We have moved toward reconstructing a dynamic pinch by tendon transfer when the BR is not needed to augment wrist extension.

References

1. Moberg E. The Upper Limb in Tetraplegia. A new approach to surgical rehabilitation. Stuttgart: George Thieme, 1978.
2. Zancolli E. Surgery for the quadriplegic hand with active, strong wrist extension preserved. Clin Orthop Rel Res 1975; 112:101–113.
3. Hentz VR, Keoshian L. Changing perspectives in surgical hand rehabilitation in quadriplegic patients. J Plast Reconstr Surg 1979; 64(4):509–515.
4. Freehafer A, Mast W. Transfer of the brachioradialis to improve wrist extension in high spinal cord injury. J Bone Joint Surg 1967; 49A:648.
5. Brand P, Beach R, Thompson D. Relative tension and potential excursion of muscles in the forearm and hand. J Hand Surg 1981; 6:209–219.
6. Freehafer A, Peckham P, Keith M. New concepts on treatment of the upper limb in the tetraplegic. Hand Clin 1988; 4:563–574.
7. Freehafer AA, Peckham PH, Keith MW. Determination of muscle–tendon unit properties during tendon transfer. J Hand Surg 1979; 4:331–339.
8. Brys D, Waters R. Effect of triceps function on the brachioradialis transfer in quadriplegia. J Hand Surg 1987; 12A:237–241.
9. Johnson DL, Gellman H, Waters R, et al. Brachioradialis transfer for wrist extension in tetraplegic patients who have fifth-cervical-level neurological function. J Bone Joint Surg 1996; 78A:1063–1067.
10. Waters RL, Grubernick LSI, Gellman H, et al. Electromyographic analysis of brachioradialis to flexor pollicis longus tendon transfer in quadriplegia. J Hand Surg 1990; 15A:335–339.
11. Waters R, Moore K, Graboff S, Paris K, et al. Brachioradialis to flexor pollicis longus transfer for active lateral pinch in tetraplegia. J Hand Surg 1985; 10A:385–391.
12. Deschodt J, Mailhe D, Lubrano J, et al. Anesthesie selective sensitive par péridurale cervicale dans la chirurgie et la rééducation de la main. Ann Chir Main 1988; 7:217–221.
13. Freehafer AA, Peckham PH, Keith MW, et al. The brachioradialis: Anatomy, properties, and value for tendon transfer in the tetraplegic. J Hand Surg 1988; 13:99–104.
14. Hentz V, Chase R. Atlas of Hand Surgery. Philadelphia: Saunders, in press.
15. Moberg E. Surgical treatment for absent single-hand grip and elbow extension in quadriplegia. J Bone Joint Surg 1975; 57A(2):196–206.
16. Keith M, Peckham P, Thrope G, et al. Functional neuromuscular stimulation neuroprosthesis for the tetraplegic hand. Clin Orthop 1987; 233:25–33.
17. McDowell CL. Tendon transfer to augment wrist extension in the tetraplegic patient. Eighteenth Veterans Administration Spinal Cord Injury Conference. 1971:78 (Abstract).
18. Hentz V, Brown M, Keoshian L. Upper limb reconstruction in quadriplegia: functional assessment and proposed treatment modifications. J Hand Surg 1983; 8(2):119–131.
19. Bryan R. The Moberg deltoid–triceps replacement and key-pinch operations in quadriplegia: preliminary experience. Hand 1977; 9(3):207–214.
20. Hiersche D, Waters R. Interphalangeal fixation of the thumb in Moberg's key grip procedure. J Hand Surg 1985; 10A:30–32.
21. Mohammed KD, Rothwell A, Sinclair S et al. Upper-limb surgery for tetraplegia. J Bone Joint Surg 1992; 74B:873–879.
22. Royle N. An operation for paralysis of the intrinsic muscles of the thumb. JAMA 1938; 111:612–615.
23. Thompson T. A modified operation for opponens paralysis. J Bone Joint Surg 1942; 24:632–6.
24. Smith AG. Early complications of key grip hand surgery for tetraplegia. Paraplegia 1981; 19:123–126.
25. Reiser T, Waters R. Long-term follow-up of the Moberg key grip procedure. J Hand Surg 1986; 11A:724–728.
26. Colyer R, Kappelman B. Flexor pollicis longus tenodesis in tetraplegia at the sixth cervical level. J Bone Joint Surg 1981; 63A(3):376–379.
27. Ejeskär A. Upper limb surgical rehabilitation in high-level tetraplegia. In: Tubiana R, ed. Hand Clinics, Vol. 4. 1988:585–599.
28. Lamb DW. Some thoughts on the current state of treatment of the upper limb in traumatic tetraplegia. Ann Chir Main 1984; 3(1):76–80.
29. House JH, Dahl A. One-stage key pinch and release with thumb carpal–metacarpal fusion in tetraplegia. J Hand Surg 1992; 17A:530–538.
30. Ejeskär A, Dahllöf A. Results of reconstructive surgery in the upper limb of tetraplegic patients. Paraplegia 1988; 26:204–208.

13

Functional rehabilitation for the stronger (International Classification Groups 3, 4, and 5) patients

Introduction

The tetraplegic patient who is graded International Classification (IC) Group 3 is characterized by normal brachioradialis (BR) strength, strong wrist extension, with both extensor carpi radialis longus (ECRL) and brevis (ECRB) muscles of Grade 4 or above in the MRC classification. The patient who is graded IC Group 4 has, in addition to BR and both ECRs, a strong pronator teres (PT, Grade 4 or above), and the patient graded IC Group 5 also has a strong flexor carpi radialis (FCR) muscle. We have gathered these three groups of patients into the same chapter because the basic recommendations for surgical rehabilitation are similar, even though there are more surgical options in IC Groups 4 and 5 secondary to the presence of one additional transferable muscle (i.e., the PT).

Evaluation of Group 3–5 patients

Motor evaluation determines the IC group to which each patient or, more precisely, each upper limb of a patient belongs. Determination of IC Group 2 versus 3 solely by manual muscle testing is probably the most challenging aspect of applying the IC system to the tetraplegic population (as emphasized in Chapters 6 and 7). The difficulty lies in assessing the strength of the ECRB in isolation. Moberg[1] stated that the only way to measure it:

'is to explore the tendon under local anesthesia. A straight needle is put through it. Then a cord is attached with a weight suspended over a pulley to the needle, and the power of the muscle is tested.'

He concludes that if the ECRB can lift at least 5 kg (11 lb), then the ECRL can be used for a transfer, that is the patient is classified as IC Group 3. Mohammed *et al.* stresses that when both ECRs are MRC Grade 4 or stronger, the two muscular masses of ECRL and ECRB are visible and separately identifiable just below the elbow.[2] Allieu states that the presence of the PT, even if weak, attests that the two ECR muscles are normal.[3] Practically, it has been our experience that when there is MRC Grade 4+ active wrist extension (i.e., extension against strong but not full resistance), the ECRB is at least MRC Grade 4. This was assessed by testing the residual strength of wrist extension after the ECRL had been transferred for another function. In the past 25 years we have experienced only one exception, a patient classified preoperatively as IC Grade 4 who, following transfer of the ECRL, exhibited only MRC Grade3+ ECRB.

In contrast, for a wrist extension graded only MRC 4 prior to surgery, using the ECRL as a transfer should not be considered:

- if it is easily fatigued (meaning that a Grade 4 level can be demonstrated only a limited number of times on successive testing, after which the muscle fatigues to produce only a Grade 3+ or 3 level); or

- if a Grade 4 can be demonstrated only if the patient is tested in the morning or after a period of muscular rest.

In each case the upper limb is considered as IC Group 2.

Sensory evaluation typically demonstrates two-point discrimination (2PD) less than 10 mm (0.4 inches) in the thumb in all three IC groups, and often in the radial border of the index finger (IC Group 4) and even of the middle finger (IC Group 5). Thus the vast majority of these patients belong to the 'Cu' sensory group (see Chapter 7 for further details).

There is a drastic difference both in presentation and in function between IC Groups 1 and 2 patients and those in IC Groups 3–5. Patients in IC Groups 3–5 have good muscular control of the shoulder girdle, with strong abductor and rotator muscles, and generally good adductor muscles. The triceps may or may not be functioning. In Moberg's experience from examining about 1000 tetraplegic patients, 25% of IC Group 3 patients have useful triceps, although usually less than MRC Grade 4.[1] On the other hand, Zancolli's experience is that the triceps is active if the FCR is active, as the upper extents of their motor columns lie at the same level in the spinal cord.[4] Often, even for cases in which the triceps is very weak, it retains enough activity to prevent the development of an elbow flexion contracture. It is our experience that a triceps graded MRC 1 (i.e., it has only a palpable or visible contraction with no motion) is usually sufficient to prevent the development of an elbow flexion contracture when the therapy is carried out appropriately.

The persistently supinated forearm, which may be present in higher levels, does not occur in these patients, because the PT is usually present, although weak, in IC Group 3 and always strong in IC Groups 4 and 5. Hence, there is no risk of contracture of the interosseous membrane and a full passive range of pronation is present, even in IC Group 3 patients.

The strong active extension of the wrist seen in IC Groups 3 and 4 is unopposed by above anti-gravity wrist flexors, but an extension contracture rarely develops because passive flexion is maintained through gravity and assisted in many IC Group 4 patients by some activity in the FCR, although less than MRC Grade 4. Finger flexion contracture may develop in these patients, since the paralyzed finger flexors are more powerful than the paralyzed ex-

tensors, and more prone to exhibit spasticity. The preoperative management of these patients should include prevention of finger contracture.

By virtue of active wrist extensors, these patients possess many more functional possibilities than do those in IC Groups 1 and 2. During the daytime the wrist does not need the support of a static splint. Active extension of the wrist produces an automatic pinch between the thumb pulp and the radial aspect of the index finger, through the so-called 'tenodesis effect' (see Chapter 9). As a consequence, the patient can grasp a number of light objects such as a telephone, small plastic bottle, or brush. However, this pinch is not strong and does not allow the patient to maintain a grasp of these light objects against resistance or to grip heavy objects. When in bed, active wrist extension helps the patients to lift their bodies out of bed using an overhead frame. When transferring from bed to chair, these patients are able to stabilize the wrist to shift the weight of the body on the closed fist rather than on the hyperextended hand, which protects the tendons and ligament from slackening and consequent instability.

Strong dynamic extension of the wrist makes the use of a manual wheelchair possible. The patient pushes on the wheels with the hypothenar eminence protected by a thick glove. Muscle power transmitted from the shoulder girdle and elbow flexors allows the patient to self-drive the chair on a flat surface and to change directions accurately, provided that both hands are at least IC Group 3.

Goals of surgery

- In IC Group 3 patients active elbow flexion is powered by three strong muscles: the biceps brachii, the brachialis, and the BR. There is also active wrist extension, powered by two strong muscles, the ECRL and ECRB. Therefore two muscles can be spared for transfer to power the fingers and thumb: the BR and one of the ECR muscles.
- In IC Group 4 patients the PT functions and is available for transfer. This brings the number of transferable muscles to three. In this group of patients it is easier to restore three different functions, namely finger flexion, finger extension, and

thumb pinch. Other options have also been advocated, and are reviewed herein.

- In IC Group 5 patients, the FCR also functions. However, this muscle should not be used as a transfer because it stabilizes the wrist and contributes to the tenodesis effect by increasing passive extension of the fingers. Furthermore, active wrist flexion enhances any future tendon transfers to the finger flexors, so bringing greater power to the hand during grasp because it stabilizes the wrist. Surgical procedures in this group parallel those for Group 4, but slightly better results can be expected because the FCR is active.

Resources for tendon transfers

Brachioradialis

The anatomy, physiology, and problems associated with transfer of the BR are discussed at length in Chapter 9. When selecting it as a donor, be aware that this is a very powerful muscle with a defined excursion. In all cases for which a surgical rehabilitation of the hand by BR transfer is planned, the triceps must be evaluated first. If no active elbow extension is present, the use of the BR as a transfer may lead to an unsatisfactory outcome, because the muscle may waste some of its excursion and power in flexing the elbow rather than performing its newly intended function. For patients in whom the triceps is absent or ineffective, it is preferable to first reconstruct active elbow extension so as to stabilize it and thus render the BR transfer optimal. Only Freehafer has reconstructed the hand before elbow extension, and he stated that it makes no difference which is performed first.[5]

Extensor carpi radialis muscles

The ECR muscles are also powerful; although they are not normally as strong as the BR they have greater amplitude, which makes them better suited for transfer to the finger flexors. One of the two muscles is left in place to retain active wrist extension. The choice is to leave the ECRB, because its wrist extensor moment is greater than that of the ECRL. Therefore it produces almost pure wrist extension, whereas ECRL also produces radial deviation.

Pronator teres

The PT is a broad muscle with a short tendon. It is the only pronator muscle in IC Group 4 and 5 patient, as the pronator quadratus is paralyzed. However, it can be transferred and yet retain most of its pronator function if the direction of the transfer does not differ much from its original direction.

Reconstructive controversies

Simple versus complex

With two or three muscles available for transfer, it is possible to be more ambitious, in terms of functional rehabilitation of the hand, in IC Groups 3–5 than in IC Groups 1 and 2 patients. In the past, some surgeons felt that to restore a pinch between the thumb and the index finger was a sufficient goal, whatever the level of injury. They felt it was too complicated, both for the surgeon and for the patient, to restore several different functions at one time.[6] However, after gaining experience and confidence, most authors (including Zancolli,[7] Freehafer et al.,[8] Lamb,[9] Hentz et al.,[10] and Moberg,[1]) became convinced that it was possible to restore both pinch and grasp in these patients following Lipscomb et al.'s earlier suggestion.[11] However, today some authors (e.g., House)[12,13] still prefer not to restore finger flexion in IC Group 3 patients, and instead perform a one-stage key pinch and release procedure.

Finger extension

A related issue was whether or not finger extension should be restored along with finger flexion. Some authors felt that this was too ambitious a goal, and relied on gravity-induced finger extension via the tenodesis effect associated with wrist flexion.[5,9,14] Freehafer recommended sparing the ECRL, retaining it as a wrist extensor, and used only the BR and PT.[5] In his scheme, the BR is transferred to the flexor digitorum profundi (FDPs) of all four fingers. The PT (or the ECRL when the PT is weak) activates the thumb through an opponensplasty derived from Royle[15] and Thompson.[16] For a few patients in whom both the PT and ECRL were considered too weak for a transfer, both the opponensplasty and the flexor tendon transfers were motored with the BR. Lamb[9] uses BR for the thumb flexor pollicis longus (FPL) and ECRL for finger flexors.

Other authors felt it was important to restore finger extension to avoid the risk of a closed-hand posture after restoration of the finger flexors, to avoid loss of the suppleness of the hand, which is so important for human contacts.[1,17] Some authors (e.g., Zancolli)[17] advocate an active restoration of finger extension using the BR, whereas others, including Moberg[1] and House[18] prefer to achieve finger extension through a tenodesis of the finger extensors to the radius. Currently, there is no consensus regarding this issue and both schemes are still advocated. We have often been dissatisfied with the transfer of BR to the finger extensors when FCR is paralyzed (IC Groups 3 and 4), as the lack of anterior wrist stabilization makes this transfer much less effective. We use it only when the FCR is strong (IC Group 5), and we prefer to restore finger extension by passive procedures in IC Groups 3 and 4, saving the BR for a more important purpose. House, who has carried out both procedures on several patients (one on each side), noted that active finger extension provided by the BR in the first method was not subjectively better than the extensor tenodesis in the other method.[18] He currently cannot justify the use of a good motor to restore finger extension.

Thumb flexion

Reconstruction of thumb flexion has generated much controversy. Contemporary surgeons agree that a lateral pinch between the thumb pulp and radial side of the index finger be carried out, but there is no consensus on how to achieve this. Moberg favored a passive tenodesis of FPL to the radius.[19] He was disappointed with the outcome of active transfers (BR to FPL), and stated on several occasions that tenodesis of the FPL to the radius activated by a good wrist extension is stronger and better. He used this tenodesis for thumb flexion, ECRL for finger flexion, and the BR for thumb and finger extension.

Zancolli favors more active procedures in which the FPL is activated either by a supernumerary ECR if present, or by a side-to-side suture between the FPL and ECRB at the distal forearm level.[4] This active tenodesis produces thumb flexion by contraction of the ECRB. An occasional problem after this procedure is a reduction in the range of active dorsi-

flexion of the wrist, probably caused by adhesions of the ECRB to the radial shaft and surrounding tissues.

Other authors have used the BR or the PT, when it is strong enough, to activate the FPL. Still others (e.g., House[18]) have used two simultaneous transfers for the thumb, one for thumb flexion (PT to FPL) and one for thumb adduction–opposition. The latter is achieved with the paralyzed flexor digitorum superficialis (FDS) to the fourth finger, left as an 'in-situ tendon graft', sutured proximally to the BR as an active donor, re-routed around a palmar fascial pulley, and sutured around the metacarpophalangeal (MP) joint of the thumb distally.

Thumb posture

There is also a lack of consensus on how to manage thumb posture, as the thumb can be activated by only one muscle (or possibly two), as opposed to its normal complement of nine or ten. Lacking a normally innervated cone of muscles, the thumb is likely to assume a pathologic posture, especially if the patient's joints are lax (whether naturally or because of repeated passive stretching through poor weight-bearing mechanics), which is likely to impair the quality and strength of the lateral pinch. The thumb needs to be stabilized either by soft tissue procedures (tenodesis) or bony procedures (fusion).

When only the FPL is to be activated, most authors prefer to fuse the thumb's carpometacarpal (CMC) joint, but some prefer stabilization by tenodesis [extensor pollicis longus (EPL) and/or abductor pollicis longus] if the CMC joint retains stability. If both FPL and thumb adduction–opposition are to be restored by tendon transfer, a tenodesis is preferred.[20] Every time the FPL is activated, interphalangeal (IP) joint stabilization is needed. As stated earlier, the preferred procedure is now a 'split' FPL-to-EPL interphalangeal stabilization, rather than an arthrodesis. Less often the MP joint needs stabilization, but if required an arthrodesis[21] or a tenodesis[10,20] can be performed.

Intrinsic substitution

For the nontetraplegic person, the multiple functions of the intrinsic muscles are made more apparent when they no longer function. The strength of grip is weakened considerably. The fingers can no longer be spread apart widely at the MP joint during finger extension. The excursion of the long flexors of the fingers is sufficient to flex all the intervening joints. However, in the absence of the synchronizing effect of the intrinsic muscles the finger tips in full flexion usually touch only to the bases of the fingers, rather than fully into the center of the palm. Digital flexion begins at the distal joint under the influence of the long flexors and the finger tip rolls into flexion, rather than sweeping broadly and expansively along the spiral that the normally innervated finger tip follows. This rolling up of the fingertip tends to push large objects out of the grasp (*Fig. 13.1*).

The second major biomechanical function of the intrinsic muscles is also manifest in their absence. In the normal hand, the extrinsic extensors lift the proximal phalanges into extension, and are assisted in extending the IP joints by the action of the intrinsic muscles. In the absence of intrinsic muscle activity, the action of the extrinsic muscles at the MP joint is unopposed. In hyperextending the MP joint, the extrinsic extensor forfeits the excursion that might allow it to extend the IP joint. Furthermore, this MP hyperextension increases the viscoelastic tone of the long flexors and induces some flexion at the IP joints. This imbalance gives rise to a particular posture termed the 'claw hand', characterized by MP hyperextension and IP joint flexion.

In the majority of tetraplegic patients, the absence of intrinsic muscle function may also result in an imbalance between the paralyzed extrinsic flexors and extensors. The preoperative tetraplegic hand of IC Groups 1–5 possesses only a residual passive tenodesis grasp and release. For these patients, the tendency for the finger to claw as the wrist is flexed may represent only a cosmetic annoyance. However, operative procedures designed to improve digital flexion and extension in IC Groups 3–5 may accentuate the clawed posture by adding tone to both extrinsic extensors and flexors. In this circumstance, the claw deformity frequently becomes a significant functional liability in addition to further detracting from the appearance of the reconstructed hand. The deformity restricts the ability of the hand to open as widely as possible and reduces the range of objects easily grasped.

House has presented convincing evidence that some type of intrinsic substitution results in a better and stronger grasp in the tetraplegic patient who

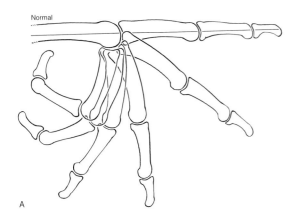

Normal

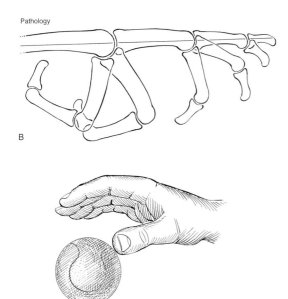

Pathology

Figure 13.1 In the absence of intrinsic function, the fingertips roll up, rather than execute a normal broad sweeping movement. This tends to push large objects out of the grasp. (Used with permission from Hentz and Chase 2001.)[22]

is a candidate for the two-stage grasp–release procedure.[13] Since most tetraplegic patients do not possess sufficient numbers of transferable muscles to allow intrinsic substitution by standard tendon transfer procedures, static procedures must typically suffice. One of two procedures, the first attributed to Zancolli[23] and termed the 'lasso procedure' and the other described by House,[20] may be utilized for the tetraplegic patient.

Zancolli's lasso procedure

In IC Groups 3–5, the FDS muscles are paralyzed, typically at the upper motor neuron level. As such, they retain some stretch reflexes through the intact spinal reflex arc and have relatively normal viscoelastic properties. Zancolli proposed using these paralyzed muscles as an elastic tenodesis to reduce MP joint hyperextension and lessen the clawed posture of the tetraplegic's hand.[23] For each finger that exhibits significantly troublesome clawing, the superficialis tendon is inserted, under some tension, into the flexor sheath at the distal margin of the A1 pulley or even slightly more distally into the proximal part of the A2 pulley. The superficialis tendon is redeployed from its role as the primary flexor of the proximal IP (PIP) joint to become the primary flexor of the MP joint. This achieves the principal goal of surgery, to provide an appropriate balance between the flexor and extensor muscles.

The mechanical basis for this dynamic tenodesis procedure is debated. Zancolli believes that the transfer must be fixed under significant tension to still provide MP flexor tone even with the wrist flexed near maximally. He believes that the transfer may help to initiate some MP flexion as a consequence of wrist extension triggering some reflexive FDS contraction. He believes that this improves the sweep of the digits as they flex by resisting the tendency of the fingers to flex first at the distal IP joint, as illustrated above.

This procedure may be performed as part of either the extensor (release) or flexor (grasp) phase of reconstruction. It is more difficult to judge the appropriate tension of the transfer if it is carried out at the time of the extensor phase. If performed as part of the flexor phase, it is preferable to perform the 'lasso procedure' before the tension of the finger flexor transfer is adjusted.

House's procedure

House's procedure[20] is a modification of Riordan's tenodesis procedure.[24] In the tetraplegic patient, it is frequently performed for only the index and middle fingers, since these fingers are the most critical in grasp-and-release functions, but it can be used for all four fingers also. In this procedure, a free tendon loop is anchored at the level of the head of the metacarpal. The free ends of the tendon graft may be anchored to one of several sites on the extensor mechanism at or proximal to the PIP joint, depending upon the findings of the preoperative examination.

Whether the flexor procedures ('flexor phase') or the extensor ones ('extensor phase') should be performed first is also still unclear. Most authors undertake the extensor phase first, because extensor procedures are easier to re-educate when the strong flexor antagonists are absent. However, the patients must understand that they will not experience any improvement until the flexor phase has been completed, otherwise they are likely to be very disappointed and may even abandon the process. A few authors (e.g., Allieu[25]) prefer to carry out the flexor phase first.

Although a very limited number of muscles are available for transfer, there is a multitude of procedures and possible combinations of the above.

Specific preparation for IC Groups 3–5

With two or three transfers available it is possible not only to restore a key pinch (between the thumb and index finger), but also the grasp and release of fingers. Therefore, the main goal of the preoperative management of the upper limb is to prevent deformities and keep all the joints supple. This is a departure from the classic recommendations that arose when reconstructive surgery of the fingers was performed infrequently (or not even available for these patients). Previously, it was considered too ambitious to restore both types of grip (pinch and grasp), so a number of authors focused on restoration of the lateral thumb-to-index (key) pinch. For this pinch to be effective, the index (and middle finger) has to assume a rather flexed position, so that the pinch is stable and the thumb does not tend to escape under the index finger. Therefore the previous therapy recommendations (see Chapter 4) included allowing the fingers to 'stiffen' somewhat. They were splinted in a position that favored a tightening of the flexor tendons, and passive range exercises were performed with this goal in mind.

More recent interest in and acceptance of the benefits of surgical procedures have led many rehabilitation teams to reassess the goals of early splinting and therapy in these patients. The main goal for IC Groups 3 and above should be to keep all the joints of the hand absolutely supple, and to maintain a normal balance between the paralyzed flexors and extensor tendons. This is achieved by passive mobilization of the joints through their entire range and by splinting, both static and dynamic, as required according to existing or potential contractures.

Another goal is to teach the patients, prior to surgery, how to protect their hands so as not to compromise the results of surgical procedures. This is especially true of passive tenodeses, which slacken with time if submitted to regular overstretching. Often these patients are taught initially to perform transfers by using the flattened palm of their hand to support their body's weight on the fully extended wrist. In this position the thumb is in retropulsion and the fingers usually hyperextended at the MP joint. This may be stable, but it does endanger tendon transfers to the thumb and digits flexors, and predictably elongates intrinsic reconstruction procedures (see below).

Therefore, patients must be taught more protective methods of transfers. One method is to roll the fingers into near-full flexion, as in forming a closed fist, and then using the dorsal surface of the flexed proximal phalanges as the platform for weight-bearing (see *Fig. 4.6B*). Another method, less protective but still better than a flat hand transfer, is to roll the fingers into flexion and use the dorsal surface of the middle and terminal phalanges and the proximal palm as a platform, with the wrist hyperextended (see *Fig. 4.6C*).

Preferred procedures

Our surgical options for IC Groups 3–5 patients have evolved over the years. In our experience some procedures have worked better than others, some have proved unnecessary, and some are mandatory. Also, some patients did not want or require sophisticated

procedures and were treated by simpler methods (e.g., usually restoration of pinch only). Finally, each patient is different both in terms of presentation and needs, so the surgical goals are adapted according to these parameters. There is no such thing as a 'standard procedure' for a specific group of patients; several options are usually discussed with the patient and the final surgical plan is matched to the patient's unique presentation and specific requirements.

Generally speaking, for patients in all three groups we plan to restore both key pinch and digital grasp-and-release, usually in two stages with the extensor phase first and the flexor phase second. Each stage requires 4 weeks of postoperative immobilization followed by physical therapy for 6–8 weeks. Therefore, the treatment of one hand is usually completed in 6 months (provided the triceps does not need prior surgical rehabilitation). The patient must be told that the first operative step does not bring any functional improvement, and that the result is achieved only after the second step.

IC Group 3

A two-stage reconstruction is performed. The first phase, referred to as the 'extensor phase', focuses on rehabilitation of the extensor tendons and includes:

- passive tenodesis of the extensor tendons of the fingers [extensor digitorum communis (EDC)] and of the thumb (EPL);
- thumb CMC joint arthrodesis; and
- intrinsic tenodesis (lasso or House procedure).

The second phase, centered on activation of the flexor tendons to the thumb (FPL) and fingers (FDP), is termed the 'flexor phase', and includes:

- transfer of the ECRL to the finger flexors;
- transfer of the BR to FPL;
- 'split' FPL-to-EPL stabilization of the thumb IP joint; and
- if there is an accessory ECR muscle, transfer it to the FPL and use the BR for another function.

Extensor phase

The whole antebrachial part of the procedure is performed through a single longitudinal incision on the lateral aspect of the forearm, running from mid-forearm down to the wrist crease, and prolonged as needed for thumb procedures. The same incision is used again during the second phase. Alternatively, multiple incisions may be used over each operative site (volar forearm, dorsal forearm, and CMC joint). The operative steps are given next in our preferred sequence.

Examine for supernumerary extensor carpi radialis muscle

The first step of the procedure is to check the dorsal wrist and forearm for the presence of a super-numerary ECR muscle. Two types of accessory tendons may be found: accessory tendinous bands, which arise from the muscular belly of either ECR, and supernumerary muscles, which have a separate muscular belly and are usually found between the bellies of the two ECR muscles (*Fig. 13.2*). We use only supernumerary muscles for transfer, as they can provide an independent function, whereas access-ory tendinous bands work simultaneously with ex-tension of the wrist. The presence and size of a supernumerary muscle is evaluated and noted in the operative report. If the muscle is of a large enough size it will be used as a transfer, usually to the FPL during the second phase. In this particular circum-stance, we may consider using the BR to activate the finger and thumb extensors during the first phase. This possibility requires that the presence and evalu-ation of a useful supernumerary muscle be performed at the beginning of the procedure.

Tenodesis of extensor tendons to radius (absence of supernumerary extensor carpi radialis)

The tendons of the EDC and EPL are dissected proximal the dorsal retinaculum, sutured together side-to-side in the appropriate digital balance with a few transfixing stitches, and then severed proximal to the suture.

Next the dorsal aspect of the radius is exposed under the severed tendons and a dorsal 15 × 15 mm (0.6 × 0.6 inches) cortical window is created with a power saw, 5–7 cm (2–2.7 inches) proximal to the wrist level. Two small holes are drilled in the radius, 1 cm (0.38 inches) proximal to the cortical window (*Fig. 13.3*). A small bone curette is used to excavate the cancellous bone underneath the window and create a channel toward the two proximal holes.

A heavy, braided nonabsorbable suture is intro-duced through one proximal hole into the cortical window, strongly fixed to the mass of the extensor tendons, and drawn back through the second proxi-mal hole. By pulling on the two ends of the suture, the tendons are progressively drawn into the window. The tension is adjusted by passive maneuvers of the wrist, and the suture is finally tied over the dorsal cortex. Tension must be such that the fingers fully extend at the MP joint when the wrist reaches 30° of flexion.

Occasionally, the contribution of the EDC to the little finger is very small and ineffective as an exten-sor. In such cases, tenodesis of the common extensor does not lead to extension of the little finger. If the fifth finger extension lags on testing, it is necessary to add the extensor digiti minimi tendon to the other

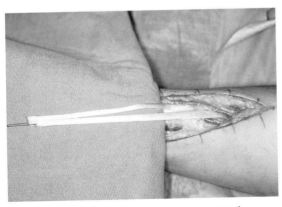

Figure 13.2 A supernumerary extensor carpi radialis muscle, harvested with extensor carpi radialis longus.

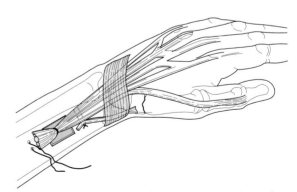

Figure 13.3 Dorsal radial window and additional proximal holes for extensor tenodesis.

tendons. This step is not routinely recommended because of the risk that the little finger will extend excessively.

Alternatively, the technique described by House may be used.[20] The plane of dissection is between the digital extensors and the two radial wrist extensors (ECRL and ECRB). By retracting the digital extensors ulnarward and the wrist extensors radially, the periostium of the distal radius is visualized. A 2 × 2 cm (0.8 × 0.8 inches) area of radius is exposed in this manner:

A fine drill point (1.1 mm) is used to pre-drill a pattern into the radius as illustrated in *Fig. 13.4A*. It is useful to take the time to drill many small holes so that the next step, elevating the C-shaped piece of dorsal cortex, can be achieved without fracturing the square-shaped ledge of bone that must remain intact. Once the holes are drilled, a fine, narrow, sharp osteotome is used to connect the holes (every effort is made to avoid fracture to the remaining bony ledge). The C-shaped bone plug is lifted out. Next, a small bone curette is used to excavate the cancellous bone and deepen the channel in the radius in preparation for placing the combined extensor tendons into the channel. Again, care is taken not to fracture the bone ledge as the cancellous bone is excavated. The several slips of EDC tendons are slid into the channel in the radius and wedged under the bony ledge. It is useful to pass a fine 0.035 Kirschner wire shallowly across the dorsal gap to help retain the tendon slips within the bone channel (*Fig. 13.4B*). The wrist is then maneuvered in flexion and extension and the appropriateness of the tension of the tenodesis is judged. If necessary, a side-to-side mattress suture is used to adjust the tension of the extensor tendons relative to one another, as illustrated in *Figure 13.4B*. This may be necessary if one or another slip of the extensor digitorum tendon becomes overstretched and if the normal cascade of the digits is lost.

Alternatively, the tendon of the EPL may be tenodesed separately, around its dorsal compartment (see 'Alternative procedures' for details).

Arthrodesis of the thumb carpometacarpal joint

The longitudinal antebrachial incision is prolonged distally, or a second incision is made. The radial artery is identified and protected, the capsule of the CMC joint is exposed, and entered longitudinally. The

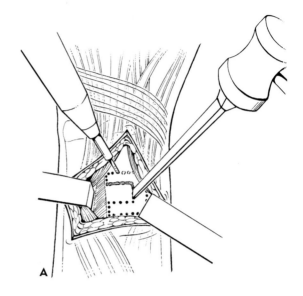

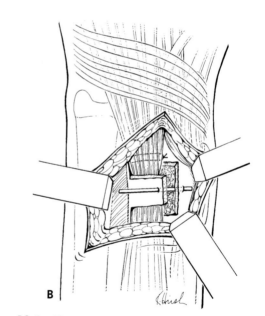

Figure 13.4 Elevating the C-shaped piece of dorsal cortex: pre-drilling of the pattern. (A) The slips of the extensor digitorum communis tendons are slid into the channel under the bony ledge. (B) A Kirschner wire helps retain the tendon slips within the bone channel. (Used with permission from Hentz and Chase 2001.)[22]

A
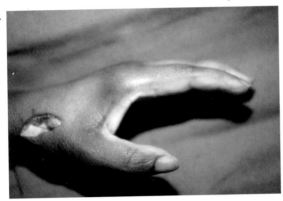

B
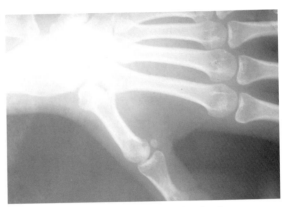

Figure 13.5 The carpometacarpal joint is fused (A) in 30° of radial abduction and (B) in 20° of palmar abduction (anteposition).

trapezial and metacarpal articular surfaces are exposed, and the cartilage of both is removed with a rongeur. Only the cartilage is removed, with care taken to keep the whole bone stock. This allows choice of the exact position in which the joint will be fixed by moving the joint around until the desired position is obtained. The joint is temporarily fixed with two Kirschner wires, and the position of the thumb evaluated throughout the whole passive range of flexion–extension of the wrist. The usual position in which the CMC joint is arthrodesed is on average at 25–30° of antepulsion and 30° of abduction (*Fig. 13.5*). However, this position is subject to modifications according to the length of the thumb and the suppleness (laxity) of the surrounding joints of the thumb and index finger, bearing in mind that the final objective is to position the pulp of the thumb facing the radial aspect of the index finger at the level of the PIP joint or distal part of proximal phalanx.

Several methods of fixation have been employed. We currently favor fixation with two or three pneumatic staples or a rectangular mini-plate (*Fig. 13.6*). This provides a strong fixation that does not require an additional period of immobilization and avoids fixation removal.

For cases in which the CMC joint is spontaneously stable, the decision may be not to fuse it. Additional tenodeses are needed in these cases to keep the thumb abducted (see 'Alternative procedures' below).

Intrinsic tenodesis

In the nontetraplegic patient, many procedures have been described to restore intrinsic balance. The tetraplegic patients who belong to IC Groups 3–5 do not possess enough transferable muscles to use these standard tendon-transfer procedures. Two passive procedures may be utilized in these patients, the 'lasso procedure' attributed to Zancolli[23] and the intrinsic tenodesis described by House.[20]

Indications

The 'lasso procedure' is indicated when tension on the digital extensors results in a good extension of the PIP joints, provided that the MP joints are not allowed to hyperextend. House's procedure is indicated when this maneuver does not effect good extension of the PIP joints. This shows that the extensor mechanism over the joint has elongated and, in this case, the lasso procedure will restrain MP joint hyperextension (prevent clawing), but will not augment IP extension.

Lasso procedure

A variety of palmar incisions may be utilized. We have used either a single longitudinal incision in or just distal to the distal palmar crease, or four longitudinal incisions centered over the midline of each finger, and extending from just distal to the proximal digital flexor crease to just proximal to the distal palmar crease.

All digital neurovascular bundles are identified and protected. The flexor sheath is cleared of the surrounding fat and fascial fibers. The proximal edge of the A1 pulley and the interval between the A1 and A2 pulleys are located. The proximal third of the A2 pulley is opened via a short L-shaped or diagonal incision (*Fig. 13.7A*).

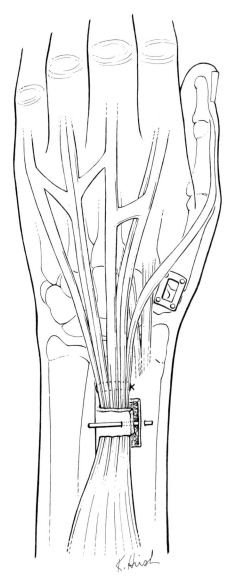

Figure 13.6 Carpometacarpal joint fusion with a rectangular plate. (Used with permission from Hentz and Chase 2001.)[22]

Next the flexor superficialis is identified. With the digit fully extended, it is superficial to the profundus tendon between the A1 and A2 pulleys. More than likely, it will have begun to decussate into two distinct tendon slips. The profundus tendon frequently exhibits a central raphe, which might be mistaken for decussation of the superficialis. One certain method to determine the identity of the tendon is to slide a small probe under the tendon slips and apply tension.

The distal IP joint should not flex, but if it does the probe has picked up the profundus tendon (*Fig. 13.7B*).

Once the superficialis tendon is identified, the first of its two tails is pulled proximally. It is sharply divided and the cut end secured with a small hemostat. The second tail is then retracted, divided, and secured within the jaws of the clamp (*Fig. 13.7C*). The divided superficialis tendon is pulled proximally around the distal margin of the A1 pulley and reflected over itself under tension. Zancolli advocated setting the tension by putting the involved finger in full extension, and pulling the FDS proximally with maximum strength. For the tetraplegic patient, we prefer to adjust the tension so that, with the wrist in neutral, the MP joint is held in about 50° of flexion. Over the years we have tended to make this tension tighter and tighter. The suture is then performed, either by weaving the two slips of the superficialis through the substance of the superficialis tendon proximal to the A1 pulley (*Fig. 13.7D*), or by suturing the tendon to itself with two stitches and to the A1 pulley with one stitch. A secure juncture using a braided synthetic nonabsorbable suture is vitally important. Equally important is to leave the flexor profundi undisturbed throughout the whole procedure so as to avoid adhesions being created between the two tendons. When multiple digits are to be rebalanced, tension of the transfer to the ulnar digits is set differently in the tetraplegic patient than in the normal hand. Normally, the goal is to recreate the normal flexor cascade by attaching the transfer more tightly to the ulnar digits than to the radial ones. This sequence is best reversed in the tetraplegic hand.

The skin is then closed with interrupted skin sutures and the MP joints are fully flexed. This tenodesis is subject to slackening if passive MP joint hyperextension is exerted inadvertently. It must therefore be protected during the rest of the procedure, as well as postoperatively.

House procedure (modified)

This procedure is often performed for only the index and middle fingers. For the two adjacent fingers, three small skin incisions are outlined, the first, a transverse incision located just proximal to the MP joint of the middle finger, and the remaining incision made over the PIP joints of the adjacent fingers (*Fig. 13.8A*). Through the proximal incision, the tendon of the

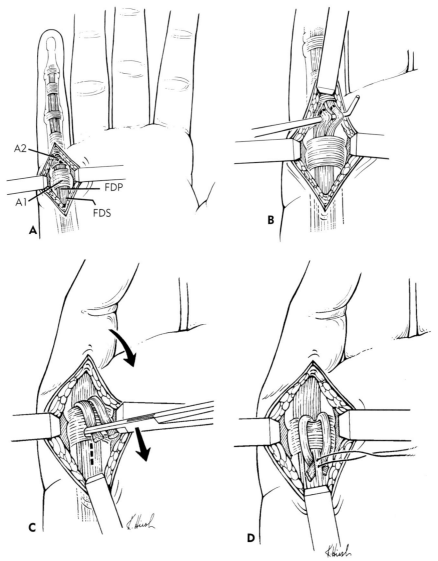

Figure 13.7 The Zancolli 'lasso' procedure (see text for details). (Used with permission from Hentz and Chase 2001.)[22]

extensor communis is exposed; through the distal incisions, the base of the middle phalanx is exposed.

The length of tendon graft needed is estimated using a heavy suture placed along the proposed course of the tendon graft. Several centimeters are added as a safety measure. A tendon graft may be obtained from the plantaris tendon, the tendon of the palmaris longus, or a strip of fascia lata.

The tendon graft is passed under the extensor digitorum tendon at the level of the metacarpal neck. By fully flexing the metacarpal, a small straight hemo-

stat or a tendon-passing forceps is gently twisted so that it passes palmar to the intermetacarpal ligament and along the course of the intrinsic muscles, to exit in the dorsal digital incision. A heavy suture is grasped within the jaws of the tendon-passing forceps and pulled proximally. The distal end of the suture is grasped with the tendon-passing forceps and, with a firm pull on the proximal end of the suture, the forceps is brought from distal to proximal into the proximal wound. The tendon is grasped and pulled distally to emerge in the distal incision site

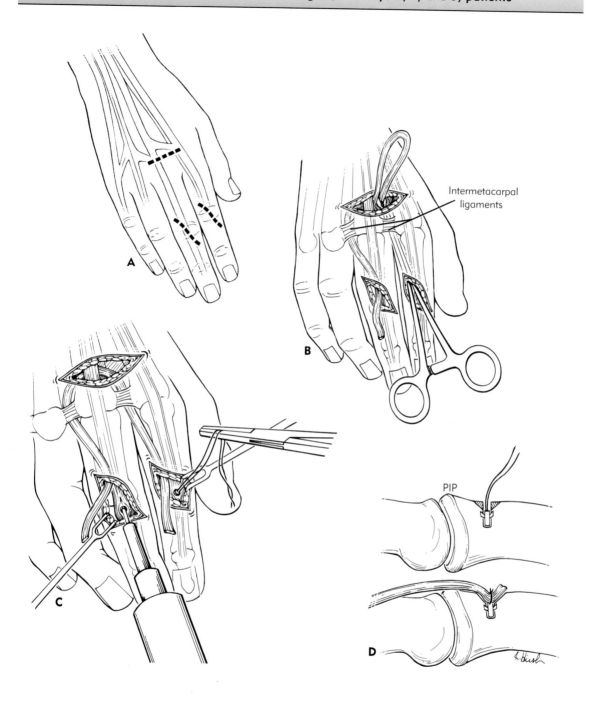

Figure 13.8(A–D) The intrinsic substitution, modified from House (see text for details). (Used with permission from Hentz and Chase 2001.)[22]

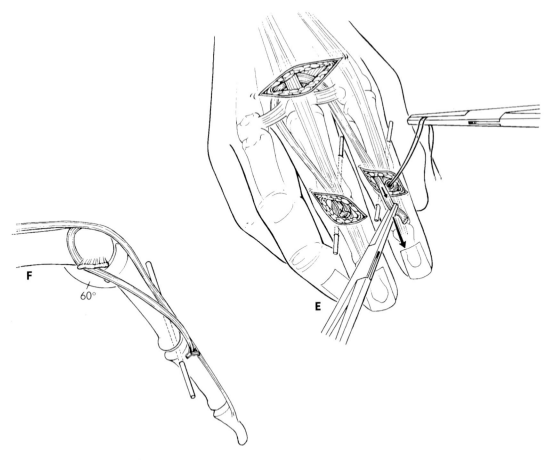

Figure 13.8(E–F) (continued)

(*Fig. 13.8B*). This maneuver is carried out on the ulnar aspect of the index finger. A scalpel is used to make a longitudinal incision into the extensor tendon at the base of the middle phalanx. A small opening is made in the periostium.

A suture anchor is used to fix the tendon graft to the bone at the base of the middle phalanx. An appropriately sized drill is used to create a hole in the bone (*Fig. 13.8C*). A 3–0 absorbable suture is threaded on to the suture anchor in place of the heavier nonabsorbable suture that comes already mounted on the disposable plunger device. The anchor is forced into the bone channel (*Fig. 13.8D*) and its security is tested by pulling on the attached suture.

A 0.035 Kirschner wire is passed across the PIP joint at this point. The wire holds the joint in near-full extension. The middle finger anchor suture is tied securely around the tendon graft. The tail of the

tendon graft is further fixed into the dorsal extensor mechanism with additional absorbable sutures. With the wrist held in a neutral posture, the opposite end of the tendon graft to be anchored into the index finger is pulled sufficiently tight to bring both the index and middle finger MP joints into about 45° of flexion (*Fig. 13.8E*). The middle finger is then pushed into slightly more flexion than the index (in an attempt to restore a more normal flexor cascade to the fingers), the tension on the tendon graft adjusted, and the final tendon anchor suture tied around the tendon graft.

The wrist is flexed gently to ensure that the MP joints do not fully extend, but are instead checkreined by the tenodesis. If the tendon graft is too attached loosely, the MP joints will fully extend. The tension of the tendon graft must keep these MP joints somewhat flexed even with the wrist fully extended.

The skin incisions are closed and the tenodesis relaxed somewhat by further flexing the MCP joints to about 60° of flexion (*Fig. 13.8F*) this posture is maintained using a dorsal plaster slab. The wrist is splinted in a neutral position, although the position of immobilization varies according to the other procedures that have been performed.

Wound closure and immobilization

At the end of this first surgical step, the wound is closed in layers over a suction drain. Absorbable sutures are used for skin sutures. The forearm and hand are then immobilized in a well-padded cast with the wrist in 45° of extension, the fingers in 60° of MP joint flexion and full extension of the IP joints of the fingers, and the thumb in the arthrodesed position with its two distal joints extended.

The thick padding we employ to protect these patients' insensate skin has resulted in some occasional sliding of the hand in the cast, which has caused the MP joints to become extended in a few cases. We now remove the first cast after a few days (within the first week), inspect the wound, and apply a second cast (usually fiberglass or plastic), tightly molded over the flexed MP joints of the fingers.

Postoperative rehabilitation

The cast is removed after 4 weeks. Postoperative rehabilitation is straightforward after this extensor phase, because only passive procedures have been performed.

If a lasso procedure was performed, a light dorsal blocking splint is applied (*Fig. 13.9*) to maintain the

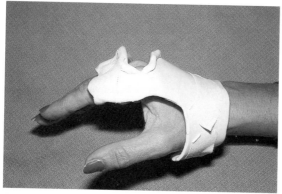

Figure 13.9   Dorsal blocking splint protects the intrinsic tenodesis.

MP joints in 60° of flexion. The MP and IP joints are gently mobilized into flexion by passive exercises, but at no time are the MP joints passively extended. The splint is worn continuously and is removed only during therapy sessions. Some of our early lasso procedures have slackened within the first few months postoperatively, so we have increased the duration of splint wear to several months, and even into the second operative phase as the splint does not interfere with either the surgery or therapy associated with the second phase.

If a House intrinsic procedure was performed, the Kirschner wires placed across the IP joints are removed at the time of cast removal. The tendon attachments need a minimum of 8 weeks of protection against stress. A dorsal blocking splint that prevents the MCP joints from fully extending is fitted and the patient begins gentle exercises to remobilize the IP joints. Once good PIP joint flexibility is restored, the blocking splint can be removed and the patient encouraged to gently extend the MP joints by passive wrist flexion exercises. The rehabilitation for this procedure must be carried out in a nonaggressive fashion to avoid overstretching the tenodesis.

Fusion of the CMC joint of the thumb is monitored with regular radiographs. It is usually sound by the time the patient is ready for the second phase, and if temporary removable fixations have been used, they are removed at this time.

The second operative step can be performed when the joints have recovered full passive motion, particularly wrist flexion (for otherwise the finger extensors' tenodesis will be ineffective). The only joints for which passive motion is not encouraged are the thumb's CMC joint, which underwent arthrodesis, and extension of the fingers' MP joints if an intrinsic substitution procedure has been performed. Active muscles must also be exercised back to their preoperative strength, especially those that are to be transferred during the second phase, namely the BR and ECRL. These muscles may have lost part of their strength because of disuse during cast immobilization, but it is mandatory that they be at their MRC initial grading before proceeding to the next phase.

Flexor phase

The flexor phase consists in activating the finger FDPs and the thumb flexor (FPL). In IC Group 3, as well as

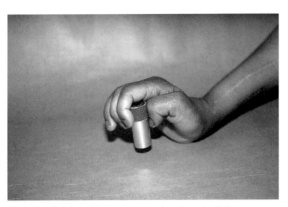

Figure 13.10 Clinical example of a pinch between the dorsal aspect of the thumb and the volar aspect of the index finger, caused by hyperflexion of the thumb interphalangeal joint.

in Groups 4 and 5, transfer of the ECRL activates the FDPs. The FPL activation is different in IC Group 3 than in Groups 4 and 5. If a supernumerary ECR muscle is available for transfer, it is employed to activate FPL. Otherwise, the BR is used for this transfer. No matter which donor muscle is utilized, the thumb IP joint needs stabilization, because the unopposed action of the new flexor tends to cause the IP joint to assume a permanently flexed position, which further increases during active flexion of the thumb. This often limits the lateral pinch, as the flexed thumb is likely to miss the lateral aspect of the index finger and to come beneath the index during an attempted pinch. This results in a pinch posture between the dorsal aspect of the thumb distal phalanx and the volar aspect of the index middle phalanx (*Fig. 13.10*), which is far less functional. Rather than performing a permanent bony fixation of the IP joint, as advocated by Moberg,[6] or a conventional arthrodesis, we adopt the procedure described by Mohammed *et al.*,[2] which is to transfer the distal radial half of the FPL to the EPL just proximal to the IP joint. This procedure, termed the 'split FPL transfer', preserves some IP joint movement while stabilizing the IP joint (see Fig. 12.9).

If no supernumerary transferable ECR is present, the operative steps include:

- transfer of the ECRL to the fingers flexors (FDP); and
- transfer of the BR to the thumb flexor (FPL).

Surgical exposure

Surgery is performed through the same incision as used in the extensor phase, prolonged proximally over the prominence of the BR muscle belly, almost up to the elbow flexor crease. Rather than complete each procedure sequentially, we dissect all the donor muscles, perform the accessory procedures such as IP joint stabilization, and then suture all transferred muscles. This allows us to set the tension of each transfer more accurately, as all the digits now rest in their appropriate pre-set position.

First the BR is dissected in the manner described in detail in Chapter 9. A heavy suture is looped through the terminal part of its tendon for further manipulations, and the muscle–tendon unit is protected and kept moistened with wet gauze throughout the rest of the procedure.

Next the ECRL is dissected (*Fig. 13.11A*). Its tendon is exposed distal to the dorsal retinacular ligament. The terminal tendon of the ECRB is identified, usually 1–2 cm (0.4–0.8 inches) ulnar to the ECRL, with the intertendinous space shaped as a triangle with a proximal apex. However, occasionally it lies close to the ECRL and can be misinterpreted as part of the terminal tendon of the ECRL. Once ECRB has been identified, the terminal tendon of the ECRL is severed as distally as possible, retracted proximal to the dorsal retinaculum, and dissected from distal to proximal. Its tendon lies radial to the tendon of ECRB and then progressively becomes dorsal, and its muscle belly lies superficial to that of the ECRB. The muscle is dissected free from its investing fascia, as far proximal as its main neurovascular bundle, to gain maximal tendon excursion. A suture is looped through its terminal tendon, and the muscle tendon unit is kept moist for the rest of the procedure.

Stabilization of the thumb interphalangeal joint

We prefer the 'split' FPL–EPL procedure described in detail in Chapter 12. We usually perform this procedure through a single longitudinal incision that runs on the radial aspect of the thumb. An oblique transarticular Kirschner wire maintains the IP joint in a neutral position. We usually leave the distal end of the Kirschner wire protruding through the skin and protected with a plastic pin cover. Either it is removed at 1 month (at the same time as the cast) and replaced by a light IP protection splint for a further month or it is removed at 2 months postoperatively.

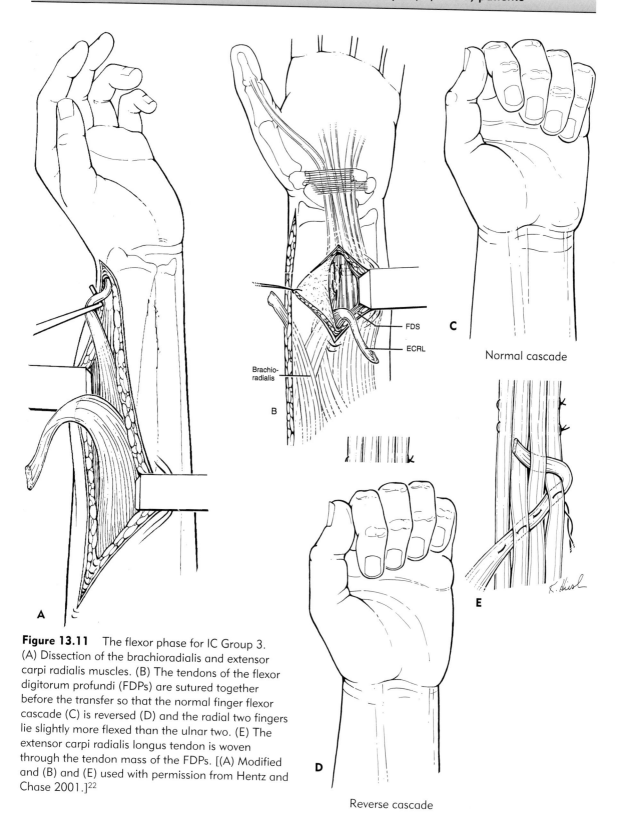

A

B

Brachio-
radialis

FDS

ECRL

C

Normal cascade

D

E

Reverse cascade

Figure 13.11 The flexor phase for IC Group 3. (A) Dissection of the brachioradialis and extensor carpi radialis muscles. (B) The tendons of the flexor digitorum profundi (FDPs) are sutured together before the transfer so that the normal finger flexor cascade (C) is reversed (D) and the radial two fingers lie slightly more flexed than the ulnar two. (E) The extensor carpi radialis longus tendon is woven through the tendon mass of the FDPs. [(A) Modified and (B) and (E) used with permission from Hentz and Chase 2001.][22]

Transfer of extensor carpi radialis longus and brachioradialis

Next the donor muscles are transferred to the recipients. The volar aspect of the forearm is approached, deep to the radial vascular bundle and the FCR. The FDPs are identified in the distal third of the forearm. Their tendons all lie in the same plane, well separated from the superficialis tendons. The tendons of all the FDPs are sutured together with a strong suture that runs obliquely to set more tension on the radial fingers than on the ulnar ones (*Fig. 13.11B*). This pre-positions the fingers in greater flexion at the radial fingers, a position that has been termed the 'reverse cascade' in reference to the normal physiological cascade of the fingers at rest (*Figs 13.11C* and *13.11D*). Some authors advise, at this stage, that the peritenon be stripped from the profundi tendons to favor intratendinous adhesions.

The ECRL is then passed palmarward in preparation for transfer to the FDPs. Rather than passing the donor tendon through each individual profundus tendon, the transfer is woven back and forth through the now combined tendons of the FDP. Multiple non-absorbable sutures are used to anchor the donor and recipient tendons together (*Fig. 13.11E*). Tension of the transfer is set with the wrist in a neutral position, such that the little finger remains in the normal resting posture, and flexion increases for each finger from ulnar to radial, displaying the reverse cascade described above. Some authors advise not to include the FDP to the little finger in the transfer, because they fear the little finger will assume a permanent hooked position. Instead, they prefer to rely on the tendinous connections between flexors to the ring and little fingers to ensure a weaker flexion of the little finger.

Finally, the BR is transferred to the FPL. After the former has been properly dissected, its tendon achieves a passive stretch excursion of 3–5 cm (1.2–2 inches). The tendon is passed palmarward toward the tendon of the FPL. This tendon may be short, in which case the BR must be inserted as proximally as possible in the FPL tendon so as to be able to interweave these two tendons once or twice.

Setting the tension of this particular transfer is probably one of the most critical elements of all the transfers in tetraplegia. If the tension is too tight, it prevents an adequate opening of the first web even with the wrist fully flexed. When the patient tries to pinch, the thumb contacts the index finger very early during wrist extension, which makes it difficult to obtain and hold larger objects. If the tension is not tight enough, the results are worse:

- either the tension is too loose for the thumb pulp to contact the index (even with a fully extended wrist) and the patient can seize large objects only; or
- the tension is a little tighter so the thumb reaches the lateral side of the index finger, but with no strength because the transferred tendon is at the maximum of its course, and thus the patient cannot hold small objects with any strength.

The appropriate tension to be given to the transfer depends upon:

- maximal amplitude of the BR, once freed from its surrounding fascia – tension should be less if the tendon's excursion is short;
- angle of radial abduction of the fused CMC joint – tension should be less if the thumb is less abducted, and more if the thumb is more abducted; and
- position of the elbow and the wrist at the time of the suture – if the tension is set with the elbow slightly flexed (40°) and the wrist in a neutral position, lateral pinch gains extra strength when the patients actively extend their elbow and his wrist.

We perform the suture in the position described above for the elbow and wrist. A first suture is inserted, all the clamps and retractors are removed from the wound, and the position of the thumb is tested through the whole range of wrist passive motion. The tension is then readjusted accordingly.

Wound closure and immobilization

The wounds are irrigated and then closed in layers over a suction drain in the antebrachial incision. A well-padded cast is applied below the elbow, maintaining the wrist in slight flexion, and for the whole length of the fingers and thumb, which are slightly more flexed than their spontaneous resting position. The pin that protrudes from the thumb IP joint is protected. As the elbow is left free, the patient and his or her attendants (including family members) must be instructed carefully to avoid strong contraction of the BR during the first 4 weeks. This is particularly important for those patients who are used to lifting their body by contracting their elbow flexors. Fearing such ruptures, some authors recommend immobilizing the elbow after transfer of the BR. However, this does not prevent inadvertent static contraction of the muscle. So even if their elbow is immobilized, patients must also be taught to avoid contracting the BR during this period.

Postoperative care

The cast is removed after 4 weeks and the patient begins to exercise his or her transfers with the therapist. The Kirschner wire in the thumb is usually left in place for 4 more weeks. Only active flexion of the fingers and thumb is encouraged for the first 2 weeks, then resisted flexion is progressively initiated, and active and passive extension are reinitialized. In our experience, it has been easier to re-educate the BR as a thumb flexor than as a finger extensor. However, for cases in which the BR fails to work in isolation and achieve its new function, it may be helpful to train it through myo-feedback, and to immobilize the elbow in 90° flexion during rehabilitation sessions.

It is important to protect the sutures against large forces for an additional 4 weeks after removal of the cast, and the patient should preferably use an electric wheelchair for this period. Also during this period, transfers and pressure relief should be restricted.

Flexor phase with a transferable accessory extensor carpi radialis muscle present

In this situation, which we have encountered six times, the accessory muscle is transferred to the FPL. Along with other authors,[12,17] we have been satisfied with the result of this transfer, which functioned as well as other motors. The BR is then available for another function. We have used it to restore active extension of the fingers, but this procedure has not been reliable in IC Group 3 patients. Perhaps the absence of a volar wrist stabilization, secondary to paralysis of the FCR, greatly reduces the efficiency of this transfer. Instead, we now tend to use the BR to restore active wrist flexion by transferring it to the FCR. The goal of this procedure is to increase finger opening through the tenodesis effect. We use it more specifically in those patients whose finger opening is not yet sufficient after the extensor phase. Otherwise, we may decide not to use the BR and save it for some other potential function at a latter stage, depending on the functional results and the patient's needs.

Surgical options in IC Groups 4 and 5

In IC Group 4 the PT is strong and available for transfer. In IC Group 5 the FCR is strong, but experience has shown that it should not be used as a transfer. Therefore, the surgical options are similar for both IC Groups 4 and 5.

The PT is the only functioning pronator muscle in these IC Group 4 and 5 patients. However, it can be transferred and yet retain most of its pronator function if the direction of the transfer does not differ much from its original direction. In this respect, it can be safely used to activate the FPL, in which case the BR is available for another function. As stated above, it can be transferred to the finger extensors provided there is enough volar stabilization of the wrist. This is achieved if FCR is MRC 3 Grade or above, otherwise the results of the transfers may be unpredictable.

Other options include fusing or leaving flexible the thumb's CMC joint and options regarding the number of transfers to strengthen the thumb function, typically carried out during the flexor phase.

Surgery is performed in two stages, as in IC Group 3, with the extensor phase performed first, and then the flexor phase.

Extensor phase

If the FCR is weak (less than MRC Grade 3, usually an IC 4 arm), the extensor phase is identical to that for Group 3 patients:

- tenodesis of the EDC and EPL to the radius;
- thumb CMC joint fusion; and
- intrinsic procedure (lasso or House) preferably on all four fingers.

If the FCR is MRC Grade 3 and above (typically an IC 4 or 5 arm), the BR can be used to activate the fingers and thumb extensors. The procedure then includes:

- transfer of the BR to EDC and EPL;
- thumb CMC joint fusion; and
- intrinsic procedure.

Brachioradialis to extensor digitorum communis and extensor pollicis longus

After fusion of the thumb's CMC joint as described for IC Group 3, the extensor tendons are exposed proximal to the dorsal retinaculum. The overlying fascia and the most proximal part of the retinaculum are widely excised. The tendon slips of the EDC are sutured together with a heavy suture that runs back and forth, and to the tendon of the EPL. Tension on the tendon of the EPL is individually adjusted, and then the BR is dissected and transferred to the extensors. The details of BR dissection are discussed in Chapter 12. Rather than passing the tendon of the BR through each individual EDC tendon slip, it is buried in the middle of the tendinous mass and sutured to it with two or three strong horizontal mattress sutures (*Fig. 13.12*). This makes tension adjustment easier.

Tension is set with the elbow in 40° flexion, the wrist in a neutral position, and the MP joint in about 20° of flexion. Tension should be such that, during passive flexion of the wrist, the MP joints start to extend when the wrist reaches neutral from an extended position. The tension on the EPL tendon should be adjusted last and its tension is typically set slightly looser than that of the EDC. The fingers should exhibit full passive flexion when the wrist is fully extended.

Associated procedures are performed as in IC Group 3 – stabilization of the thumb with CMC joint fusion (or abduction tenodesis if the joint is stable) and intrinsic tenodesis (lasso or House procedure).

Postoperative immobilization and rehabilitation

Postoperative immobilization requires some thought if the extensor phase includes an active extensor transfer and an intrinsic substitution procedure (lasso or House), because the typical position of immobilization for one procedure may compromise the other.

For example, the wrist and MP joints should be extended to relieve tension on the suture of the BR to the EDC, but they should be flexed to protect the lasso procedure. A mid-position is thus required, with the wrist in 30° of extension, the thumb fully extended at the MP joint, and the finger MP joints flexed to 60°.

After 4 weeks the cast is removed and rehabilitation is initiated. This phase is a challenging one, as again the goals sought seem to be irreconcilable. Rehabilitation of active finger extensors is directed toward developing active extension of the MP joints, whereas protection of the intrinsic substitution procedure precludes early or vigorous MP joint extension. As a result of this apparent antagonism, some authors prefer to perform the intrinsic substitution procedure during the second operative step. However, the problem is usually satisfactorily addressed if the therapist prevents full extension of the patient's MP joints, either manually during rehabilitation sessions, or with a dorsal MP splint (called a 'lumbrical bar') between sessions. As stated earlier, patients must not thereafter transfer their body weight on their extended MP joints.

Flexor phase

The second stage is performed once the patient has been able to demonstrate active thumb and finger extension. The operative steps include:

- transfer of the ECRL to finger flexors (FDP);
- transfer of the PT to FPL; and
- 'split' FPL-to-EPL thumb IP stabilization.

Transfer of extensor carpi radialis longus to flexor digitorum profundi

Transfer of the ECRL to finger FDPs is performed as described for IC Group 3.

Transfer of pronator teres to flexor pollicis longus

The PT is a broad muscle that inserts around the shaft of the radius with a very short, large, and thin tendon. It is detached from the radius together with a strip of periosteum so as to extend the length of its short tendon. Two parallel incisions are made alongside the tendon at its distal insertion, and the periosteal strip is elevated in continuity with the tendon (*Fig. 13.13A*).

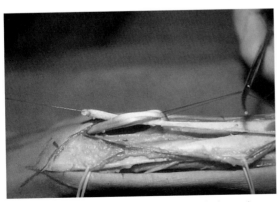

Figure 13.12 Suture of the brachioradialis to the extensor digitorum communis.

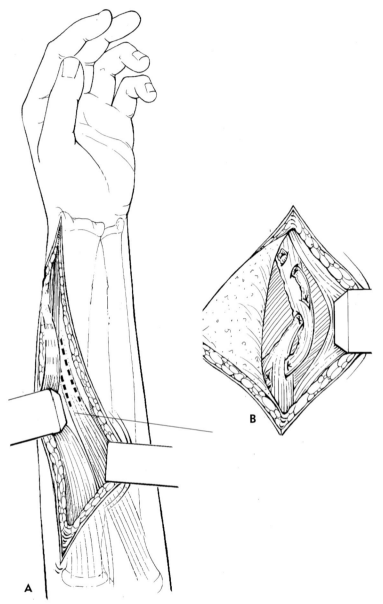

Figure 13.13 Flexor phase, pronator teres (PT) to flexor pollicis longus (FPL). (A) Dissection of the PT. (B) Interweaving of the tendons of PT and FPL.

The muscle is mobilized proximally from out of its investing fascia, after which the muscle–tendon junction of the FPL is identified. As much tendinous material as possible is dissected out of the muscle–tendon junction in an attempt to make a direct suture with the PT. In a number of cases the tendon of the FPL is short and, in spite of this dissection, its proxi-

mal end does not reach the periosteal strip used to prolong the transferred PT. In such cases, an interpositional tendon graft is needed. The palmaris longus may be used, but if this risks further weakening of the weak wrist flexors (such as in IC Group 4) an alternative is to use the paralyzed extensor indicis or extensor digiti minimi. The tendons are woven through each other (*Fig. 13.13B*). The tension is adjusted so that, with the wrist in neutral, the thumb rests against the lateral aspect of the index finger.

'Split' flexor pollicis longus to extensor pollicis longus thumb interphalangeal stabilization

The 'split FPL-to-EPL transfer' is performed before adjusting the tension of all the transfers, so the thumb assumes its final position and the tension can be set accordingly.

Postoperative immobilization and rehabilitation

Postoperatively, the wrist and fingers are immobilized with the wrist in slight flexion and the fingers in 60° of MP and 45° of PIP flexion. At 4 weeks the cast is removed, and physical therapy is conducted in the

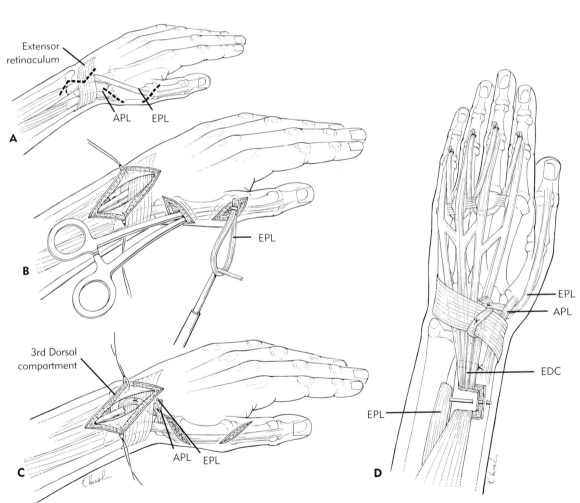

Figure 13.14 An alternative extensor phase for the IC Group 5 patient with a stable thumb carpometacarpal (CMC) joint. (A) Incisions. (B) The extensor pollicis longus (EPL) is divided at its muscle–tendon junction and withdrawn into the incision made over the thumb metacarpophalangeal joint. It is passed subcutaneously to the level of the abductor pollicis longus (APL) insertion and then passed under this tendon and (C) wrapped around the extensor retinaculum at the third compartment and anchored to itself. (D) The tendons of the extensor digitorum communis (EDC) are tenodesed to the radius, as illustrated in *Figure 13.4*, and the final tension adjusted. This maneuver with the EPL gives the thumb an extension-radial abduction vector as the wrist is flexed, which provides some additional CMC stability.

same manner as for IC Group 3 patients. The use of a manual wheelchair and shifting of the body weight on to the hands are restricted for 1 month more.

Alternative procedures

Alternative procedures for IC Groups 4 and 5 include various combinations of the procedures already described. Since patients differ, it is important to be able to plan for variations in patient presentation and individual functional objectives. For example, it has been our experience that patients who have had different procedures performed for each arm are pleased with their differences. They preferentially use one hand for certain activities, such as grasping large objects, and the other for different tasks (e.g., manipulating smaller objects). The greatest variation in hand use is a consequence of the management of the thumb's CMC joint. A fused CMC joint, while predictably prepositioning the thumb, does limit the size of objects easily grasped within the first web space. If the CMC joint is left mobile, the postoperative position of the thumb ray is less predictable, sometimes significantly so, but larger objects can be pushed into the first web space and held.

We have based decisions regarding these alternatives in large part on the preoperative presentation of the thumb's CMC joint. If the joint is completely unstable (time and poor transfer mechanics have resulted in slackening of all the CMC ligaments), we prefer to fuse the CMC joint and carry out the reconstruction as just described. Occasionally, we alter the method used to obtain finger and thumb extension or alter the time of intrinsic substitution or thumb IP joint stabilization (extensor versus flexor phase). These variations seem to make no difference in terms of outcome.

Stable thumb carpometacarpal joint

The surgical objectives for the extensor phase include fingers that extend and a first web space that widely opens when the wrist is flexed. For the flexor phase, these include active flexion of the fingers and thumb and a strong lateral pinch between the thumb pulp and radial side of the index finger, which becomes even stronger as the wrist is extended.

Extensor phase

For this patient, the extensor phase typically includes the following operative steps (*Fig. 13.14*):

- tenodesis of the EDC to the radius;
- tenodesis of the rerouted EPL (see *Figure 13.14* for details); and
- 'split' FPL-to-EPL thumb IP stabilization.

Postoperative immobilization, rehabilitation, and precautions are addressed above. A detailed discussion of the course of rehabilitation is included in Appendix VI.

Flexor phase

The flexor phase can be carried out once passive mobility and muscle strength have recovered to their maximum potential. The goals of this phase include transfers to provide both positional control and a powerful thumb pinch, a transfer to restore active finger flexion, and intrinsic balance. The operative steps include:

- transfer of the ECRL to FDP (fingers in reverse cascade position);
- transfer of the PT to FPL;
- BR, extended with the ring finger FDS tendon, transferred across the palm to restore thumb flexion and/or abduction; and
- intrinsic substitution procedure, either lasso or House method, if not performed in the extensor phase.

Since all these procedures (except the BR modification) are described earlier in this chapter, only the BR modification is discussed in detail. It is essentially House's[20] modification of the transfer described by Royle[15] and refined by Thompson.[16] Alternative locations for the incisions are illustrated in *Figure 13.15A*.

Brachioradialis transfer for thumb flexion and abduction

This BR transfer is performed after dissection and passage of the ECRL and PT transfers. The motor tendon is interwoven through the recipient, awaiting the final adjustment of tension. The BR tendon must be elongated to accomplish its goal, and one of the paralyzed superficialis tendons is used for this purpose. Note that if the lasso procedure is chosen it requires modification for this step of intrinsic substitution. In this case, the FDS tendon to the middle finger is split into two strips, one of which is attached to the A1 pulley of the middle, while the other is passed to the ring finger where it is attached to this finger's A1 pulley.

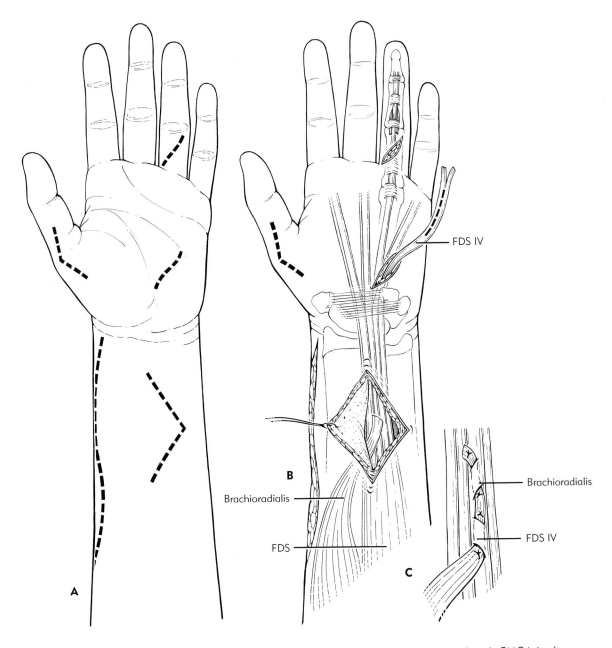

FDS IV

Brachioradialis

FDS

B

Brachioradialis

FDS IV

C

A

Figure 13.15(A–C) An alternative flexor phase for IC Group 5 patients with a stable thumb CMC joint (see text for details). [(B)–(E) used with permission from Hentz and Chase 2001.][22]

The BR is passed, as were the tendons of the ECRL and the PT, into the palmar forearm wound (*Fig. 13.15B*). The superficialis tendon to the ring finger is identified and the muscle-tendon junction divided. In the forearm, the BR tendon and the cut end of the ring finger's superficialis tendon are joined together by a weaving technique and anchored firmly with nonabsorbable sutures (*Fig. 13.15C*).

The small incision at the base of the ring finger is made to allow exposure of the superficialis tendon, the A1 pulley at this level is opened somewhat to allow access, and the two tails of the superficialis are

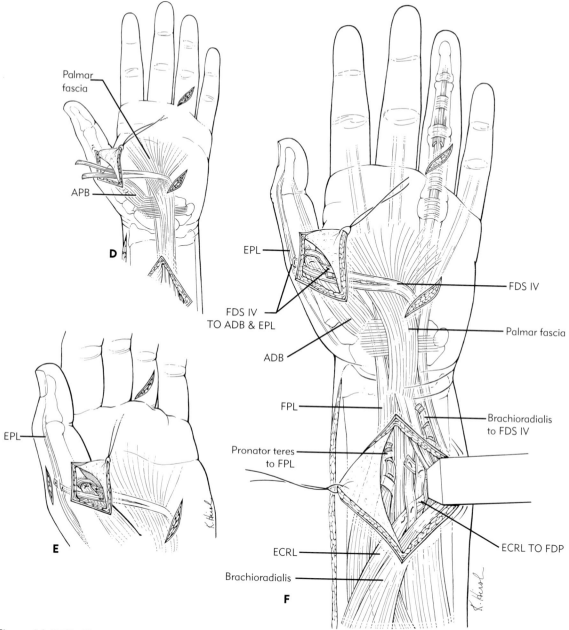

Labels in figure:
Palmar fascia
APB
D
EPL
FDS IV TO ADB & EPL
ADB
FPL
Pronator teres to FPL
EPL
E
ECRL
Brachioradialis
F
FDS IV
Palmar fascia
Brachioradialis to FDS IV
ECRL TO FDP

Figure 13.15(D–F) (continued)

divided (*Fig. 13.15B*). The palm incision is made just distal to the distal edge of the transverse retinaculum and over Guyon's canal. The tendon of the superficialis to the ring finger is located within the depths of this incision and the cut ends of the tendon are withdrawn (*Fig. 13.15B*). The final incision is made on the radial aspect of the thumb at the MP joint. The tendon of the abductor pollicis brevis (APB) is identified as it will be used as one of the anchor points for the transfer (*Fig. 13.15D*). A subcutaneous tunnel is created from this incision to the palmar incision. In this way, the palmar fascia becomes the pulley for this tendon. The vector for this transfer is one of flexion and abduction as opposed to the more proximal abduction vector of a standard opponens transfer. The superficialis tendon is passed through the subcutaneous tunnel to exit at the thumb incision. Two points of attachment are prepared. The first is the tendinous insertion of the APB, and the second is the tendon of the EPL over the proximal phalanx of the thumb (*Figs 13.15D* and *13.15E*). One slip of the split insertion of the superficialis tendon of the ring finger is passed through the tendon of the APB tendon. The second slip is passed dorsally and through the tendon of the EPL to await the final adjustment of tension. If this transfer is carried out in isolation, the appropriate tension is obtained by pulling first on the slip that passes through the APB, so that the thumb ray lies over the index finger as viewed from the palmar perspective. This slip of the flexor superficialis is anchored to the APB at this tension. Next, the tendon of the EPL is pulled proximally with enough tension to lift the IP joint to the neutral position. While this tension on the EPL is maintained, the other slip of the superficialis is anchored to the EPL.

Final adjustment of the tension

Final adjustments are made to the tension on the three transfers. The initial step is to adjust the tension of the ECRL to profundus transfer. This tension is judged according to the posture of the fingers. An appropriate goal is to have the fingers well flexed with the wrist in neutral. The fingers should extend almost fully when the wrist is flexed, however. Next, the tension on the PT to FPL is adjusted. This tension pulls the thumb against the side of the index finger with the wrist in neutral. Thirdly, insertion of the BR to thumb transfer is carried out. One slip of the superficialis is anchored into the tendon of the APB. The tension is adjusted so that the thumb abducts to the point where the pulp of the thumb lies over the distal IP joint of the now partially flexed index finger. Nonabsorbable sutures are used to anchor this superficialis slip into the tendon of the APB. As a final adjustment the other half of the superficialis tendon is woven into the tendon of the EPL and the tension adjusted to cause the thumb to extend slightly from its previous posture. This last step helps to prevent hyperflexion of the thumb during pinch (Froment's sign) and makes it more likely that the broad pulp surface of the thumb will be used in the pinch.

Tension is assessed by passively flexing the wrist gently to determine that the fingers and thumb can be opened almost fully, and by extending the wrist gently to judge the cascade of the fingers and posture of the thumb. The tourniquet is deflated and bleeding is controlled. The wounds are irrigated and the various incisions closed. The wrist and fingers are splinted with the wrist in very slight flexion; the fingers are nearly fully flexed at the MP joints and the thumb relatively widely abducted, with the tip of the thumb touching the tip of the index finger. Immobilization is maintained for approximately 4 weeks followed by rehabilitation.

The tendon junctures must be protected against any large force for some additional weeks, particularly in the wheelchair-bound patient. Transfers and pressure relief activities are restricted for a full 8 weeks.

Common complication and salvage procedures

Suture breakage and rupture of transfer

It is difficult to draw conclusions from published reports regarding complications after these surgical procedures, as there is no 'standard' procedure and each author uses a number of procedures during each surgical step that vary with each patient according to the anatomy, exact motor level, and desires and/or needs. Also, most published series are based on a small number of operations so any attempt at a statistical analysis is futile.

From our personal experience and from the data gathered from the literature suture breakage occurs regularly. This complication can be a technical problem, such as an inadequate suture technique (terminoterminal, or too few stitches) or inadequate suture material (fine thread, absorbable sutures). It can also result from inappropriate positioning of the involved joint(s) postoperatively, or from removal of the cast too early. We believe that it is also associated with an inadvertent contraction of the transferred donor muscle, which places the suture area under such great tension that it gives way. In our experience and in that of others this occurs mainly with the BR transfer. As the elbow is not immobilized, all the elbow flexors, including the BR, may contract freely. If the patients and their attendants have not been warned to avoid strong contraction of the elbow flexors, the suture is likely to rupture in any situation in which the patients lift their body weight with their elbow flexors. Even if the patient has been instructed not to do so, it may happen inadvertently. One of our patients experienced such a rupture while his attendant was carrying him to bed. The patient had his operated arm around the attendant's neck and inadvertently tried to help the attendant by lifting his body with his flexed elbow. Although the patient did hear a 'popping' sound and felt the BR retract proximally, the correct diagnosis was not made until 2 weeks later. The delayed secondary repair led to a mediocre result. Another patient reported experiencing a similar event while being placed in a cast following the extensor phase. Immediate re-exploration and resuturing of the BR to EDC transfer led to an exceptionally good outcome.

It would seem an easy solution to immobilize the elbow within a cast during the first 4–6 weeks. However, this would further impair function and nursing of the patients during this period in which they are already much more dependent on others and immobilization of the elbow does not prevent isometric contraction of the muscle, which may also lead to a rupture.

Early in our experience one patient disrupted a split FPL–EPL tenodesis a few days after cast removal. For this reason we fix the IP joint with a Kirschner wire for a period of 8 weeks (*Fig. 13.16*). Thus, when the cast is removed at 4 weeks, patients may start exercising their transfer to the FPL without

any restriction and yet without any risk to the FPL–EPL tenodesis.

A serious complication has been described by Revol after active tenodesis of the FPL with the ECRB.[26] In four cases, his patients experienced rupture of the ECRB after side-to-side suture to FPL. Secondary repair led to suboptimal results in all cases, especially as the ECRL had been transferred during the same operative phase to the FDP. This resulted in a weak residual wrist extension.

Breakage of the suture between the donor muscle and individual flexor tendons has also been reported. This is always related to a technical problem. We have encountered this complication several times, especially with the FDP to the index finger after ECRL transfer. In one patient the suture gave way progressively over several months. However, he was very satisfied with the cosmetic result (*Fig. 13.17A*) and the functional result was still satisfactory, as the wrist tenodesis produced enough flexion of the index finger for a satisfactory lateral pinch (*Fig. 13.17B*). Two other patients requested that the side-to-side FDP tenodesis be adjusted at a second procedure; the ultimate outcome was satisfactory.

Another cause of failure of the transferred tendon to activate the recipient tendon may be tendon adhesions. This usually occurs at the suture site, and is more likely to happen if the part has been immobilized for longer. We have performed secondary tenolysis of the BR to EDC donor–recipient tendon unit in two patients with satisfactory results, as reported by Gansel *et al.*[14] Whenever a transfer fails to demonstrate any distal activity, despite a good proximal contraction of the muscle belly, an early revision of the suture site it is worth considering. Whether the transfer is adherent to the local tissues or has undergone rupture, the sooner it is revised the more likely is a satisfactory outcome.

Loosening of transfers

A more subtle complication of these procedures is tendon and/or suture slackening. This is more often related to the patient's lack of education or deleterious habits than to the operative procedure itself. It is more likely to occur with tenodeses than with tendon transfers, and with flexion procedures than with extension procedures. A typical example of this complication is slackening of the intrinsic substitution

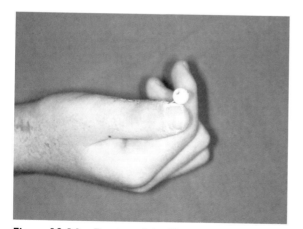

Figure 13.16 Fixation of the IP joint in extension with an oblique transarticular Kirschner wire to protect the 'split-FPL' procedure.

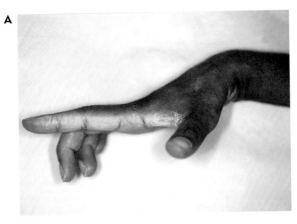

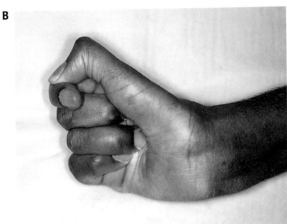

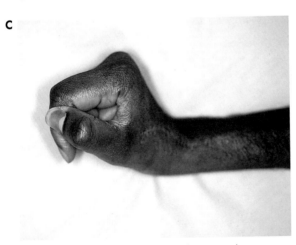

Figure 13.17 Suture breakage between the extensor carpi radialis longus and flexor digitorum profundus to the index finger. (A) Full active extension. (B, C) Full active flexion.

procedures. The lasso and House procedures, as applied to tetraplegic patients, are passive procedures (e.g., in the lasso procedure the FDS muscles are paralyzed). These tendons are thus subject to slackening if submitted to repeated stretching. If patients have not been taught or do not comply with the specific maneuvers to protect their transfer, then the tendons will stretch, probably at the level of the loop around the A1 pulley for the lasso procedure or at the tendon-to-tendon or tendon-to-bone juncture for the House procedure. After a variable period of time (usually a few months) the initially flexed posture of the MP joints moves toward full extension, and then to hyperextension (*Fig. 13.18*). As soon as the MP joints begin to fully extend, clawing of the fingers is likely to occur, which leads to a functional impairment of grasp. It is therefore critical to teach patients, prior to upper limb surgery, how to protect their future operations. This training does take some time, but by the time surgery is undertaken the patients must be familiar with these protective measures. The MP joints should never be pushed by force into passive extension. At rest the hands should not lie flat on the thighs or chair arms; rather, the fingers should be rolled into flexion. Most importantly, during transfers and any weight shifts, the weight of the body should never be borne on the flattened palm of the hand. Rather, the fingers must be rolled into flexion, as in forming a fist, and the weight supported either by the dorsal aspect of the proximal phalanges or, if the wrist is not stable enough, by the dorsal aspect of the flexed middle and distal phalanges and the proximal palm. The first method protects the finger flexors more efficiently, but puts the thumb more at risk of passive hyperextension at the MP and IP joints. The second method protects the thumb better, but has been reported by some patients to produce pain in the thumb CMC area if a CMC joint fusion has been performed.

Thumb position and carpometacarpal fusion

Problems can also arise with the thumb CMC joint fusion. The fusion is usually achieved in 2–3 months; if temporary fixations, such as Kirschner wires, have been used they can usually be removed during the second phase. However, evolution of the fusion to a nonunion has been described (House reported this to be as frequent as 24%.)[12] It does not seem to be

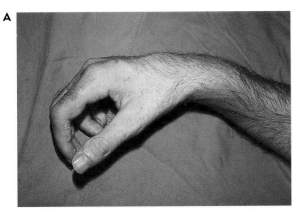

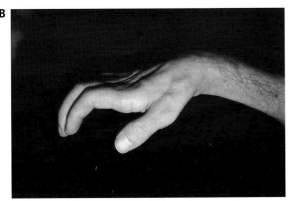

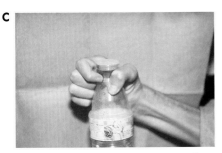

Figure 13.18 Slackening of a lasso procedure led to recurrence of metacarpophalangeal hyperextension and a poor opening of the hand.

related to the type of fixation used. We have observed nonunion in six of the 45 CMC joint arthrodeses we performed, of which two had been fixed with pneumatic staples, two with tension bands, and two with plates.

In our experience and in that of others[12] these fibrous unions do not cause pain. They prove stable with time on successive radiographs and do not seem to create any impairment of pinch strength or func-

tion compared to those patients in whom fusion was sound. As stated above, CMC joint fusion can also create pain when the patient leans on this area for pressure relief or to shift body weight. In our experience this pain, when it occurs, has always been temporary, and disappears after a few months.

Thumb positioning remains one of the most challenging technical parts of these procedures. The thumb is a complicated articular complex made of three joints (one of which has a wide range of motion) and activated by four extrinsic and four intrinsic tendons and/or muscles. Although in tetraplegic patients attempts are made to restore only a simple type of motion (lateral pinch), all the joints must be either activated or stabilized, and sometimes both, to make this complex chain into a simple one.

Interphalangeal joint hyperflexion

Interphalangeal joint hyperflexion occurred regularly in our early experience after FPL activation, but is now effectively prevented by either IP fusion or, preferably, by stabilization with the so-called 'split-FPL' transfer.

Carpometacarpal joint hyperlaxity

Hyperlaxity requires a fusion. If it is not performed, it is very difficult to predict and control the final position of the thumb pulp after activation has been achieved. The EPL extends and adducts the thumb dorsally and tends to create an inefficient lateral pinch between the thumb and proximal phalanx of the index finger. Activation of the FPL tends to adduct the first metacarpal, which closes the first web and may lead to MP joint hyperextension.

Metacarpophalangeal joint stabilization

The MP joint may be or become unstable both in excessive flexion or in hyperextension. Occasionally, thumb MP hyperextension is functionally beneficial, even if esthetically unbecoming, as it allows a wide opening that facilitates grasping larger objects. An excessively flexed MP joint may cause the thumb tip to pass under the index, a circumstance that requires intervention – either fusing the joint or passive stabilization by dorsal tenodesis of the extensors just proximal to the MP joint.

Tension of flexor pollicis longus transfer

The tension of the transfer to the FPL is critical, as stated above. Excessive tension leads to inability to open the first web and seize large objects. Lack of tension reduces pinch strength drastically, and may even prevent thin objects being seized. Only experience can help to adjust the tension properly during surgery. Suture of this transfer must be performed last, after all the other procedures have been completed, so that all fingers assume their final position. Temporary stitches and gentle passive motion of the wrist help to determine which position is most appropriate for the thumb. The surgeon must be able to take the time to change the tension of a transfer if the positioning of the thumb is not satisfactory at the end of the procedure.

Illustrative case

An 18-year-old male sustained a spinal cord injury in a diving accident. At age 25 years he sought surgical rehabilitation. At that time his ASIA motor injury level was right C7–C8, and left C8. His left upper limb was classified IC Group 5, with a triceps of MRC Grade 2. His triceps on the right side was MRC Grade 3. His 2PD was rated 8 on the thumb, 10 on the radial aspect of the index, and 12 on the ulnar index and the radial middle fingers.

Prior to surgery, he had a satisfactory tenodesis effect in the left hand, with a lateral pinch between the thumb pulp and the lateral aspect of the index finger. However, this pinch was not efficient, and could not hold 5 g (0.01) of weight (*Figs 13.19A* and *13.19B*). This patient had satisfactory functional performances for his spinal cord lesion level. He also had a good sense of position and a good body balance. He was well motivated for surgical improvement of his upper limb, had good family support, and realistic expectations regarding surgical improvement. We felt he was a good candidate for hand surgery. He was not interested in activation of his left elbow extension, being already able to relieve buttock pressure and reach overhead with his right arm.

A two-stage procedure was performed for the left hand. During the extensor phase, the BR was transferred to the EDC and EPL. Associated procedures included arthrodesis of the thumb IP joint, and a lasso

procedure of all the fingers. After 3 months, the flexor phase was carried out and involved transfer of the ECRL to the finger FDPs, and active tenodesis of the FPL to ECRL.

At review 2 years later, all the transfers were functioning. He had attained excellent active finger extension and flexion (*Figs 13.19C* and *13.19C*). Lateral pinch, measured in full forearm pronation without any compensation, was 500 g (1.1 lb, *Fig. 13.19E*) and finger grasp was 15 kg (33 lb, *Fig. 13.19F*). There was no analytic or functional loss as a result of harvesting the donor muscles. His functional performances, on a functional independence measure scale, had improved from 156 to 201. His satisfaction, measured on a 0–10 linear scale, ranked 8.2. Surgery was beneficial, and although his functional performances were still far from normal, he had gained a much more efficient left upper limb.

Long-term outcomes

From our experience with surgical reconstruction in 68 IC Group 4 and 5 patients, 18 patients have been re-examined at least 10 years after surgery. Almost all had undergone two stage procedures, and half had elected bilateral reconstruction. Flexor power was by active transfer of the ECRL, BR, PT, or accessory wrist extensor, always in some combination to the thumb and digital flexors. Extension was by tenodesis in 12 cases, by active transfer in six cases, and four patients did not undergo intrinsic substitution. Six patients had undergone some type of additional surgery in the period between their initial surgery and the date of long-term evaluation, typically adjustment of the flexor to one or another finger (usually the index) or release of a contracted PIP joint (usually the ring or little finger). Grip power [average 60 N (13.5 lbf)] had not deteriorated in these patients compared to that at the 6–12 month evaluation after their initial surgery. Pinch force, measured with a modified pinch gauge, averaged 34 N (7.6 lbf). Typically, two muscles were devoted to thumb function in these patients. We found, as did House, that those patients who had had some type of intrinsic stabilization, either by Zancolli lasso or by House's intrinsic reconstruction procedure, had a more powerful grasp [76 N (17.1 lbf) versus 40 N (9.0 lbf)]. This may be a product of pre-selection, however, with

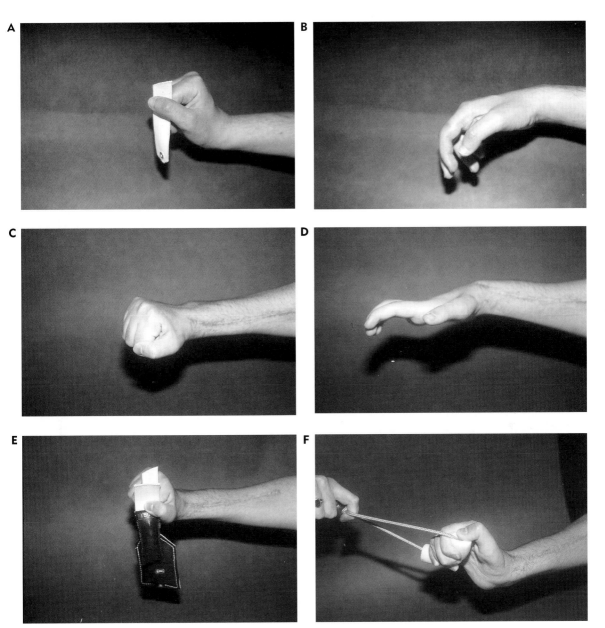

Figure 13.19 Clinical case of an IC Group 5 patient. Preoperative function: (A) attempted grasp through the tenodesis effect, with which the patient can hold a strap if it is very light; (B) attempted release. Clinical result 2 years after operation: (C) active grasp; (D) active release. (E) Lateral pinch at review; (F) grasp at review.

the stronger patients selectively chosen for intrinsic substitution.

We conclude from this long-term analysis that carefully chosen upper limb reconstructive procedures in appropriately educated and compliant patients are both effective and durable. Systematic postoperative re-evaluation of these patients upper limbs should become a standard part of their interval examinations, more typical of the more generally studied systems, for renal and bladder function, blood pressure, and pulmonary status. Aside from their brain, the upper limbs remain the most important residual resource for tetraplegic patients. Frequent re-evaluation of their upper limbs ultimately makes good sense.

As mentioned earlier, few of our patients perform many new activities. Typically, a good or excellent result means that the patient performs many of the same functions, but with much greater efficiency. The rewards for surgeons, rehabilitation medicine specialists, and therapists are best expressed by one of our patients who replied to a question requesting his feelings on his outcome:

It's not as much as I hoped for, but it's much more than I ever had.

References

1. Moberg E. Upper limb surgical rehabilitation in tetraplegia. In: Evarts CM, ed. Surgery of the Musculoskeletal System, Vol. 1. New York: Churchill Livingstone, 1990:915–941.
2. Mohammed KD, Rothwell A, Sinclair S, et al. Upper-limb surgery for tetraplegia. J Bone Joint Surg 1992; 74B:873–879.
3. Allieu Y. Réhabilitation Chirurgicale du Membre Supérieur du Tétraplégique. Cahiers: SOFCOT, 1988:233–255.
4. Zancolli E. Surgery for the quadriplegic hand with active, strong wrist extension preserved. Clin Orthop Rel Res 1975; 112:101–113.
5. Freehafer A. Tendon transfers in patients with cervical spinal cord injury. J Hand Surg 1991; 16A:804–809.
6. Moberg E. Surgical treatment for absent single-hand grip and elbow extension in quadriplegia. J Bone Joint Surg 1975; 57A(2):196–206.
7. Zancolli E. Structural and Dynamic Basis of Hand Surgery. Philadelphia: JB Lippincott, 1968.
8. Freehafer A, Vonhamm E, Allen V. Tendon transfers to improve grasp after injuries of the cervical spinal cord. J Bone Joint Surg 1974; 56A:951–959.
9. Lamb D, Chan K. Surgical reconstruction of the upper limb in traumatic tetraplegia. J Bone Joint Surg 1983; 65B(3):291–298.
10. Hentz V, Brown M, Keoshian L. Upper limb reconstruction in quadriplegia: functional assessment and proposed treatment modifications. J Hand Surg 1983; 8(2):119–131.
11. Lipscomb P, Elkins E, Henderson E. Tendon transfers to restore function of hands in tetraplegia, especially after fracture–dislocation of the sixth cervical vertebra on the seventh. J Bone Joint Surg 1958; 40:1071–1080.
12. House JH, Dahl JCA. One-stage key pinch and release with thumb carpal-metacarpal fusion in tetraplegia. J Hand Surg 1992; 17A:530–538.
13. House J. Two stage reconstruction of the tetraplegic hand. In: Strickland J, ed. Master Techniques in Orthopedic Surgery. Philadelphia: Lippincott, 1998:229–255.
14. Gansel J, Waters R, Gelman H. Transfer of the pronator teres tendon to the tendons of the flexor digitorum profundus in tetraplegia. J Bone Joint Surg 1990; 72A:427–432.
15. Royle N. An operation for paralysis of the intrinsic muscles of the thumb. JAMA 1938; 111:612–615.
16. Thompson T. A modified operation for opponens paralysis. J Bone Joint Surg 1942; 24:632.
17. Zancolli E. Structural and Dynamic Basis of Hand Surgery, 2nd edn. Philadelphia: JB Lippincott, 1979.
18. House JH, Shannon MA. Restoration of strong grasp and lateral pinch in tetraplegia: a comparison of two methods of thumb control in each patient. J Hand Surg 1985; 10A(1):22–29.
19. Moberg E. Traitement chirurgical des tétraplegies dues a des lesions cervicales medullaires hautes. In: Tubiana R, ed. Traité de Chirurgie de la Main. Paris: Masson, 1991.
20. House JH, Gwathmey FW, Lundsgaard DK. Restoration of strong grasp and lateral pinch in tetraplegia due to cervical spinal cord injury. J Hand Surg 1976; 1(2):152–159.
21. Zancolli E, Zancolli E. Tetraplegies traumatiques. In: Tubiana R, ed. Traite' de Chirurgie de la Main. Paris: Masson, 1991.
22. Hentz V, Chase R. Hand Surgery: A Clinical Atlas. Philadelphia: WB Saunders, 2001.
23. Zancolli E. Correccion de la 'garra' digital por paralisis intrinseca. La operacion del 'lazo'. Acta Ortop Latinoam 1974; 1:65.
24. Riordan D. Tendon transplantation in median nerve and ulnar nerve paralysis. J Bone Joint Surg 1953; 35A(2):312–320.
25. Allieu Y. Le membére supérieur du tétraplegique. Conferences d'enseignment du GEM. Paris: L'expansion Scientifique, 1994:1–17.
26. Revol M. Personal Communication.

14

Rehabilitation for the strongest (International Classification Group 6) patients

Introduction

International Classification (IC) Group 6 patients are a minority of tetraplegic individuals (less than 5% of our operated series). The IC defines such patients as possessing a strong extensor digitorum communis (EDC) muscle (graded MRC 4 and above). Functional assessment of their hands, however, reveals that these patients are not significantly better performers than those in IC Groups 4 and 5, and sometimes may perform less well, because active digital extension without active antagonistic finger flexion is more a handicap than a benefit. This group of patients usually benefits directly and greatly from surgical rehabilitation of their upper limbs, which results in a tremendous improvement in their ability to grasp and pinch, and indirectly because they have a greater potential to make use of these improvements.

Assessment of IC Group 6 patients

These patients are unique in that they have much more muscular potential than the IC Group 5 patients, and yet the functional capacities of their hands are often lower. This results from the increased tone of the digital extensors, which is not balanced by any active digital flexors. This imbalance leads to a characteristic posture of the hand, with the fingers in full extension at the metacarpophalangeal (MP) and interphalangeal (IP) joints, which is often referred to as the 'flat hand' (*Fig. 14.1*).

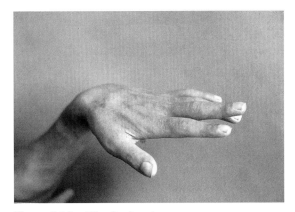

Figure 14.1 The flat hand.

This posture is not improved much by wrist extension; the tenodesis effect does not take place, because the tone of the active extensors at rest is much greater than the viscoelastic tone developed by the paralyzed flexors. Therefore these patients have very little prehensile capacity. A lateral pinch may be produced in full wrist extension, between the palmar aspect of the extended IP joint of the thumb and the radial side of the index MP joint. If present, this pinch is very weak and of little functional value. A grasp cannot be obtained with the fingers only, even in full wrist extension; the tenodesis effect produces some MP flexion, but the IP joints remain extended (*Fig. 14.2*). However, these patients have extensive muscle resources, with many muscles available for transfer. Besides the brachioradialis (BR), the extensor carpi radialis longus (ECRL and ECRB), and the pronator

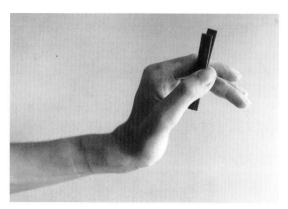

Figure 14.2 Wrist extension produces a poor lateral pinch, and no finger grasp.

teres (PT), which are usually available in IC Group 5 patients, additional muscles may be present and strong. In order of their appearance along the motor level, these include the extensor digiti minimi (EDM), the extensor carpi ulnaris (ECU), and the extensor indicis proprius (EIP). According to Barthes[1] (see Chapter 7), the flexor carpi ulnaris (FCU) may also be strong in these patients.

In IC Group 6 patients, other muscles in the upper limb and around the shoulder are strong, but in IC Group 5 they are weak or paralyzed. The triceps is usually strong enough not to need augmentation; in all Group 6 patients from the authors' Centers, it was graded MRC 5. Consequentially, IC Group 6 patients can reach overhead and widen what is referred to as the 'space of prehension', which is the area surrounding their body in which their hands can reach for objects, that is their working environment. (However, as they have an ineffective grip, this 'space of prehension' is little utilized, unless a better grip is restored.) These patients typically spend many hours a day sitting in their wheelchair and, as a rule, propel the chair manually. If the triceps is strong bilaterally, patients can efficiently relieve buttock pressure points and increase their performances with their manual wheelchair. However, restoration of the grasp allows the patient to grip the rims of the wheels and propel the chair in a far more efficient manner than by pushing the rims with the hypothenar eminence. Push-gloves are then no longer necessary, and the patient is able to propel the wheelchair much faster, change directions more efficiently, ride on uneven

ground, and climb gentle slopes, small steps, and even 'pop a wheelie'.

At the level of the shoulder, the latissimus dorsi and the pectoralis major are also very strong. This muscular potential notably improves the functional capacities of these patients. The major step forward is to achieve complete independence for body transfers from the bed and chair, usually with no need for an intermediate board and with no help from the patient's attendant. Also, these patients have a better trunk balance when sitting in their wheelchair and so they are less likely than patients from lower IC groups to fall forward. Even if they do, their triceps are strong enough to prevent the fall and therefore their day-to-day security is improved. They can reach for things on the floor, lean sideways, and thus further increase their functional environment.

IC Group 6 patients usually have a good proprioception in the thumb and index fingers, and two-point discrimination that averages 8–10mm in the middle finger. The fourth and fifth fingers have little or no epicritic sensation. They are categorized O/Cu in the international classification scheme.

Goals of surgery

The primary goal, in IC Group 6 patients, is to restore strong pinch and grasp, as well as thumb extension and intrinsic balance. Many muscles are available for transfer, and usually the strongest donor muscles are chosen for finger and thumb flexion, typically the ECRL, BR, or PT, and a muscle of lesser strength for thumb extension. Donors are insufficient in number to restore independent flexion of each finger, or to restore both flexor profundi and flexor superficialis. The choice is, as in lower IC groups, to activate the profundi. The remaining potential donors are used to restore some intrinsic function, not only in the fingers, but also in the thumb.

Substitution of finger intrinsics may be performed either with the 'lasso' procedure,[2] or with House's procedure.[3] The 'lasso' procedure is indicated when tension on the digital extensors results in good extension of the proximal IP (PIP) joints, provided that the MP joints are kept from hyperextending. House's procedure is indicated when this maneuver does not produce good extension of the PIP joints.

Good extension of the PIP joints occurs more often in this group of patients, because the active digital extensors have kept the PIP joints from flexing, and thus the extensor mechanism does not become over-stretched with time. Therefore, a 'lasso' procedure is the intrinsic substitution performed most often, in our experience.

For the IC Group 6 patients, the 'lasso' procedure may be performed in the same manner as for lower groups (see Chapter 13). However, in a number of cases enough donor muscles are available to motor the 'lasso'. For this purpose, an active donor may be transferred proximally to the paralyzed flexor superficialis tendons, and a typical lasso procedure performed distally. Potential donors are usually the BR, ECU, or FCU.

For the thumb, some form of opposition can be restored to provide a stronger pinch; alternatively, some antepulsion, commonly referred to as palmar abduction, can be restored to achieve a pulp to pulp (subterminal) pinch. This pinch, which is neither as strong nor as stable as the lateral pinch, is very useful, as a complement to the precision pinch (*Fig. 14.3*). With a lateral pinch only, to pick up small objects is a challenge as it requires that the object be pushed to the edge of the table (or support) with the extended thumb, then seized between the lateral aspect of the index and the thumb. A subterminal pinch, can seize the object directly, wherever it is.

Thumb stabilization in this group of patients can usually be achieved through tendon transfers and tenodeses, rather than arthrodesis. At the carpometacarpal (CMC) level, stability is usually achieved through various tendon transfers performed around the thumb. An arthrodesis would be considered only for cases in which the trapeziometacarpal joint is very unstable, but if it is needed it will no longer be possible to restore any form of adaptable opposition, adduction, or abduction of the thumb. Rather, if it seems mandatory to stabilize one joint, in cases when the thumb is very lax, we prefer to fuse the MP joint.

In some patients, the MP joint of the thumb may be unstable in extension or in flexion. Hyperextension is the most frequent situation and is directly related to the lack of active intrinsics in the presence of some activity, though less than that in MRC Grade 4 of the extensor pollicis longus (EPL). This hyperextension must be recognized and treated, otherwise it is likely to increase when the extrinsic muscles of the thumb are activated. The result is not only hyperextension of the MP joint, but also compensatory hyperflexion of the IP joint, and progressive closure flexion and adduction of the thumb's CMC joint. This abnormal posture, sometimes referred to as the 'thumb swanneck' deformity, results in a poor, unstable pinch, so some form of volar stabilization is necessary. This can be achieved through different means:

A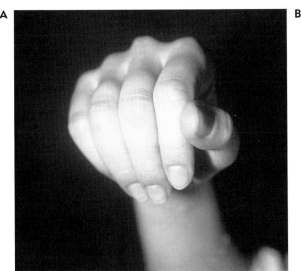
B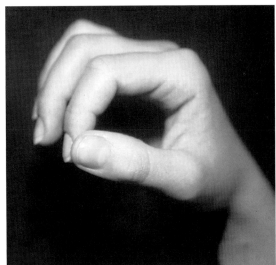

Figure 14.3 A normal hand demonstrates (A) lateral pinch and (B) subterminal pinch.

- The most elegant method is to stabilize the joint using the same tendon transfers used to power the thumb, which are brought around the MP joint. The procedure described by Brand[4] (see next paragraph) is very effective in that respect.
- Anterior capsulodesis of the MP joint is not an easy procedure because of the presence of the two sesamoid bones. It is also likely to loosen with time.
- Rather than a conventional arthrodesis, the procedure utilized by Zancolli,[5] which involves a sesamoidometacarpal arthrodesis, may be helpful. It usually results in an effective volar stabilization, and the joint retains active flexion.

Excessive passive flexion of the joint may be detrimental to function when active flexion of the thumb is restored, resulting in an hyperflexed MP joint. As a consequence the thumb pulp is likely to miss the lateral side of the index finger, and a dorsal stabilization is necessary. This can be achieved by anchoring the tendon of the extensor pollicis brevis (EPB) more distally into the proximal phalanx, or by a strong tenodesis of the EPB into the metacarpal just proximal to the MP joint.

The necessity to stabilize the distal joint of the thumb if the flexor pollicis longus (FPL) is to be motored is stressed in previous chapters. Failure to do so results in a hyperflexed IP joint after the FPL is activated (Froment's sign). This induces a poor lateral pinch with the very tip of the thumb facing the radial side of the index finger (*Fig. 14.4*) or, even worse, with the dorsal aspect of the thumb facing the volar aspect of the index. The best procedure to achieve stability is the 'split-FPL' transfer described in previous chapters.

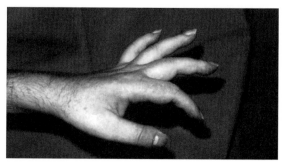

Figure 14.5 This patient demonstrates strong extension of the ulnar fingers, and weak extension of the radial fingers.

To achieve an ideal result, in IC Group 6 patients a two-stage procedure is still necessary, as both the EPL and the FPL need to be motored. These two procedures are not readily compatible as postoperative immobilization requires opposite positions, and their physical therapy is contradictory. However, in some IC Group 6 patients who have pre-existing thumb extension that is nearly MRC Grade 3, we have chosen to perform the procedure (including enhancing thumb extension) in one stage, explaining to the patient that a second stage to further power thumb extension may be necessary.

A specific group of patients has strong extensors to the ulnar fingers (IV and V, or III, IV, and V), and weaker extensors in the radial fingers (I and II, or I, II, and III; *Fig 14.5*). These patients, who might be classified as intermediate IC Groups 5–6, are included in Group 6 as their treatment scheme is similar.

Our preferred procedures

Surgery is usually performed in two stages. The first stage, referred to as the extensor phase, consists of:

- activation of EPL (and radial finger extensors if needed) with EDC;
- alternatively, EPL with EDM;
- tenodesis of abductor pollicis longus (APL); and
- finger intrinsics substitution (activated lasso if possible).

During the second stage, we perform either:

- ECRL to flexor digitorum profundus (FDP), BR to FPL, and EDM to abductor pollicis brevis (APB); or

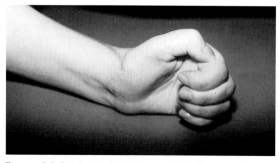

Figure 14.4 Lack of IP joint stabilization, resulting in a poor lateral pinch.

- transfer of three muscles to the fingers and thumb namely ECRL to finger flexors, PT to FPL and BR for thumb opposition; and IP joint stabilization by the 'split' FPL–EPL transfer (Fig. 12.9).

Extensor phase

Surgery is performed through a lateral antebrachial incision, which is used again during the second step. Alternatively, a dorsal incision may be used during the first phase, and an anterior one during the second.

Complementary incisions may be needed for specific transfers.

Thumb (and radial fingers) extension

If the radial extensors are somewhat weak, and need augmentation, a side-to-side suture is performed between all the tendons of the EDC. The tendons are exposed 2 cm above the dorsal retinaculum, and stripped of their peritendinous tissues. A heavy non-absorbable transverse mattress suture is then passed through each of the tendons. Ensure that all the fingers are kept parallel in the same balanced extended position throughout the suturing; failure to do this might result in some fingers extending more than others.

The tendon of EPL may or may not be included in the suture. If it is, tension should be slightly less on the thumb than on the finger extensors.

If only the thumb extensor (EPL) needs augmentation, two methods can be used. One is as described above, with a side-to-side suture to the tendons of the EDC. Although this provides active thumb extension, the thumb extends automatically at the same time as the fingers are actively extended. Therefore, extending the thumb to release the pinch is dependent on simultaneous grasp and release.

Another method is to restore the thumb extension by transferring the EDM to the EPL. Motor innervation of EDM is usually at the same level as that of EDC, so in most cases it is strong enough to be used as a transfer in IC Group 6 patients. A small longitudinal or transverse incision is made on the dorsal aspect of the fifth MP joint. The tendons are checked for anatomical variations, knowing that in a limited number of cases the little finger has no EDC tendon. In such cases, the EDM ensures MP joint extension and cannot be utilized as a transfer, unless it consists of several distinct tendon slips.[6,7]

If there are several individual EDM tendons, the most ulnar one is detached at the level of the MP joint, dissected subcutaneously, and retrieved proximal to the dorsal retinaculum through a small incision. An additional incision may be necessary at the level of the distal wrist extensor crease if the tendon cannot be retrieved, usually because of small connecting bands between the different tendons of EDM or between the EDM and ECU.[8]

The EDM tendon is then rerouted subcutaneously toward the EPL. Its muscular belly is dissected far enough proximally to direct its muscle and tendon in a straight line toward the EPL, and it is tunneled under the dorsal retinaculum. This can be achieved through the third or the second compartments, depending on the thumb's spontaneous position. Routing it in the same direction as the original EPL (third compartment) usually produces some adduction of the thumb at the same time as extension, which ultimately may prevent the patient from seizing large objects. If the tendon is routed through the second compartment, some abduction is produced at the same time as extension. On occasion, we have simply routed the tendon subcutaneously toward the insertion of the APL and have used the tendon of the APL just beyond the distal edge of the extensor retinaculum as a pulley, as illustrated in Figure 13.14.

The EDM tendon is then woven through the EPL distal to the dorsal retinaculum. The tendon juncture must be made distal enough to ensure it does not impinge on the distal edge of the retinaculum in full extension. The suture tension is set by moving the wrist passively: the thumb should start to extend when the wrist starts to flex from the neutral position.

Thumb stabilization

Abductor pollicis longus tenodesis

The various transfers performed during the first or second surgical stage typically stabilize the CMC in flexion, extension, and opposition. However, there remains the need for stabilization in radial and perhaps palmar abduction to avoid a progressive contracture of the first web space. This is best performed with a passive tenodesis of the APL, which, besides contributing to stability, maintains the thumb in a slightly abducted posture. This further improves thumb opening, and helps in grasping large objects.

The tendon of APL is approached through the lateral antebrachial incision. It is severed proximally, at the muscle–tendon junction, the proximal end is looped around the distal edge of the extensor retinaculum distalward, and the tendon is sutured to itself around the retinaculum. Tension is adjusted so that the thumb assumes a mild radially abducted position. As this tenodesis lies along the flexion–extension axis of wrist, it is not influenced by the position of the wrist. If some degree of palmar abduction is to be added, the tenodesis can be done as recommended by Zancolli.[5] After transection of the APL tendon at its muscle–tendon junction, the tendon is split into two strips, one of which is left in its original pathway. The other strip is withdrawn near its insertion, passed deep to the flexor carpi radialis, and back into its extensor compartment. Both tendon halves are looped around the extensor retinaculum as described previously. Tension of each strip is adjusted individually so as to induce both radial and palmar abduction (antepulsion).

For cases in which the CMC joint is particularly unstable, an arthrodesis might be considered. However, as stated earlier, this prevents restoration of intrinsic function to the thumb.

Intrinsic substitution

This step can be performed either during the extensor or the flexor phase. We prefer to include it here for reasons related to the duration of each procedure. Usually more procedures are performed during the flexor phase and tourniquet time may become a limiting factor, whereas usually plenty of time is available to perform the intrinsic substitution procedure during the extensor phase. As stated earlier, a 'lasso' procedure is indicated more often than the intrinsic substitution described by House *et al.*[3]

If no donor muscle is available, the procedure is performed as described in Chapter 13. If extra donors, such as the EC, FCU, or even BR, are available they may be used to produce an 'active' lasso.

Active lasso by transfer of ECU

The distal part of the procedure is performed first, with each flexor superficialis severed distally and looped around the A1 pulley in the same manner as in a passive lasso. Tension of the suture should not be as tight as in the passive procedure (for details, see p. 171). Next, the ECU is dissected. For cases in

which a long, single, radially based longitudinal incision has been made, a second longitudinal incision is needed over the ECU at its insertion onto the dorsoulnar base of the fifth metacarpal. The dorsal sensory branch of the ulnar nerve is first identified at the wrist and the ECU tendon is divided at its insertion. The ECU tendon is passed through a capacious window created in the interosseous membrane to the volar aspect of the forearm, where it is sutured to the four tendons of the paralyzed flexor digitorum superficialis. Rather than passing the donor through each individual recipient tendon, it is buried in the sutured mass of the recipient tendons, and a heavy braided nonabsorbable suture passed back and forth through all tendons, including the ECU. Tension of the transfer is set so that the resting position of the finger MP joints, with the wrist in neutral, averages 30° of flexion after the suture has been completed.

Postoperative regimen

The thumb and wrist are protected in a cast for 4 weeks, with the wrist extended and the thumb extended and abducted. If a lasso procedure has been performed, the MP joints of the fingers are also immobilized in 60° of flexion. Re-education is usually brief when only passive procedures have been performed (side-to-side activation of the extensors, passive lasso).

If the EDM was transferred, the second step is carried out once the transfer has demonstrated satisfactory excursion.

If an active lasso was performed, a dorsal splint of the 'intrinsic bar' type is used to protect the sutures for another 4 weeks. This is less time than for the passive procedure, because the risk of elongation is much less for an active transfer than for a tenodesis.

As with many of the two-stage procedures performed to restore function in the tetraplegic patient, he or she must be aware that no functional gain will occur until the second phase has been completed.

Flexor phase

Besides restoration of finger and thumb flexion, as described in Chapter 13, some intrinsic function of the thumb can and should be restored. Among the many procedures available, we have used two different techniques in tetraplegic patients to restore somewhat different functions.

Restoring palmar abduction of the thumb

Restoring palmar abduction of the thumb is best carried out on patients in whom the EDM has not been utilized during the first phase. We prefer to use the ECRL tendon to activate the FDP, and the BR to activate the FPL. These procedures are fully described in Chapter 13. Alternatively, if an active 'lasso' is possible and no other muscle is available, the PT may be used to activate the FPL, thus saving the BR to activate the lasso.

The EDM is utilized to restore palmar abduction (antepulsion) of the thumb. The tendon is harvested as described above, taking care to divide it as far distally as possible. It is then retrieved proximal to the dorsal retinaculum, passed around the ulnar border of the forearm, and transferred subcutaneously to the thumb, with a direction parallel to the APB.

If the thumb MP joint does not need stabilization, the tendon is woven into the distal tendon of the APB. If stabilization is needed, the distal part of the EDM is divided into two equal strips, and inserted as described by Brand.[9] The proximal slip is not fixed to APB; rather, it is passed dorsally around the metacarpal neck and sutured ulnar to the terminal tendon of the adductor muscle. The second slip is woven through the APB, passed dorsally, and sutured to the

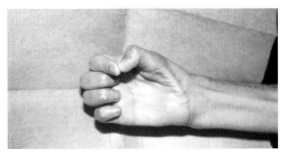

Figure 14.7 Transfer of EDM to APB to produce a subterminal pinch.

EPL, distal to the MP joint (*Fig. 14.6*). The tendon is sutured with a slight flexion of the MP joint. Tubiana has slightly modified the distal insertion by passing the two strips through the extensor tendon, one proximal and one distal to the MP joint.[10]

Alternatively, if the EDM has been used during the first stage, the palmaris longus may be transferred, if this is strongly active, and elongated with a strip of the superficial palmar fascia, as advocated by Camitz.[11] However, the palmar fascia may be disappointingly thin and frail, and it may be technically difficult to perform the double insertion distally.

As stated earlier, this technique provides, through active anteposition, the possibility that the thumb will produce a pinch anywhere on the radial aspect of the index finger, including a subterminal pinch (*Fig. 14.7*). This greatly improves pinch precision, but it does not provide greater strength.

Restoring thumb opposition

Restoring thumb opposition, often referred to as the 'triple transfer', uses the ECRL for finger flexion, PT for thumb flexion, and BR for thumb opposition (conjoint flexion–abduction), as advocated by House et al.[3] It is described fully in Chapter 13. This technique provides an increase in pinch strength, but this pinch remains essentially a lateral one. However, the BR, when attached (via the superficialis tendon graft) into the tendon of the EPL as part of the thumb intrinsic substitution procedure, has proved strong enough to stabilize the thumb's IP joint against excessive flexion (Froment's sign) of the thumb's IP joint. This is so even when the FPL is strongly motored (e.g., by PT transfer). By whatever means, intrinsic extension of the IP joint must be substituted for, to avoid a Froment's sign, either by the transfer

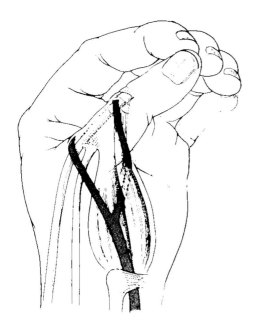

Figure 14.6 Distal insertion of EDM around the MP joint, as performed by Brand.

A

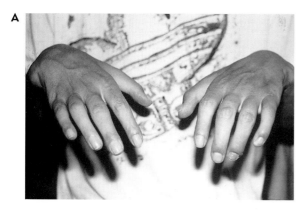

B

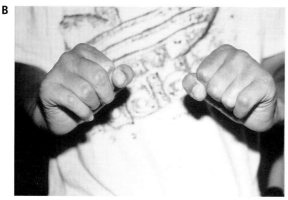

C

described above or by the 'split' FPL to EPL procedure, as described in Chapter 13.

In a bilateral Group 6 patient it may be useful, to perform a different technique on each side, to provide the patient with two different types of pinch, one for precision and one for strength.

Results

Patients from IC Group 6 usually benefit greatly from surgery. Their hands evolve from a poor and weak pinch and no grasp to a strong lateral pinch (usually with a precision subterminal pinch on one side) and a strong and effective grasp.

These patients usually make the best of these transfers, as they also possess strong wrist stabilizers, which potentiate the strength of the transfers, and a number of proximal muscles around the shoulder and elbow, which allow them to reach out into a much greater functional space. Following restoration of grasp and pinch in IC Group 6 patients, they begin to function more as a high-level paraplegic than a tetraplegic. Our patients refer to themselves as 'para-quads'.

Illustrative case

A 24-year-old man had sustained a C8 spinal cord injury in a motor vehicle. His upper limbs were classified as bilateral IC Group 6, with a triceps graded MRC 5 bilaterally. A two-stage procedure was performed on each side. The left hand was operated 12 months post-injury, and the right hand 17 months post-injury. His results in flexion and extension are shown, respectively, at 7 months (*Fig. 14.8A*) and 2 months (*Fig. 14.8B*) postoperatively. *Figure 14.8C* shows pinch strength, which was 700 g (true lateral pinch, with forearm fully pronated, and weight hooked to a thin piece of material) on each side at final review, 2 years postoperatively.

He was very satisfied (8.5 on a visual linear scale of 0–10) with both procedures, and has acquired complete independence for essentially all activities of daily living, including personal hygiene, dressing, feeding, and body transfers.

Figure 14.8   Results of a two-stage procedure in an IC Group 6 patient, at 7 months postoperatively (A) and 2 months postoperatively (B). (C) Pinch strength of the same patient.

References

1. Barthes G. Contribution a l'étude de la métamérisation motrice medullaire, Paris, Thesé, 1964.
2. Zancolli E. Correccion de la 'garra' digital por paralisis intrinseca. La operacion del 'lazo'. Acta Ortop Latinam 1974; 1:65.
3. House JH, Gwathmey FW, Lundsgaard DK. Restoration of strong grasp and lateral pinch in tetraplegia due to cervical spinal cord injury. J Hand Surg 1976; 1(2):152–159.
4. Brand P, Beach R, Thompson D. Relative tension and potential excursion of muscles in the forearm and hand. J Hand Surg 1981; 6:209–219.
5. Zancolli E. Structural and Dynamic Basis of Hand Surgery. 2nd edn. Philadelphia: JB Lippincott; 1979.
6. Rupnik J, Leclercq C. Extensor tendons to the little finger: anatomy and classification (in French, English summary). La Main 1997; 2: 3–9.
7. Blacker G, Lister G, Kleinert H. The abducted little finger in low ulnar nerve palsy. J Hand Surg 1976; 1:190–196.
8. Mestdagh H, Bailleul JP, Vilette B, et al. Organization of the extensor complex of the digits. Anat Clin 1985; 7:49–53.
9. Brand. 189–234.
10. Tubiana R. Paralysies motrices du pouce. In: Tubiana R, ed. Traité de Chirurgie de la Main, Vol. 4. Paris: Masson; 1991:211–288.
11. Camitz. 81.

15

Surgical rehabilitation of refined hand function (International Classification Groups 7, 8, and 9)

Introduction

Even patients who are classified as International Classification (IC) Group 7, 8, or 9 [American Spinal Injury Association (ASIA) level C8] may experience increased upper limb function from surgical procedures for their upper limbs. Few will benefit from or accept orthoses because, compared to the majority of tetraplegic patients, they already function at a high level. Most possess normal shoulder, elbow, and wrist control and, by definition, they have strong thumb and finger extension. Many IC Group 7 patients also have some useful finger flexion. The IC Group 8 patients have strong finger flexion and typically some active but weak thumb flexion also. The IC Group 9 patient has strong thumb flexion in addition to strong finger flexion. Their hands are very similar to the hands of those who suffer a distal laceration of the median and ulnar nerves and lose all intrinsic muscle function in the hand. This is referred to as the 'intrinsic minus hand'.

Since these patients function at relatively high levels, they are more likely to be involved in full time employment or school. It may be difficult for them to set aside enough time to undergo surgery and the follow-up therapy. They are typically using a manual wheel chair and do not like the idea of having to use a powered chair, even for a short period of time. They are far more independent and see even a short period of time in a more dependent state (i.e., having one arm in a cast) as a huge liability. Finally, because they already function at a relatively high level, compared to the IC Groups 3, 4, 5, and 6 patients discussed in previous chapters, decisions regarding surgery must be considered carefully. These patients require more analysis and discussion regarding the risks and potential benefits of surgery. They frequently want to 'think' about surgery for longer periods of time.

As IC Groups 7, 8, and 9 patients all possess functionally adequate finger and thumb extension, they rarely require multi-stage procedures. Appropriate surgical procedures include tendon transfers to restore or strengthen finger (IC Group 7) and thumb flexion (IC Groups 7 and 8) and dynamic intrinsic substitution procedures (IC Groups 7–9) to provide digital balance.

Reconstructive options – International Classification Group 7

The IC Group 7 patient, by definition, possesses at least MRC Grade 4 finger and thumb extension. The actual number of Grade 4 or 5 muscles varies from patient to patient. Some may retain strong function in accessory wrist or digital extensors, such as the extensor carpi ulnaris and/or the extensor indicis. The variety of potential reconstructive surgery options differs accordingly. The most basic surgical plan should include provisions for:

- finger flexion;
- thumb flexion and/or adduction and abduction; and
- digital intrinsic balance.

This plan is similar to those described in Chapters 13 and 14 for the flexor phase for IC Groups 4, 5, and 6 patients.

Finger and thumb flexion

These patients possess a number of potentially transferable synergistic muscles with which to restore finger and thumb flexion. The muscles most typically transferred to achieve these goals include the extensor carpi radialis longus (ECRL), the brachioradialis (BR), and the pronator teres. Usually, one donor muscle is transferred to the tendons of the flexor digitorum profundus to restore finger flexion. Another donor muscle is transferred to restore thumb flexion. Rarely, function of both superficial and deep flexors can be restored. For example, some IC Group 7 patients have MRC Grade 3 deep flexor strength. In such cases, the choice may be to restore power to the superficial flexors. The operative steps for many of these transfers are discussed in Chapters 9 and 13.

Thumb intrinsic reconstruction

The IC Group 7 patient benefits from reconstruction of thumb opposition, either by standard opponensplasty procedures or various modifications thereof. There may be several sources for a muscle–tendon transfer to restore this function and more than one effective method of routing the transfer. Surgical choices must be made for each individual according to the specific presentation of the thumb and available accessory muscles, such as the extensor indicis, extensor digiti minimi (EDM), or flexor carpi ulnaris. We have significant experience with House's method using the BR muscle lengthened with a tendon of one of the superficial flexors (see Chapter 13) for the IC Group 7 patient who lacks any of these accessory muscles.

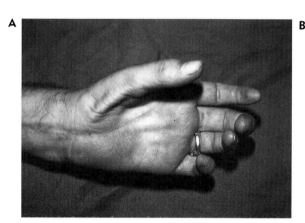

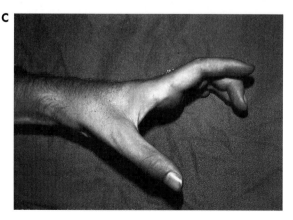

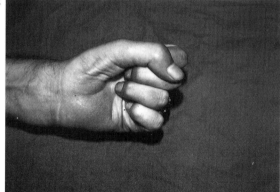

Figure 15.1 The left hand of an IC Group 7 tetraplegic patient is pictured. He had undergone multiple tendon transfers in one stage some months before. At surgery, the extensor carpi radialis longus (ECRL) was used to power the deep finger flexors (flexor digitorum profundus), the brachioradialis was used to strengthen the long thumb flexor (flexor pollicis longus), and the extensor indicis was passed around the ulnar side of the distal forearm and attached into the tendinous insertion of the abductor pollicis brevis and also into the extensor pollicis longus tendon over the proximal phalanx. He maintained (A) a good opening, (B) a powerful grasp, and (C) excellent palmar abduction.

If the independent extensor of the index finger, the extensor indicis, is functioning at MRC Grade 4+, we prefer to transfer this muscle. The procedure involves division of the extensor indicis tendon as far distal as possible, withdrawal of the tendon via a distal dorsal forearm incision, and then routing the tendon around the ulnar side of the distal forearm and across the base of the palm. Typically, a small incision is required at the ulnar aspect of the distal forearm to assist in passing the tendon from dorsal to palmar. An additional palmar incision may be needed to pass the tendon across the base of the palm. A final incision is made over the radial aspect of the thumb's metacarpophalangeal joint for attachment of the transferred extensor indicis tendon. We have found it

useful to split the terminal 2 cm (0.8 inches) of the tendon of the extensor indicis and perform a two-tailed insertion. The first tail is woven into the tendon of the abductor pollicis brevis muscle, near its insertion into the thumb's proximal phalanx. The second tail is passed dorsally over the thumb and is woven into the tendon of the extensor pollicis longus. This tail is attached in a snug fashion to provide some interphalangeal joint stabilization for the thumb. *Figure 15.1* shows the postoperative result in an IC Group 7 patient after transfers of the ECRL to the profundus finger flexors and the BR to flexor pollicis longus (FPL), and the extensor indicis was transferred for thumb opposition (just described).

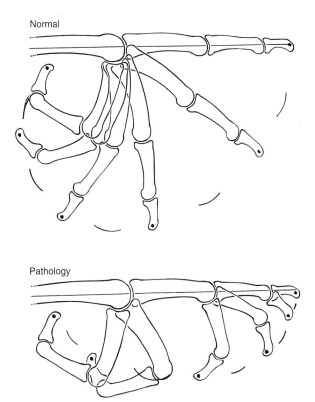

Normal

Pathology

Figure 15.2   In the normal hand, flexion is initiated at the metacarpophalangeal joints, next at the proximal interphalangeal joints, and finally at the terminal distal interphalangeal joints. (A) The fingers sweep through a large arc. The hand is then able to grasp objects of large or small diameter equally well. (B) In the tetraplegic hand that lacks intrinsic function but retains or has reconstructed active profundus muscles, flexion of the fingers is initiated at the terminal distal interphalangeal joint. This causes the fingers to roll into flexion as opposed to broadly sweeping into a closed position. As the fingertips roll up, they push larger objects out of the hand, but smaller objects are held securely. Restoring intrinsic function enables the hand to again grasp both large and small objects with security.

An alternative is to stabilize the interphalangeal joint of the thumb against hyperflexion (Froment's sign) by performing Mohammed *et al.*'s 'split FPL transfer', as described in Chapter 11, and make only a single insertion into the tendon of the abductor pollicis brevis.[1]

Other potential sources of motor power for restoring thumb flexion and/or abduction or opposition include the extensor carpi ulnaris, the flexor carpi ulnaris, the palmaris longus, and the EDM. The first two of these require an interpositional tendon graft, which can be obtained from one of several sources, such as one-half of the two-part EDM tendon, the palmaris longus tendon, the plantaris tendon, or by harvesting a section of the tendon of the flexor carpi radialis.

Reconstruction of digital intrinsic function

When the strong digital extension enjoyed by these patients is combined with transfers for restoring strong finger flexion, a significant risk is created of troublesome metacarpophalangeal joint hyperextension and a 'claw' finger deformity as the patient attempts to open the hand. Therefore, these patients are candidates for one or another intrinsic substitution procedure. Restoring the function of the intrinsic muscles of the digits improves both opening and closing of the hand. It improves the opening posture by enhancing interphalangeal joint extension, and so preventing the claw deformity. It improves the closing posture of the hand by assisting the initiation of flexion at the metacarpophalangeal joints, as opposed to finger flexion beginning at the terminal distal interphalangeal joint (*Fig. 15.2*). The biomechanical basis for this improvement is discussed in greater detail in Chapter 13. House demonstrated improved function and strength of grasp in his patients when he performed an intrinsic substitution at the time of restoring finger flexor power.[2] He hypothesizes that having intrinsic function allows the surgeon to place the finger flexor transfer under greater tension. He believes that this provides increased flexor power on the part of the donor muscle's length–tension curve, which is most useful to the tetraplegic patient's manner of grasp.[2]

Many surgical procedures have been described as effective in restoring intrinsic function. These include static procedures, such as various tenodesis or cap-sulodesis procedures, and many active muscle–tendon transfer procedures. The tenodesis procedure described by House *et al.*[3] and the 'lasso' procedure described by Zancolli[4] are discussed and illustrated in detail in Chapter 13. The useful criteria in deciding which procedure might be most beneficial for a particular patient are also discussed in Chapter 13. It has been our experience that the majority of IC Groups 7, 8, and 9 patients retain good interphalangeal extension when metacarpophalangeal joint hyperextension is prevented and the 'lasso' procedure is more often performed. Furthermore, in contrast to IC Group 4 and 5 patients, for whom only the index and middle finger may need intrinsic substitution, IC Groups 7, 8, and 9 patients benefit from intrinsic substitution to all four digits.

Some IC Group 7 patients may have sufficient numbers of transferable motor resources to enable an active intrinsic substitution procedure. For example, the pronator teres *could* be used to power the thumb by transfer to the FPL and the BR could be passed into the volar forearm and its tendon woven into one or several of the paralyzed flexor digitorum superficialis tendons in the forearm. In the hand, the superficial flexor tendons could be re-deployed as prime flexors of the metacarpophalangeal joints by Zancolli's 'lasso' procedure, described in detail in Chapter 13.

Single-stage reconstruction of strong finger and thumb flexion, combined with intrinsic substitution procedures, can lead to a dramatic improvement in hand function. Such patients may obtain pinch power exceeding 20 N and digital grasp power exceeding 100 N. *Figure 15.3* illustrates one such IC Group 7 patient. This 52-year-old man worked full-time as an executive administrator of a chapter of the Paralyzed Veterans of America. As an IC Group 7 level tetraplegic, he had strong finger and thumb extension but only MRC Grade 1–2 finger flexion, primarily through the flexor digitorum superficialis muscle. His digital extension strength was such that he was able to carry his briefcase on his outstretched fingers (*Fig. 15.3A*). Functional reconstruction involved transfer of the ECRL to the combined flexor digitorum profundus tendons, transfer of the BR to the thumb flexor, and transfer of the extensor indicis to the abductor pollicis brevis. A Zancolli 'lasso' procedure was performed since he had some MRC Grade 3 flexor digitorum superficialis strength.

A

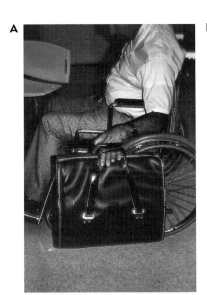

B

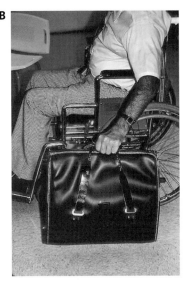

Figure 15 3 (A) Preoperatively, this IC Group 7 patient used his strong digital extensors to carry his briefcase. (B) Postoperatively, after reconstruction of a strong grasp, he could carry his case in a more secure and normal manner. (C) He could vary the posture of his thumb depending on the task.

C

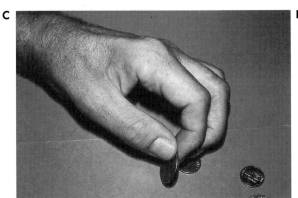

D

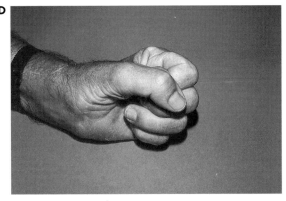

Postoperatively, he achieved strong finger and thumb flexion power. He now could carry his briefcase in a more normal manner (*Fig. 15.3B*). He regained refined pinch function and could handle objects with varying thumb postures, including small objects using the true thumb opposition (*Figs 15.3C* and *15.3D*).

Reconstructive options – International Classification Groups 8 and 9

An exceedingly small percentage of tetraplegic patients fit this category. Therefore, we have had much less experience in performing surgical reconstruction in these two groups than in the other functional categories. However, in a very practical sense, these patients are very much more like a paraplegic patient since they typically have strong shoulders and arms and very useful hand function. The IC Group 8 patient lacks only strong thumb flexion (typically they possess some thumb flexor power) and the IC Group 9 patient lacks only hand intrinsic function. These two groups of patients have many potentially transferable muscles and, aside from reinforcing thumb power, would benefit most from intrinsic reconstruction. In this sense they can be considered much like someone who suffers a low median and ulnar nerve palsy from some type of peripheral nerve trauma. As discussed in Chapter 6, the difficult decisions are not technical in nature but rather whether or not to recommend surgery for an individual already functioning at a high level. The IC Group 8 or 9 individual requires a great deal of counseling and discussion before undergoing surgery. Since they are functioning well, their expectations regarding the outcome of surgery may be greater than can be achieved.

Many potential combinations of procedures might be considered. In principle, dynamic rather than static procedures should be the first choices, that is muscle–tendon transfers rather than tenodesis procedures. A useful combination for an IC Group 8 patient who already possesses some thumb interphalangeal joint flexion, but less than MRC Grade 4, might include:

- A thumb opposition transfer (e.g. using the extensor indicis, routed as discussed for the IC Group 7 patient).
- Reinforcing the power of the thumb in a strong pinch and grasp by extending the extensor carpi

radialis brevis with a tendon graft and then passing the tendon graft from dorsal to palmar via the second intermetacarpal space. In the palm, the graft parallels the course of the transverse head of the adductor pollicis, passing dorsal to the nerves and flexor tendons and toward the ulnar aspect of the metacarpophalangeal joint of the thumb. The tendon graft is split and one slip is attached into the stout ulnar collateral ligament of the metacarpophalangeal joint of the thumb, whereas the other slip is brought onto the dorsum of the thumb and attached into the tendon of the extensor pollicis longus over the proximal phalanx.

- Attaching one of the tendon slips of the abductor pollicis longus (if not already functioning) into the tendon of the flexor carpi radialis. This helps

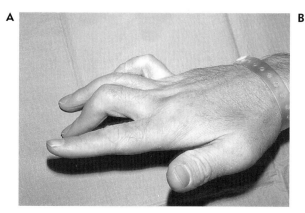

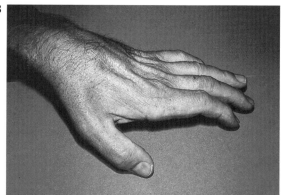

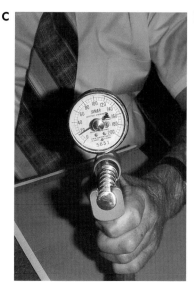

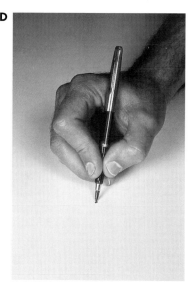

Figure 15.4 This IC Group 8 patient required strengthening of the thumb flexor by pronator teres transfer to the flexor pollicis longus, transfers for opposition (extensor indicis), and intrinsic substitution using brachioradialis extended by a plantaris tendon graft. (A) Preoperatively, he demonstrated marked clawing of his hand when he tried to extend his fingers. (B) Postoperatively, he achieved a good opening posture with little tendency toward 'clawing', (C) a strong grasp exceeding 80 N, and (D) excellent thumb control and strength.

stabilize the thumb when the wrist is flexed as part of the opening posture of the hand.

- Digital intrinsic substitution procedure, using the BR as the motor and the tendon of the flexor digitorum superficialis to the ring finger as an interpositional tendon graft. Another option is to harvest the plantaris tendon and use it to create a four-tailed tendon graft. The ring-finger flexor digitorum superficialis tendon is detached at its insertion and the tendon is split into four tails. These are passed, as recommended by Brand *et al.*,[5] palmar to the intermetacarpal ligament of the second, third, and fourth web spaces and sutured into the lateral bands along the radial side of the middle, ring, and little fingers, and into the ulnar-sided lateral band of the index finger.

Figure 15.4 shows the operated hand of an IC Group 8–9 patient. The patient had intrinsic transfers for both thumb and fingers. He achieved almost 80 N of grip, 40 N of pinch power, and excellent balance both in extension and when handling small objects, such as a normal pen.

There are many potential combinations of active muscle–tendon transfers that might be considered for thumb and digital intrinsic substitutions for the IC Group 8 or 9 patient. Technical details regarding these procedures can be found in most general hand surgery texts and in specific articles in the hand, orthopedic, and plastic surgery literature.

References

1. Mohammed KD, Rothwell A, Sinclair S, et al. Upper-limb surgery for tetraplegia. J Bone Joint Surg 1992; 74B:873–879.
2. House JH, Shannon MA. Restoration of strong grasp and lateral pinch in tetraplegia: a comparison of two methods of thumb control in each patient. J Hand Surg 1985; 10A(1):22–29.
3. House JH, Gwathmey FW, Lundsgaard DK. Restoration of strong grasp and lateral pinch in tetraplegia due to cervical spinal cord injury. J Hand Surg 1976; 1(2):152–159.
4. Zancolli E. Correccion de la 'garra' digital por paralisis intrinseca. La operacion del 'lazo'. Acta Ortop Latinoam 1974; 1:65.
5. Brand P, Beach R, Thompson D. Relative tension and potential excursion of muscles in the forearm and hand. J Hand Surg 1981; 6:209–219.

16

Surgical rehabilitation for the unusual, incompletely injured, or pediatric-age tetraplegic patient (International Classification Group X)

Introduction

Many cervical spinal cord injuries do not fit into the relatively homogeneous categories of the International Classification (IC) system. This classification was developed to categorize primarily complete cord injuries. Individuals with incomplete cervical cord injuries exhibit greater upper limb variability than the complete cord injury groups. Their limbs defy easy categorization and are appropriately, but inefficiently, placed in an 'all others' category, designated IC Group 10 or X. Within this classification are very inhomogeneous types of patients, such as patients with so-called 'central cord' or 'Brown–Sequard' syndromes and other incomplete cervical cord injuries or afflictions, such as syringomyelia. A discussion of the methods to improve hand function in this disparate group of patients can only deal in principles, since these patients have such individualized presentations and pathology.

These patients frequently present with pathological postures as a consequence of their sensory or motor disturbances. They deserve a great deal of study and thought because correcting the deformity and restoring some function to their hands may require multiple operative stages to gain much functional benefit. The initial procedures are designed to overcome dysfunctional postures, such as depicted in *Figure 16.1*. These procedures include the release of contracted muscles, tendons, and joint capsules.

The patient who presents with metacarpophalangeal joints fixed in hyperextension represents a significant surgical challenge. To bring the joints into a more functional, flexed position, the collateral ligaments must be incised or excised. As most patients lack any functioning intrinsic muscles, release of the collateral ligaments renders the joint completely unstable. The fingers are free to rotate into dysfunctional positions and the ultimate finger posture is unpredictable. For such patients, we have carried out very judicious ligament releases through a volar approach, so that the dorsal capsule and extensor mechanisms remain undisturbed. Following release, the fingers are exercised in an outrigger type orthosis, and the splint controls any tendency for the digit to rotate.

Another common deformity is a wrist fixed either in flexion or extension. We have utilized excision of the proximal row of carpal bones to overcome both flexion and extension contractures of the wrist.

Surgical release of contractures is followed by a period of intensive therapy and appropriate splinting. Once the gains from therapy have reached a plateau, the patient is re-examined. Occasionally, releasing a contracted joint unmasks a useful muscle unappreciated at the initial examination. Further surgery is designed to assist the patient in achieving a functional grasp. Common procedures include both tendon transfers and tenodeses, as described in the preceding chapters.

A

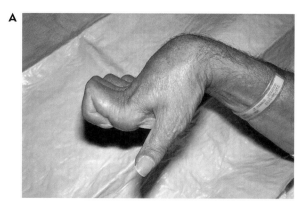

B

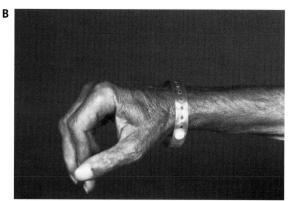

C

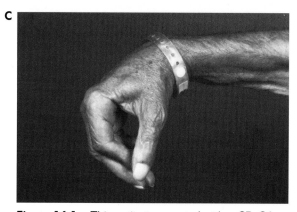

Figure 16.1   This patient presented with a C5–C6 incomplete 'central cord' lesion. (A) Both shoulder and elbow control were limited and the hand had become severely contracted. Following release of the contractures, including proximal row carpectomy, tendon transfers were performed to restore finger extension. (B, C) Subsequently, he developed a useful grip.

Management of the upper limb in children with cervical spinal cord injury

Introduction

Of the approximately 10,000 individuals who sustain spinal cord injuries each year in the USA, 3–5% are younger than 12 years of age and 20% are younger than 20 years of age. The incidence of cervical spine injuries increases from about 30% in the 0–8 years of age group to 53% in the 9–15 years of age group. Motor vehicle accidents are the most common etiology, followed by violence, including child abuse and sports injuries.

The pediatric spinal cord population is characterized by unique anatomical features that distinguish it from injured adults. Cord injury is frequently unassociated with radiological abnormalities and the onset of neurological abnormalities may be delayed. Growth and development are responsible for complicating factors such as the development of spinal and hip deformities. The direct costs of lifetime care for a child injured at 10 years of age are estimated at nearly two million dollars. There is an equal indirect cost, the result of lost wages, benefits, and productivity.

The pediatric upper limb

The goal of upper extremity management in children with spinal cord injury is to prevent deformities and pain, to promote arm and hand use for ambulation, wheeled mobility, and performance of play, school, and self-care activities, and to maintain a pliable and pleasing appearance for social contact. Similar to the interventions used in adults with spinal cord injury, management of the pediatric arm and hand includes appropriate positioning and range of motion exercises, early application of orthoses, and surgical reconstruction in the form of tendon transfers, tenodeses, and arthrodeses. For some children the application of functional neuromuscular stimulation may be beneficial.

Children with tetraplegia are prone to the same upper limb deformities as seen in adults. Elbow flexion and forearm supination contractures can be particularly troublesome in younger children who are unable to understand the importance of range of motion exercises or of compliance with splint programs. Unlike adults with spinal cord injury, young children with tetraplegia often develop severe metacarpophalangeal joint extension contractures that can preclude the acquisition of a functional wrist-extension, finger-flexion tenodesis posture and complicate the successful outcomes of functional neuromuscular stimulation and reconstructive surgeries. While few published reports exist, experiences with stretching, serial casting, and surface stimulation programs for the remediation of metacarpophalangeal joint extension contractures have been disappointing; the results of surgical capsulotomies have also been somewhat disappointing. The rehabilitation team should educate family members and school therapists on the importance of maintaining a pliable hand, since failure to do so can be devastating not only for socialization but also for the long-term function of the hand.

Orthoses

Orthotic use by adults with spinal cord injury in home and work environments is dependent upon the cosmesis and reliability of the orthosis, simplicity to don and doff it, effective training, the opportunity to perform activities, preference, and the ability to use an alternative method.[1] While these factors also influence the use of orthoses by children, critical factors in the successful employment of orthoses by children and in long-term use also appear to be:

- size and weight of the orthosis;
- child's understanding of the purpose of the orthosis;
- parental support; and
- independent ability of the child to employ it in school.

In the acute injury period, all tetraplegic children should have their hands placed in resting hand splints, as described in Chapter 4. Once they have entered early rehabilitation, they may benefit from light, easily donned orthoses to provide some independence in tabletop activities. Depending on the residual strength of the upper limbs, palmar (universal) cuffs, mobile arm supports, balanced forearm orthoses, and wrist-driven flexor-hinge orthoses are all available in children's sizes and may be prescribed. Importantly, teachers and other school personnel should be educated about the type of orthosis and trained in the donning and doffing process. Lastly, frequent growth spurts require local vendors who are able to modify the orthoses in an expeditious and affordable manner.

Surgical indications

There are few indications for upper limb surgical rehabilitation prior to 4 years of age. For children younger than this, conventional therapy should be provided to maintain joint motion and pliability and to strengthen the muscles for future hand surgery or the application of functional neuromuscular stimulation.

Surgical reconstruction to improve arm and hand function should be considered for all children with tetraplegia who are 4 years of age and older. By this age a child is generally more able to cooperate with splint wear and directed hand therapy in the postoperative period. Functional upper limb surgery should first be performed on a child's dominant hand, if possible prior to the child entering formal schooling. This means usually by 6 years of age. It is at this time that at least one functioning hand is most needed for school activities such as writing, coloring, pasting, and cutting.

The indications, techniques, and outcomes of surgical reconstruction for arm and hand function in the adult spinal cord population are well documented. More recently, indications, techniques, rehabilitation, and outcomes of tendon transfers for upper extremity function in children with spinal cord injury have emerged.[2–4]

Indications for and techniques of surgical reconstruction with children reflect the practices in the adult population, with some notable differences, particularly the effect of surgical procedures on the growth of the limb and the effect of growth on the residual functional outcome. For example, there is concern that an arthrodesis may traumatize a nearby growth plate and result in premature closure of the epiphysis. However, it has been demonstrated clearly that the wrist or other more distal joints can be fused successfully in the child without endangering the growth potential of the limb. A different technique is employed in the child to that in the adult. Powered saws and burrs are avoided to minimize the risk of overheating adjacent tissues. Hand tools are preferred when denuding joint surfaces of articular cartilage. The articular cartilage is carefully shaved away in fine layers until the ossification center of the metaphysis is encountered. A single Kirschner wire is passed across the joint as longitudinally as possible, again to avoid unnecessary injury to the physes.

Experience has demonstrated that tendon transfers can be performed safely in the rapidly growing child and that the transferred muscle–tendon unit will adapt to growth in a manner similar to a normal muscle–tendon unit. These procedures have been performed successfully for many years in children with cerebral palsy, brachial plexus injuries, and other conditions. Less experience has been gained in tenodesis procedures, such as flexor pollicis longus tenodesis to restore key pinch in the rapidly growing limb. Unyielding scar tissue causes a growing bone to curve in the direction of the scar. The same may occur when a stout tendon is anchored across several intervening joints. However, tenodesis procedures have been performed in a few young children with no problems such as growth arrest reported to date. Until more experience has been gained, tenodesis procedures in the child with significant growth potential should be approached with caution.

Postsurgical rehabilitation

Healing of surgically attached tissues, such as tendon transfers, takes place more rapidly in children than in adults. However, in general children have a more difficult time in adhering to precise exercise schedules and in following restriction guidelines, so that a longer period of immobilization is a more prudent course. Rehabilitation following tendon transfers and other procedures is modified for children with respect to their developmental age, ability to cope, and family needs and abilities. However, children are naturally active and enthusiastic, and after tendon transfers their play activities can be adapted to facilitate muscle re-education, active range of motion exercises, and strengthening activities.

Functional neuromuscular stimulation

A functional neuromuscular stimulation device, the FreeHand System, has recently been approved by the Food and Drug Administration for use in children. This system is described in greater detail in Chapter 17. Studies with adults[5] and adolescents[6] show that the device increases grasp and pinch force, improves performance during a standardized test of hand function, and improves abilities during activities of daily living. Much of the current research using functional

neuromuscular devices in the pediatric population is on usage patterns in home, school, and work environments, and on user satisfaction. Wider application of such devices holds promise for many spinal cord injury adolescents who desire improved hand function, but who are not candidates for more traditional tendon transfers. Research applications of functional neuromuscular stimulation in youngsters with tetraplegia have been equally positive,[7] and preliminary studies of the effect of growth on stimulated muscle responses suggest that young growing children with spinal cord injuries may also benefit from totally implanted functional neuromuscular stimulation systems.[8] There are differences in some of the implantation techniques to accommodate for longitudinal growth of the implanted limb. For example, the electrode leads are implanted as loose loops to provide redundancy.

References

1. Allen V. Follow-up study of the wrist-driven flexor-hinge splint use. Am J Orthotic Res 1971; 25:420–426.
2. James M. Surgical treatment of the upper extremities: indications, patient assessment and procedures. In: Mulcahey RBM, ed. The Child with Spinal Cord Injury. Rosemont: American Academy of Orthopedic Surgeons, 1996:393–404.
3. Weiss A. Tendon transfers in tetraplegia: surgical technique. In: Mulcahey RBM, ed. The Child with Spinal Cord Injury. Rosemont: American Academy of Orthopedic Surgeons, 1996:405–418.
4. Mulcahey M. Rehabilitation and outcomes of upper extremity surgery. In: Mulcahey RBM, editor. The Child with Spinal Cord Injury. Rosemont: American Academy of Orthopedic Surgeons, 1996.
5. Woulle KS, Van Doren C, Thrope G, et al. Development of a quantitative hand grasp and release test for patients with tetraplegia using a hand neuroprosthesis. J Hand Surg 1994; 19A:209–218.
6. Triolo R, Betx R, Mulcahey M, et al. Application of functional neuromuscular stimulation to children with spinal cord injuries. Candidate selection for upper and lower extremity research. Paraplegia 1994; 32:824–843.
7. Mulcahey MJ, Smith B, Betz R, et al. Functional neuromuscular stimulation: Outcome in young people with tetraplegia. J Am Paraplegia Soc 1994; 17:20–35.
8. Akers J, Triolo R, Betz R. Motor responses to implantable electrodes in growing limbs. J Spinal Cord Med 1996; 19:301–306.

17

Upper limb functional neuromuscular stimulation

Introduction and history

The use of electric currents to overcome neuromuscular disorders has led to the development of a variety of devices and applications. The initial research and development was directed at overcoming electrical disorders of the heart with implanted pacemakers. Other implantable neuromuscular stimulators were designed to stimulate the diaphragm. The earliest applications of electric currents for spinal cord injury patients were directed more toward conditioning exercises,[1-3] or to assist the surgeon in determining the appropriate tension of a muscle–tendon transfer at surgery.[4]

Early interest in the application of electric currents to restoring limb function in patients who have suffered spinal cord injuries led to the pioneering work of Peckham and Marsolais.[1,5,6] While the initial thrust of functional neuromuscular stimulation (FNS) research was to enable paraplegic patients to stand and walk, other researchers began to consider the application of these technologies to the paralyzed upper limb of the tetraplegic population.[2,7-10] These investigators have advanced the application of FNS to the upper limb much more rapidly than their colleagues have been able to apply FNS to the goals of standing and walking. Currently, FNS technology to activate the hand has been commercialized, and this technology is being investigated to assist shoulder function in the higher C4 level tetraplegic[11] and to restore elbow flexion.[12]

Initial concepts involved the chronic use of percutaneously inserted electrodes and multi-channel external stimulators controlled by a programmable computer;[13,14] patient-specific stimulation sequences could be programmed to affect various grasp patterns. The programmed stimulation sequences were themselves activated and modulated by a controller mounted externally on a part of the body still under voluntary control, typically the contralateral shoulder.[15] Other control systems used the patient's voice[16] or respiration.[17]

Complications inherent in a system based on a series of percutaneous electrodes,[18] including infection, electrode migration, and breakage, led to the search for less problematic designs.[14,19,20] Today, the near-fully implantable FNS system developed by scientists and engineers from Case Western University in Cleveland, USA,[21] has been approved for use in tetraplegic patients by the Food and Drug Administration (FDA) and its European corollary, and has been commercialized through the Neurocontrol Corporation as the 'Free-Hand System'.

Current concepts

The FNS approach takes advantage of the existence of muscles no longer under voluntary control but with spinal reflex arcs that still remain intact. These upper motor neuron injury muscles can be directly stimulated with relatively weak direct electric currents, or can be made to contract by stimulation of their motor nerve. These muscles may undergo disuse atrophy, but are not subject to the essentially complete denervation atrophy of a muscle whose motor nerve has been cut or whose anterior horn cell has been destroyed, as in poliomyelitis (lower motor neuron paralysis.)

Investigators[5,20] have found that in the upper limb of the tetraplegic patient there exist, in the same limb, muscles completely under normal voluntary control and innervated well rostral to the zone of injury, and muscles completely affected by an upper motor neuron paralysis, typically located well below the spinal injury. In addition, there are muscles that have segments under voluntary control, segments that are totally denervated (lower motor neuron paralysis), and segments that are upper motor neuron paralyzed. These are typically muscles for which the medullary source of innervation is closer to the actual spinal cord injury.

If, in the same arm and hand, sufficient numbers of key upper motor neuron paralyzed muscles exist, these muscles can be recruited via FNS to perform useful functions, and so a patient might benefit from the application of this technology. Such patients also need a way to control the stimulation parameters, that is which muscles contract, when, and at what proportion of their potential contractile force. Therefore, a candidate for such a device must have adequate numbers of electrically stimulatable muscles and, currently, adequate voluntary control of the movement of some upper limb joint, now typically the contralateral shoulder.

Also, FNS has led to an interesting and natural conceptual leap. If a key muscle [e.g., the extensors of the digits (EDC)] has a lower motor injury and is not electrically stimulatable, any other non-key muscle in proximity [e.g., the extensor carpi ulnaris (ECU)] may be identifiable and its function substituted. This substitution is generated via FNS for the worthless key muscle by combining an old procedure, muscle–tendon transfer, with this new technology. In such cases, the tendon of the ECU is detached from the base of the fifth metacarpal and woven into the combined tendons of the EDC. Electrical stimulation of the ECU now brings about digital extension.

Additional key concepts derived from rigorous research include better proportional stimulation by placing the stimulating electrode near to but not over the motor point of the muscle. This permits better modulation of the stimulus parameters of the individual muscle, rather than an all or nothing contraction of the muscle. Since the total number of muscles that can be stimulated is limited by the number of available stimulation channels, and the potential number of muscles that might respond to stimulation vastly

greater, it has been necessary to simplify the mechanics of the hand. For example, eight muscles are normally employed to flex the fingers, four superficial and four deep flexor muscles. By suturing together all of the profundus tendons, stimulation of one of the profundus muscles effects flexion of all the digits. Muscle independence is sacrificed for simplicity. This

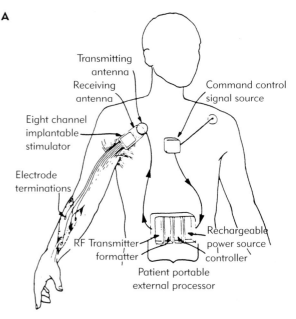

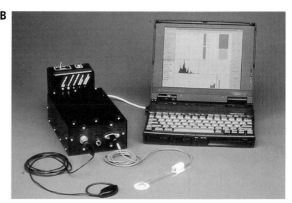

Figure 17.1 (A) The components of the current upper extremity functional neuromuscular system. The implanted components include the eight-channel stimulator package, electric leads, and muscle electrodes. External components include a transmission coil and a shoulder–chest mounted controller. (B) The wheelchair-mounted interface device and computer that is used to program the individual grasp and release patterns.

same simplification can be carried out for the tendons that effect extension of the fingers.

We have had recent experience with implanting a system of electronics, including a programmable stimulator that controls an array of eight epimyseal electrochannels. This system (*Figs 17.1A* and *17.1B*), developed by surgeons and engineers from the Case Western Reserve University and the Cleveland Veterans Administration Medical Center, has the ability to allow a patient with a very high spinal injury to activate and control a pre-programmed sequence of muscle contractions and thus achieve a useful grasp for one hand. Two different grip and release patterns can be programmed and the patient can switch between the two patterns. These include a lateral or key-pinch pattern useful for grasping smaller objects in a secure grip (*Figs 17.2A* and *17.2B*) and a tip-to-tip pinch or opposition pinch useful for acquiring and holding larger objects (*Figs 17.3A* and *17.3B*). The control mechanism is mounted externally about the opposite shoulder, and allows active and volitional shoulder movement to open and close the grip and modulate the force. Some additional movements can lock the grip in a closed position at the desired force of closure (*Fig. 17.4*). This system of electrodes placed on predetermined upper motor neuron paralyzed muscles has the potential to restore useful function in limbs heretofore deemed useless and unreconstructable by standard surgical techniques.

Current indications

The current indication for FNS for the tetraplegic upper limb is a patient for whom standard surgical procedures or orthotic devices cannot provide useful and improved (over current) function. Today, this system has been implanted in patients at several International Classification (IC) levels, including IC Groups 1, 2, and 3. The device is expensive to purchase, the surgical procedure is extensive, and the rehabilitation is somewhat complex. Time will allow us to determine its true place in the reconstructive armamentarium.

Patient preparation

Once a potential candidate has been identified, a systematic assessment protocol begins. This includes an assessment of the physical parameters of the upper limbs and the patient's abilities, motivation, and support. The patient must be able to sit for long periods in the wheelchair and to control more proxi-

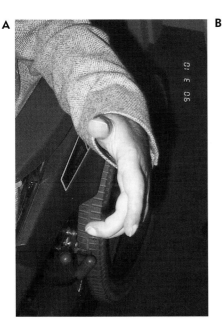

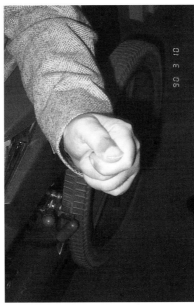

Figure 17.2 The key or lateral grasp pattern is shown in its (A) fully opened phase and (B) fully closed phase.

A

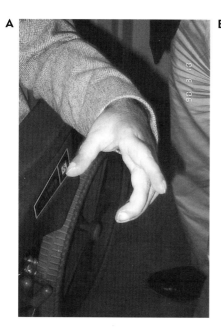

B

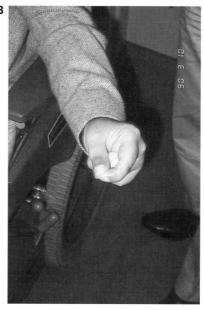

Figure 17.3 The palmar grasp pattern is shown in its (A) fully opened phase and (B) fully closed phase.

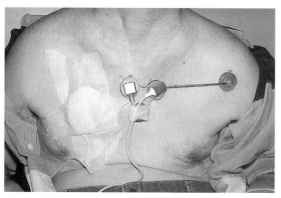

Figure 17.4 The shoulder–chest mounted 'joystick' controller and the transmitting coil. These external devices are applied every day.

mal joints (such as the shoulder and the elbow), as well as have the resources to stabilize the wrist when the fingers are stimulated to contract (otherwise the wrist will flex and the grasp will be weaker). We have found that patients complain if they must wear an external wrist splint to stabilize the wrist and have begun to recommend wrist fusion for the FNS candidate who lacks resources for wrist stabilization. The patient must possess adequate motivation to endure

preoperative conditioning exercises, one or more difficult surgical procedures, and complex post-operative therapy, and must also have adequate support from family or attendants since the system employs external devices that must be attached to the patient on a daily basis.

Physical assessment includes a standard manual muscle test to determine residual motor resources still under voluntary control, assessment of passive

Table 17.1 Key muscles for FNS lateral and palmar pinch

Opening the hand	
1.	Extensor digitorum communis
2.	Extensor pollicis longus
3.	Flexor digitorum superficialis (used as active 'lasso' for intrinsic substitution
4.	Abductor pollicis brevis
Grasp	
5.	Flexor pollicis longus
6.	Flexor digitorum profundus
7.	Abductor pollicis

and active joint mobility and sensation, and identification of significant pathological conditions such as severe spasticity, joint contractures, or hypersensitivity. The final assessment involves identifying which muscles respond to external direct current (DC) stimulation to determine which of the seven or eight key muscles are suitable. The key muscles are listed in *Table 17.1*. Knowledge of all these factors allows suitability for the procedure to be determined and surgical strategies to be developed.

Once the operative strategy has been determined, the patient undergoes a period of conditioning of the muscles to be implanted. This is helpful, as these muscles will be de-conditioned to some extent. Pre-surgical conditioning has many aims. Occasionally, a period of conditioning by external electrical stimulation may lead to increased strength of one or another muscle so that the surgeon may confidently plan on using this muscle as part of the grasp–release sequence. More importantly, pre-surgical conditioning makes the muscles less fatigable during surgery. Since the muscles to be implanted will be stimulated frequently during surgery, a muscle that fatigues easily becomes difficult to assess.

Current operative techniques

The common functional goals include provisions for elbow stabilization (by deltoid-to-triceps or biceps-to-triceps transfer, see Chapter 10), carried out as a separate procedure or at the time of device implantation, or by implantation of an electrode on the triceps as part of the procedure to implant the device.[22] Which of these is carried out is established early in the assessment scheme. A second key goal is wrist stabilization to prevent wrist flexion during grasp. This may pre-exist (as in the IC Group 2 or 3 patient) or is provided by:

- traditional muscle–tendon transfers (e.g., brachioradialis to extensor carpi radialis brevis);
- transfer of an upper motor neuron paralyzed 'spare' muscle to be activated by one of the implanted stimulation channels; or
- wrist fusion if no other means is available.

With these goals met, the remainder of the implantation procedure is directed by the results of the preoperative assessment.

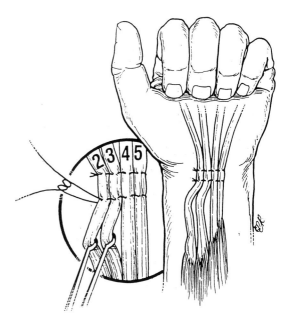

Figure 17.5 Synchronization of the flexor profundus tendons (FDP). The goal is to establish the flexor pattern for the hand in response to electrical stimulation of any one or more of the FDP muscles. Note that the normal flexor cascade is not the goal. Rather, it is preferable to have a somewhat greater flexion of the radial two digits.

Typically, both the tendons of the common digital extensors and the deep (profundus) digital flexors are sutured, one to another (side-to-side tenodesis) so that only one electrode is needed for extension and one for flexion (*Fig. 17.5*). If any muscle–tendon transfers are required, these are performed. Other predetermined specific procedures are carried out, such as the split FPL transfer to stabilize the interphalangeal joint of the thumb,[23] or transfers for intrinsic stabilization (e.g., the Zancolli 'lasso'[24] or the House procedure[25]). Next, the best position to locate each of the eight electrodes is determined by trial stimulation. Once determined, the electrodes are sutured to the epimysium of the muscle and the leads from the electrodes are tunneled proximally such that they cross the elbow joint close to the lateral or medial axis of rotation. Recently, intramuscular electrodes have become available, and may perform better than epimyseal electrodes for some muscles.

The stimulator package is inserted into a subclavicular subcutaneous pocket and the leads from the stimulator package are connected to the leads from the electrodes via an incision close to the axilla. Using specially designed external controllers, each of the eight channels is tested and its characteristic stimulation parameters assessed. This testing may show that one or another electrode needs to be relocated to provide the optimum functional position of the thumb and fingers. Finally, a trial of grasp and release in both the lateral and the opposition patterns is attempted. Wounds are closed and the arm and hand immobilized.

Postoperative protocol

Several weeks later, the patient begins another period of muscle conditioning, this time using the implanted system. The precise time of immobilization depends on the procedures performed in addition to electrode placement. Once the muscles are conditioned to offset the deconditioning that accompanies surgery and postoperative immobilization, the patient and therapist work together to program the computer that interprets the signals from the mechanical shoulder position sensor and controls the stimulation hardware. Several periods of programming are necessary to optimize the grasp and release patterns. The patient acquires experience in the use of the device and typically recognizes shortcomings and this interplay is necessary to arrive at the best control and stimulation parameters for each patient. Depending on the circumstances, some patients require frequent updating of their program, while others require little.

As a daily routine, the patient's attendant must attach the shoulder control 'joystick' to the patient's chest and shoulder, and attach the external transmitting coil over the implanted stimulation package. These external pieces are connected to the wheelchair-mounted computer. The computer's batteries, which are recharged nightly, generate all the power required by the implanted stimulators. Transcutaneous inductive coupling through the transmitting coil charges the eight stimulation channels. The benefit of this source of power, compared to an on-board battery, is obvious.

Investigators have, to date, reported few significant complications. One system was totally explanted because of infection. A few electrodes that have become exposed have required removal, with or without replacement.

Current results

At the time of writing, more than 200 tetraplegic patients have been implanted worldwide,[26,27] including several tetraplegic children.[28] The functional outcome from the use of these devices is well-documented by means of specifically designed functional tests and by subjective patient assessment.[26,27] There is general agreement among clinicians that the device extends the possibility for improved upper limb function to groups of patients, such as the IC Group 0 or 1 patient, for whom standard surgery or braces offers little in the way of functional gain. Patient acceptance has been high. Unfortunately, the expense of the device and the associated implantation costs restrict its application. In the USA, insurers have been reluctant to approve the necessary expenditures. Very recently the commercial provider, Neurocontrol Corporation has decided to discontinue selling new units because of lack of profitability. Other methods to make this technology available are being sought.

Future possibilities

For patients who retain strong active wrist extension, such as the IC Group 2 or 3 patient, investigators are experimenting with less cumbersome control hardware. On an investigational basis, several patients with retained wrist extension have had electromagnetic sensors implanted on either side of the wrist joint. This device recognizes wrist movement, which becomes the basis for commanding the opening and closing of the grasp. This is a very natural and easily learned method.

Provisions to add additional channels of stimulation are being investigated. Using small intramuscular electrodes, it may be possible to implant many intrinsic muscles of the hand, and thus offer more refined hand functions.

Additional future possibilities involve extending the device to more proximal paralyzed muscles such as biceps and deltoid muscles. This may allow higher level C4–C5 tetraplegics to become more functional.

References

1. Hansen G. EMG-controlled functional electrical stimulation of the paretic hand. Scand J Rehabil Med 1979; 11:189–193.

2. Kiwerski J, Weiss M, Pasniczek R. Electrostimulation of the median nerve in tetraplegia by means of implanted stimulators. Paraplegia 1983; 21:322–326.

3. Bajd T, Kralji A, Turk R, et al. Use of functional electrical stimulation in the rehabilitation of patients with incomplete spinal cord injuries. J Biomed Eng 1989; 11:96–102.

4. Kelly CN, Freehafer AA, Stroh K. Postoperative results of opponensplasty and flexor tendon transfer in patients with spinal cord injuries. J Hand Surg 1985; 10A:890–894.

5. Peckham P, Mortimer J, Marsolias E. Upper and lower motor neuron lesions in the upper extremity muscles of tetraplegics. Paraplegia 1976; 14:115–121.

6. Simard T, Ladd H. Hand orthotic device influence on fine neuromuscular control. Arch Phys Med Rehabil 1976; 57:258–263.

7. Peckham P, Mortimer J. Restoration of hand function in the quadriplegic through electrical stimulation. In: Hambreck FT, Resnick JB, eds. Functional Electrical Stimulation: Applications in Neural Prostheses. New York: Dekker, 1977:543–550.

8. Brucker BS. Combining biofeedback and FES to improve function. Paraplegia News 1985;39:32–35.

9. Petrofsky J, Phillips C, Stafford D. Closed loop control for restoration of movement in paralyzed muscles. Orthopedics 1984; 7:1289.

10. Rose EH. The high-tech hand surgery interface. Lewinn L, ed. Clinics in Plastic Surgery, Vol. 13. St Louis: CV Mosby, 1986:333–344.

11. Carroll S, Meeney C. Electrical stimulation for restoring independent feeding in a man with quadriplegia. Am J Occup Ther 1993; 47:739–742.

12. Betz R, Mulcahey M, Smith B, et al. Bipolar latissimus dorsi transposition and functional neuromuscular stimulation to restore elbow flexion in an individual with C4 quadriplegia and C5 denervation. J Am Paraplegia Soc 1992; 15:220–228.

13. Peckham P. Functional electrical stimulation: current status and future prospects of application to neuromuscular systems in spinal cord injury. Paraplegia 1987; 25:279–288.

14. Peckham P, Keith M, Freehafer A. Restoration of functional control by electrical stimulation in the upper extremity of the quadriplegic patient. J Bone Joint Surg 1988; 70A:144–148.

15. Johnson M, Peckham P. Evaluation of shoulder movement as a command control source. IEEE Trans Biomed Eng 1990; 37:876–885.

16. Handa Y, Hoshimiya N. Functional electrical stimulation for the control of the upper extremities. Med Prog Tech 1987; 12:51–63.

17. Hoshimiya N, Naito A, Yajima M, et al. A multichannel FES system for the restoration of motor functions in high spinal cord injury patients: A respiration controlled system for multijoint upper extremity. IEEE Trans Biomed Eng 1989; 36:754–760.

18. Smith B, Betz R, Mulcahey M, et al. Reliability of percutaneous intramuscular electrodes for upper extremity functional neuromuscular stimulation in adolescents with C5 tetraplegia. Arch Phys Med Rehabil 1994; 75:939–945.

19. Keith M, Peckham P, Thrope G, et al. Functional neuromuscular stimulation neuroprosthesis for the tetraplegic hand. Clin Orthop 1987; 233:25–33.

20. Keith M, Peckham P, Thrope G, et al. Implanable functional neuromuscular stimulation in the tetraplegic hand. J Hand Surg 1989; 14A:524–530.

21. Kilgore K, Peckham P, Thrope G, et al. Synthesis of hand grasp using functional neuromuscular stimulation. IEEE Trans Biomed Eng 1989; 36:761–770.

22. Miller L, Peckham P, Keith M. Elbow extension in the C5 quadriplegic using functional neuromuscular stimulation. IEEE Trans Biomed Eng 1989; 36:771–780.

23. Mohammed KD, Rothwell A, S Sinclair, et al. Upper-limb surgery for tetraplegia. J Bone Joint Surg 1992; 74B:873–879.

24. Zancolli E. Correccion de la 'garra' digital por paralisis intrinseca. La operacion del 'lazo'. Acta Ortop Latinoam 1974; 1:65.

25. House JH, Gwathmey FW, Lundsgaard DK. Restoration of strong grasp and lateral pinch in tetraplegia due to cervical spinal cord injury. J Hand Surg 1976; 1(2):152–159.

26. Stroh-Woulle K, Van Doren C, Thrope G, et al. Common objects test: a functional assessment for quadriplegic patients using an FNS hand system. RESNA 12 Annual Conference. New Orleans, 1989:387–388.

27. Smith B, Mulcahey M, Betz R. Quantitative comparison of grasp and release abilities with and without functional neuromuscular stimulation in adolescents with tetraplegia. Paraplegia 1996; 34:16–23.

28. Triolo R, Betz, R, Mulcahey M, et al. Application of functional neuromuscular stimulation to children with spinal cord injuries. Candidate selection for upper and lower extremity research. Paraplegia 1994; 32:824–833.

18

Assessing post-treatment improvement in upper limb function in the tetraplegic patient – evaluating function

Introduction

The ability to determine the outcome of one treatment versus another has become extremely important as clinicians strive toward outcomes-based decision-making. Critical evaluation of the tetraplegic's hand and upper limb function is of particular value to the clinician because the choice of treatment today is very dependent on perceptions of the resultant hand and arm function, and perception is not always reality. Unless a 'gold-standard' already exists, all outcome instruments must possess sufficient validity, feasibility, acceptability, sensitivity, and reliability.

Physiologic measurements

Force of grip

The simplest tests of presumed function measure purely physiological parameters. Manual muscle testing, with the observer testing resistance, represents the most unsophisticated of the commonly used physiological evaluations. Various commercially available devices to measure the force of grip and pinch are commonly used. However, as designed, they are less than ideal for the tetraplegic patient since most devices that purport to measure grasp are very insensitive at the lowest range. For example, the Jamar dynamometer is too insensitive to measure accurately the small but functionally significant changes in grasp strength that might follow a tendon transfer in a tetraplegic hand. It is difficult to read small changes since the registrations on the dial are in 5 lb and 1 kg increments. Additionally, the device must typically be placed in the subject's hand and supported by the examiner. This introduces an uncontrollable variable if results obtained by one examiner need to be compared with those obtained by another. While many studies of normal subjects exist, there are no protocols for using the device for tetraplegic patients.

A standard blood pressure cuff can be tightly rolled into a cylinder and partially inflated. The patient is asked to squeeze the cuff and the increase in manometer pressure over baseline is used as an objective measure. This is economical, but many authors question its reliability. It measures a pressure rather than a force and different manometers may be used. Different grasp patterns are used by patients and the sensitivity to low grasp forces is unknown.

Force of pinch

The commercially available devices to measure the strength of pinch require the patient to grasp the instrument in a more or less standard manner so that the force is directed perpendicular to the force plate of the device. Many tetraplegic patients cannot easily move the device into the space between the thumb and index finger and, even if able to do this, frequently cannot control the direction of force because of lack of stability at the multidirectional carpometacarpal joint of the thumb. Either the device spins out of their grip, or the force they exert is not perpendicular to the force plate and the device registers an artificially low force. Patients who have had this joint fused may be able to control the direction of force somewhat more readily. In addition, such pinch gauges are usually constructed with surfaces so smooth that the frictionless fingers of the IC Group 1–3 tetraplegic (who lack sweat-gland activity in their finger tips) easily slip off the device.

Various investigators have tried to modify commercially available devices or create unique ones. Taping the smooth surface of the pinch gauge with sandpaper may increase the coefficient of friction between finger and device, which reduces the tendency of the fingers to slip off the contact surfaces.

In addition to the lack of any standardization in measuring the force generated, there is no standardization in terms of position of the hand or arm during measurements. Our recent research into how nonoperated patients use passive tenodesis to generate small but still useful forces has demonstrated the many tricks and adaptations used by patients to effect a grip. For example, if the examiner holds the device used to measure force, the patient, using more proximal muscles such as the elbow flexors, can generate a greater force against a rigidly held device than against a 'free-floating' device. To avoid this possible bias, for several years we have measured the patient's ability to pinch a ribbon of rough fabric and lift a known weight attached to the ribbon. The patient must perform this activity with the thumb and index finger held more or less perpendicular to the table so that only the pressure they exert between their thumb and index fingers is used to grasp the ribbon. We thus measure their ability to resist the slippage of the weighted ribbon.

Joint motion

A change in the range of active and/or passive motion of a joint can be measured to represent the effect of treatments such as reconstructing elbow extension by deltoid-to-triceps transfer or augmenting wrist extension by brachioradialis transfer. More sophisticated instruments are needed to measure true joint torque.

Sensation

Sensation is typically assessed by testing various sensory modalities, such as presence or absence of light touch or sharp–dull discrimination (as described in Chapter 7), or by the two-point discrimination tests described in Chapter 6. All provide objective data of variations in sensitivity, specificity, and significance that can document a change in status between pre- and post-treatment dates.

Task-oriented assessment

In addition to the standard physiological measurements of such parameters as range of motion, strength, and sensitivity, a number of standardized functional testing methodologies designed to provide objective, valid, reliable, and reproducible data have been introduced to measure functional gains in the tetraplegic patient's upper limbs. Some methods directly measure the individual's ability to perform a standard set of tasks in a prescribed manner or within a prescribed period of time. All require the individual to grasp and move objects (e.g., the Perdue Peg-board test). Some measure only fine dexterity (e.g., the O'Conner Finger Dexterity test) or measure the ability to use tools, (e.g., the Bennett Hand-tool test). Some permit bimanual use, whereas others restrict the activity to be performed to one hand only. The most commonly applied tests include the protocol described by Jebsen et al.[1] and that described by Sollerman.[2,3] None were designed specifically for the tetraplegic patient and all have recognizable shortcomings when so applied.

Ejeskar and Sollerman published their experience with the Sollerman test as an outcomes instrument for a large series (59) of tetraplegic patients.[4] The test is based on seven of the eight most common normal grasp patters and consists of 20 activities of daily living (ADLs). Test scores correlated well with the International Classification (IC) level of the patient's arm, more so for patients in IC Group 3 or higher and less well for those classified at greater IC levels.

Recently, Woulle et al. analyzed the instruments currently used and defined areas of deficiency for the Jebsen and Sollerman tests.[5,6] Their criticisms were based primarily on the inability of most tetraplegic patients, certainly before but usually also after surgery, to produce the type of grasp called for by the test. They opined that a more ideal instrument must include tasks that can be performed preoperatively by some of the patients, either unassisted or wearing an orthosis, and following surgery. The tasks should not require extensive use of the arm or trunk (i.e., they should focus mostly on the function of the hand and not the arm). The tasks should be performed using grasp patterns appropriate, that is possible, for the tetraplegic patient, such as lateral prehension. They have developed and utilized a tetraplegia-specific ADL-based 'pick and place' instrument as part of their investigation of the practical benefits of functional neuromuscular stimulation systems. Their test requires the use of both lateral and palmar prehension and involves objects of different weights and shapes.

Functional capacity measurements

The major goal of rehabilitation for the tetraplegic patient is to maximize the functional and physical skills and resources, and move the individual toward a greater level of independence. Another category of assessment instrument examines the individual's level of independence in performing a variety of tasks that represent the broad range of ADLs. These are termed 'functional indices'. Several have been used to measure function and post-treatment functional gains in tetraplegic patients. These include the modified Barthel index (MBI)[7] and the Quadriplegia Index of Function (QIF).[8] The most common functional index applied to the tetraplegic patient today is termed the 'Functional Independence Measure' (FIM).[9,10] Of these, the only functional index designed specifically for the tetraplegic patient is the QIF.

The QIF (*Table 18.1*) uses 10 weighted activities (transfers, grooming, bathing, feeding, dressing, wheelchair mobility, bed activities, bladder program, bowel program, and understanding of personal care, and scores may range from 0 to 100.

The FIM is an ADL-based assessment of independence (see *Figure 18.1*). Six general categories are scored, on a one to seven scale, according to the level of assistance, if any, required to carry out the task(s). Currently, the FIM is being used in the USA by the Model Spinal Cord Injury System. *Table 18.2* compares the scoring of the QIF and FIM systems. *Table 18.3* shows a representative patient score pre and post upper limb surgery (see Appendix III).[8]

The QIF is felt by some authors to be somewhat more sensitive since more than a general category of activities (e.g., communication skills) is scored, which

may allow a finer discrimination of functional ability. Marino *et al.* compared FIM and QIF scores using only three of the seven functional categories (feeding, grooming, and bathing) and found that both correlated well with upper extremity muscle strength.[11] No difference was found between FIM and QIF for the bathing and grooming tasks, but QIF exhibited a closer correlation to upper extremity strength for the feeding tasks. Appendix VIII contains the patient outcome questionnaire developed by Dr James House at the University of Minnesota.

Recommendations for tetraplegia-specific upper limb tests

No single instrument (or set of instruments) that measures the outcome of treatments to improve the function of the upper limb in tetraplegic patients is widely accepted. An ideal assessment scheme should, by necessity, incorporate key elements of physiological, task-oriented, and functional measurements. It must possess a good appearance and construct validity so that both the examiner and patient view it as appropriate and comprehensive. It must also permit measurement of the patient's subjective assessment of change of experience as a consequence of the treatment. Finally, it should recognize the development of avoidable pathological factors, such as loss of joint movement or torque (e.g., elbow flexion torque following biceps-to-triceps transfer). It should be accomplished in a relatively brief period of time, and the patient him- or herself must appreciate the test as relevant.

The key reconstructable functions for the tetraplegic patient include elbow extension, wrist extension, pinch and grasp, and for each a tetraplegic-specific evaluation can be constructed, keeping in mind the original goals of reconstruction and how the tetraplegic patient uses the limb.

Elbow extension

The goal of elbow extension restoration in the tetraplegic patient is to improve the patient's ability to use his or her upper limb in various limb postures, including reaching overhead (i.e., extend the elbow against gravity with the shoulder abducted greater than 90°), and also in transfers where the shoulder is adducted.

Table 18.1   The Quadriplegia Index of Function (QIF)

Category	Component activities (each scored separately)	Relative weights of category (%)
I. Transfers	1. Bed-chair	8
	2. Chair to bed	
	3. Chair to toilet or commode	
	4. Toilet or commode to chair	
	5. Chair to vehicle	
	6. Vehicle to chair	
	7. Chair to shower or tub	
	8. Shower or tub to chair	
II. Grooming	1. Brushing teeth/managing dentures	6
	2. Brushing/combing hair	
	3. Shaving (men)	
	4. Managing tampon (women)	
III. Bathing	1. Wash/dry upper body	4
	2. Wash/dry lower body	
	3. Wash/dry feet	
	4. Wash/dry hair	
IV. Feeding	1. Drink from cup/glass	12
	2. Use spoon/fork	
	3. Cut foods (meat)	
	4. Pour liquids out	
	5. Open carton/jar	
	6. Apply spreads to bread	
	7. Prepare simple meals	
	8. Apply adaptive equipment	
V. Dressing	1. Upper indoor clothes on/off	10
	2. Lower indoor clothes on/off	
	3. Upper outdoor (heavy) clothes on/off	
	4. Socks on/off	
	5. Shoes on/off	
	6. Fasteners	
VI. Wheelchair mobility	1. Turning corners	14
	2. Reverse directions	
	3. Lock wheelchair brakes	

Table 18.1 (*continued*)

Category	Component activities (each scored separately)	Relative weights of category (%)
	4. Propel wheelchair on rough/uneven surfaces	
	5. Propel wheelchair on an incline	
	6. Move and position in chair	
	7. Maintain sitting balance	
VII. Bed activities	1. Supine to prone	10
	2. Supine to long sitting	
	3. Supine to side	
	4. Side to side	
	5. Maintain long sitting balance	
VIII. Bladder program	Separate sets of scoring criteria for:	14
	A. Voluntary voiding:	
	1. Toilet	
	2. Commode	
	B. Intermittent catheterization program	
	C. Autonomic bladder program	
	D. Indwelling catheter	
	E. Ileal diversion	
	F. Credé	
IX. Bowel program	Separate sets of scoring criteria for:	12
	A. Complete control:	
	1. Toilet	
	2. Commode	
	B. Suppository:	
	1. Toilet	
	2. Commode/bed/Chux pad	
	C. Digital disimpaction:	
	1. Toilet disimpaction	
	2. Commode/bed disimpaction	
	D. Digital or mechanical stimulation:	
	1. Toilet	
	2. Commode/bed	

continued

Table 18.1 (*continued*)

Category	Component activities (each scored separately)	Relative weights of category (%)
X. Understanding personal care	1. Skin care	10
	2. Diet/nutrition	
	3. Medications	
	4. Equipment	
	5. Range of motion	
	6. Autonomic dysreflexia	
	7. Upper respiratory infection	
	8. Urinary tract infection	
	9. Deep venous thrombosis	
	10. Obtaining human services	

An outcome device should recognize improvement of function in various arm positions, and not simply measure the ability of the patient to reach overhead.

Physiological tests

Physiological tests should include measurements of:

- Passive elbow flexion and extension.
- Active elbow extension in different positions of the shoulder. A standardized active anti-gravity test involves the patient lying prone, close to the edge of the examining table or bed. The upper arm is supported parallel with the body in an adducted position. The elbow is flexed to 90° by gravity. The range of active elbow extension is then measured. The next measurement of active elbow extension should be taken with the arm fully and internally rotated at the shoulder and horizontally abducted to 90° and with the elbow flexed to 90°. The final measurement of active elbow extension is made with the patient seated in the wheelchair, the shoulder abducted to 120°, and the elbow flexed so that the patient's forearm rests on the top of his or her head.
- Maximum weight that the patient can move from the elbow in the flexed to the extended position in

Table 18.2 Scoring of self-care tasks

Quadriplegia Index of Function items	Level	Functional Independence Measure
4	Independent	7
3	Independent with devices	6
2	Supervision	5
1	Physical assistance:	
	Minimum	4
	Moderate	3
	Maximum	2
0	Dependent	1

Functional Independence Measure (FIM)

LEVELS		
7 Complete Independence (Timely, Safely) 6 Modified Independence (Device)	No Helper	
Modified Dependence 5 Supervision 4 Minimal Assist (Subject = 75%+) 3 Moderate Assist (Subject = 50%+)	Helper	
Complete Dependence 2 Maximal Assist (Subject = 25%+) 1 Total Assist (Subject = 0%+)		

                                    ADMIT   DISCH

Self Care
A. Eating
B. Grooming
C. Bathing
D. Dressing-Upper Body
E. Dressing-Lower Body
F. Toileting

Sphincter Control
G. Bladder Management
H. Bowel Management

Mobility
Transfer:
I. Bed, Chair, Wheelchair
J. Toilet
K. Tub, Shower

Locomotion
L. Walk/wheelChair
M. Stairs

Communication
N. Comprehension
O. Expression

Social Cognition
P. Social Interaction
Q. Problem Solving
R. Memory

Total FIM

NOTE: Leave no blanks; enter 1 if patient not
testable due to risk.

Figure 18.1   The Functional Index Measure (FIM).
See *Table 18.3* for an example of the scale used.

these same three shoulder positions. As well as the maximum weight tests, repetitive tests using a weight that is 50% of the maximum that can be moved may be used to assess the muscle's resistance to fatigue.

Subjective tests

Subjective tests should include questions regarding changes in ADL skills that are a consequence of the reconstruction of elbow extension and questions that focus on tasks that require elbow control or movement. This includes ADLs associated with reaching, such as dressing the body, transfers, and wheelchair mobility.

Wrist extension

Physiological tests

Physiologic assessment should include measurement of:

- Passive range of wrist flexion and extension.
- Active range of motion, with gravity eliminated and against gravity. For the former, the forearm is maintained in neutral rotation and the active extension is measured. For the latter, the forearm is pronated and active wrist extension measured.
- The maximum weight that can be lifted by wrist extension with the forearm pronated and the elbow flexed at 60°. Repetitive tests using a weight that is 50% of the maximum that can be moved may be used to assess the muscle's resistance to fatigue.

Subjective tests

Subjective assessment should include questions regarding changes in ADL skills that are a consequence of the reconstruction of wrist extension and questions that focus on tasks that require wrist control or movement (e.g., the ability to perform ADLs without the splints previously needed).

Pinch and grasp

For patients in IC Groups 1 and 2, and for some IC Group 3 patients, only the thumb is powered, either directly by muscle transfer or by augmented (flexor pollicis longus) tenodesis. For patients in the other Groups, both finger flexors and extensors are powered. No standard tetraplegic-specific instrument to assess improvement in hand function following functional upper limb surgery is accepted uniformly, but the principles on which to base such an instrument seem clear:

- For hand function to be improved, the surgical procedure and assessment instrument must recognize

Table 18.3 The Functional Index Measure (FIM) as modified by the occupational therapists at Craig Rehabilitation Hospital, Denver, Colorado, and used to chart progress between pre- and postoperative periods. See *Figure 18.1* for a description of the scale used.

Activity		Presurgery	Usual routine, postsurgery	If time allows, postsurgery
Dressing	Upper extremities	1	3	4
	Lower extremities	1	1	1
Communications	Typewriter/computer	1	1	7
	Write	1	7	7
	Telephone	1	7	7
	Turn pages	1	7	7
Housemaking	Cold food	1	4	6
	Stove top	1	1	1
	Oven/microwave	1	1	4
	Marketing	1	1	1
	Light cleaning	1	1	1
	Heavy cleaning	1	1	1
	Laundry	1	1	1
Bladder management	Empty leg bag	1	6	6
	Put on leg bag	1	1	1
	Leg bag connection	1	1	1
	Clothing/clean up	1	1	1
Feeding	Spoon/fork	4	7	7
	Cup/glass	1	7	7
	Cup/food	1	1	1
Grooming	Brush/comb hair	1	4	7
	Brush teeth	4	5	7
	Shave	1	3	7
	Wash face and hands	1	7	7
Bathing	Bathing/showering	1	4	4

the patient's need to grasp and release objects using the thumb (always powered) and the fingers (sometimes powered). Simply stated, the hand must open (to obtain an object) and also must close (around the object).

- For the tetraplegic patient most objects are grasped within the first web space.
- Opening the hand is a positional activity, one that does not require or even necessarily benefit from greater strength.

- In contrast, grasp requires strength and, particularly for the thumb, function is improved and increased strength is associated with an improved ability to direct the force.

Physiology-based outcome instruments must assess these two reciprocal functions, although any scoring system should be weighted toward the more important grasping functions.

Physiological tests

Hand opening

Physiological assessment of grasp and release should include measurement of the hand opening, or release, in terms of the ability of the first web space to open in preparation to grasp. Tetraplegic patients grasp both supported (either by virtue of their own weight or by some other means of support, such as by their opposite hand) and unsupported objects. The heavier or supported object is generally easier to surround as the supported object pushes open the first web space (i.e., passive opening). The unsupported or light object must be surrounded by the actively opened first web, since the object is neither heavy enough nor fixated sufficiently to open the first web space passively. Therefore, a standardized physiological based system to assess opening should consist of two tests:

- maximum size of a supported object that can be accommodated between the patient's thumb and fingers; and
- maximum size of an unsupported object that can be accommodated between the patient's thumb and fingers.

For those patients who have had procedures to assist opening digits other than the thumb, some measure of digital opening should be included. For example, the distance from the center of the finger pulp to the midpalmar crease of the least extended digit could be measured. The rationale for this measurement rests on the observation that usually the least extended digit limits the ability of the patient to maneuver the hand around the largest objects.

Hand closure

Physiological assessment of hand closure or grasp should recognize the several ways a tetraplegic patient uses his or her hands for grasp, that is the preferential use of the first web space for key pinch as opposed to grasping objects using only the second to fifth fingers. For the patient who has had only the key pinch reconstructed an appropriate system should evaluate, in addition to measurement of hand opening discussed above, how successful the procedure was in providing

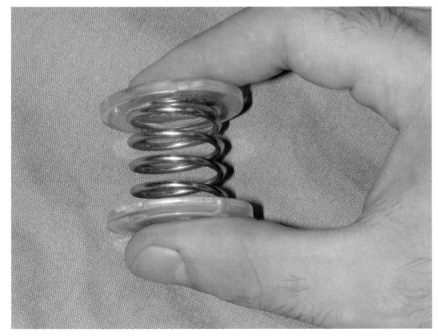

Figure 18.2
A compressible spring. The resistance increases uniformly as the spring is compressed.

a stable platform for the thumb to work against and in improving the force of the thumb pinch.

How stable the platform is can be assessed by determining whether the fingers provide a stable platform:

- in all wrist positions;
- only with the wrist fully extended; and
- only with assistance (e.g., the patient must use his or her other hand to roll the fingers into position).

We propose the force of thumb pinch can be measured using a simple, reliable, reproducible, and economic instrument that consists of a series of compressible springs of various resistances (*Fig. 18-2*). These springs can be fashioned to mimic a very stable task, one in which control of the direction of force is not important to achieve the task. They can also be constructed to mimic a very unstable task in which control of the force is essential to success. By varying the length of the spring, it can mimic grasping large or small objects. Several potential end-points are possible, such as the heaviest grade of spring that can be compressed to 50% or 100% of its length.

For IC patients who have undergone more extensive two-stage grasp-release procedures, a more comprehensive set of physiological measurements are needed to measure thumb and digital grasp. These should include:

- force of the thumb using both stable and unstable springs as described above;
- force of the active finger flexion using similar springs; and
- measuring the resistance of the flexed digits to being extended, termed resisted pull.

All patients who have undergone procedures to improve hand function should have, in addition to these physiological measures, object-oriented and patient-centered assessments.

An object-oriented task assessment consists of four tasks:

- insert and/or remove an automated teller machine card;
- insert and/or remove a videocassette;
- insert and/or remove a key; and
- push a fork into a known resistance.

A patient assessment questionnaire to evaluate the patient's sense of change following surgery includes:

- new tasks now possible following surgery;
- lost abilities; and
- pre- and postsurgical comparison of efficiency in performing presurgical ADLs (a standard analog scale is used).

Figure 18.3 is an example of a typical question that such a questionnaire might contain.

Conclusions

Unless a standardized assessment instrument is developed and validated, and then used to measure outcomes, it will be impossible to determine whether one procedure or one tendon transfer is better than another, especially because the subject population presents such a wide range of preoperative variability.

References

1. Jebsen R, Tatlor N, Trieschmann R. An objective and standardized test of hand function. Arch Phys Med Rehab 1969; 50:311–319.
2. Jacobson-Sollerman C, Sperling L. Grasp function of the healthy hand in a standardized hand function test. Scan J Rehab Med 1977; 9:123–129.
3. Sollerman C. Assessment of Grip Function – Evaluation of a new test method. Goteborg: , 1980.
4. Sollerman C, Ejeskar A. Sollerman hand function test. Scand J Plast Reconstr Surg 1995; 29:167–176.
5. Stroh-Woulle K, Van Doren C, et al. Common objects test: a functional assessment for quadriplegic patients using an FNS hand system. RESNA 12th Annual Conference. New Orleans: , 1989:387–388.
6. Woulle KS, Thrope G, Keith M, et al. Development of a quantitative hand grasp and release test for patients with tetraplegia using a hand neuroprosthesis. J Hand Surg 1994; 19A:209–218.

Patient assessment questionnaire

Bathing (compare your post surgical level of effort or efficiency to carry out this task to your preoperative state)

More difficult	No change	Much easier
-10	0	+10

Figure 18.3   An analog scale to assess pre- and postsurgical activities of daily living tasks.

7. Mahoney FI, Barthel DW. Functional evaluation: The Barthel index. Md State Med J 1965; 14:61–65.

8. Gresham GE, Labi M, Dittmar S, et al. The quadriplegic index of function (QIF): sensitivity and reliability demonstrated in a study of thirty quadriplegic patients. Paraplegia 1986; 24:38–44.

9. Hamilton B, Granger C. Guide for the Use of the Uniform Data Set for Medical Rehabilitation. Buffalo: Research Foundation of State University of New York, 1990.

10. Schindler L, Robbins G, Hamlin C. Functional effect of bilateral tendon transfers on a person with C-5 quadriplegia. Am J Occup Ther 1994; 48:750–757.

11. Marino R, Huang M, Knight P, et al. Assessing self-care status in quadriplegia: a comparison of the quadriplegic index of function (QIF) and the functional independence measure (FIM). Paraplegia 1993; 31:225–233.

I

Standard neurological classification of spinal cord injury

Sample chart for indicating neurological classification of spinal cord injury. (Courtesy of the American Spinal Injury Association, Atlanta.)

STANDARD NEUROLOGICAL CLASSIFICATION OF SPINAL CORD INJURY

MOTOR

KEY MUSCLES

C2
C3
C4
C5 Elbow flexors
C6 Wrist extensors
C7 Elbow extensors
C8 Finger flexors (distal phalanx of middle finger)
T1 Finger abductors (little finger)
T2
T3
T4
T5
T6
T7
T8
T9
T10
T11
T12
L1
L2 Hip flexors
L3 Knee extensors
L4 Ankle dorsiflexors
L5 Long toe extensors
S1 Ankle plantar flexors
S2
S3
S4-5 Voluntary anal contraction (Yes/No)

0 = total paralysis
1 = palpable or visible contraction
2 = active movement, gravity eliminated
3 = active movement, against gravity
4 = active movement, against some resistance
5 = active movement, against full resistance
NT= not testable

TOTALS { } R + L = MOTOR SCORE
(MAXIMUM) (50) (50) (100)

SENSORY

KEY SENSORY POINTS

C2
C3
C4
C5
C6
C7
C8
T1
T2
T3
T4
T5
T6
T7
T8
T9
T10
T11
T12
L1
L2
L3
L4
L5
S1
S2
S3
S4-5

0 = absent
1 = impaired
2 = normal
NT= not testable

LIGHT TOUCH R L   PIN PRICK R L

• Key Sensory Points

Any anal sensation (Yes/No)

TOTALS
(MAXIMUM)

LIGHT TOUCH R + L = (56) (56) (56)
PIN PRICK R + L = (56) (56) (56)

PIN PRICK SCORE (max: 112)
LIGHT TOUCH SCORE (max: 112)

NEUROLOGICAL LEVEL
The most caudal segment with normal function

SENSORY R L
MOTOR R L

COMPLETE OR INCOMPLETE?
Incomplete = presence of any sensory or motor function in lowest sacral segment

ZONE OF PARTIAL PRESERVATION
Partially innervated segments

SENSORY R L
MOTOR R L

Version 4d
GHC 1992

This form may be copied freely but should not be altered without permission from the American Spinal Injury Association

Sample chart for indicating neurologic classification of spinal cord injury. (Courtesy of the American Spinal Injury Association, Atlanta.)

Hand surgery evaluation (tetraplegia)

Hand Surgery Evaluation (Tetraplegia)

Hospital:

Patient's name: _____

Date of examination: Born: Sex:

_____   Home address: Telephone number:

Examiner's signature: Ward: Doctor:

_____   Occupation before accident:
Occupation now, if any:

Date of injury: Type of accident: Car accident
Level of skeletal injury: Diving
Leading arm-hand before: Gunshot
Leading arm-hand now: _____

Use of wheelchair: Handdriven   Can raise seat in wheelchair?
                    Electric   Can turn over in bed without help?
                    Other   Can transfer without help from bed to wheelchair?
                               Can transfer without help from wheelchair to car and back again?

Functional C level: Eating with?   Grip?   Tools?

Right   Left   Method of grooming? (Shaving, make-up)

                         Method of writing?

                         Stabilization in wheelchair?

Contractures?
Previous amputations?
Unusual lack of joint stability?

Group: Right   Left

      [O] [Cu] : [ ]   [O] [Cu] : [ ]

       Tr [ ]   Tr [ ]

Delete as necessary.

Spasticity (significant)   Shoulder   Wrist

                                    Elbow   Hand

Muscles available:
(Highets scheme)

	Right	Left
Trapezius Latissimus dorsi Deltoid Serratus anterior		
Rotators out Rotators in Pectoralis muscles: Sternoclavicular part Costal part		
Triceps Biceps + Brachialis Brachioradialis Radial carpal extensors (together) Pronator		
Finger extensors Long thumb abductor Thumb extensor Flexor carpi radialis Flexor pollicis longus Extensor carpi ulnaris Finger flexors Intrinsics		

Passive range of flexion
Thumb metacarpophalangeal
joint in degrees:

    R   L

Patient's understanding:

Cooperation expected:

Sensibility: (only two-point discrimination
test with paperclip of value;
includes proprioception)

	R.	L
Thumb pulp Index Middle Ring Little		
Dorsal radial area Dorsal ulnar area		

Unusual features and remarks:

Patient's main hand and arm problems:

Suggestions for improvement by splinting or
surgery:

III

Expected functional outcomes

Level C5

Functionally relevant muscles innervated: deltoid, biceps, brachialis, brachioradialis, rhomboids, serratus anterior (partially innervated)

Movement possible: shoulder flexion, abduction, and extension; elbow flexion and supination; scapular adduction and abduction

Patterns of weakness: absence of elbow extension, pronation, all wrist and hand movement; total paralysis of trunk and lower extremities

Functional independence measure (FIM)/Assistance data: Exp = Expected FIM score; **Med** = National Spinal Cord Injury Statistical Center (NSCISC) median; **IR** = NSCISC interquartile range

NSCISC sample size: FIM = 41; Assist = 35

Expected functional outcomes	Equipment	FIM/Assistance data	Exp	Med	IR
Respiratory		Low endurance and vital capacity secondary to paralysis of intercostals; may require assist to clear secretions			
Bowel	Total assist	Padded shower/commode chair or padded transfer tub bench with commode cutout	1	1	1
Bladder	Total assist	Adaptive devices may be indicated (electric leg bag emptier)	1	1	1
Bed mobility	Some assist	Full electric hospital bed with Trendelenburg feature with patient control			
	Side rails				
Bed/wheelchair transfers	Total assist	Transfer board	1	1	1
	Power of mechanical lift				
Pressure relief/positioning	Independent with equipment	Power recline and/or tilt wheelchair			
	Wheelchair pressure-relief cushion				
	Hand splints				

Expected functional outcomes	Equipment	FIM/Assistance data	Exp	Med	IR
	Specialty bed or pressure-relief mattress may be indicated				
	Postural support devices				
Eating	Total assist for setup, then independent eating with equipment	Long opponens splint	5	5	2.5–5.5
	Adaptive devices as indicated				
Dressing	Lower extremity: total assist	Long opponens splint	1	1	1-4
	Upper extremity: some assist	Adaptive devices as indicated			
Grooming	Some to total assist	Long opponens splints	1–3	1	1–5
	Adaptive devices as indicated				
Bathing	Total assist	Padded tub transfer bench or shower/commode chair	1	1	1–3
	Handheld shower				
Wheelchair propulsion	Power: independent	Power: power recline and/or tilt with arm drive control	6	6	5–6
	Manual: independent to some assist indoors on noncarpet, level surface; some to total assist outdoors	Manual: lightweight rigid or folding frame with handrim modifications			
Standing/ambulation	Total assist	Hydraulic standing frame			
Communication	Independent with some assist after setup with equipment	Long opponens splint			
Transportation	Independent with highly specialized equipment; some assist with accessible public transportation; total assist for attendant-operated vehicle	Highly specialized modified van with lift			
Homemaking	Total assist				
Assist required	Personal care: 10 hours/day		16*	23*	10–24*
	Homecare: 6 hours/day				
	Able to instruct in all aspects of care				

*Hours per day.

Level C6

Functionally relevant muscles innervated: clavicular pectoralis supinator; extensor carpi radialis longus and brevis; serratus anterior; latissimus dorsi
Movement possible: scapular protractor; some horizontal adduction, forearm supination, radial wrist extension

Patterns of weakness: absence of wrist flexion, elbow extension, hand movement; total paralysis of trunk and lower extremities
FIM/Assistance data: Exp = Expected FIM score; **Med** = NSCISC median; **IR** = NSCISC interquartile range
NSCISC sample size: FIM = 43; Assist = 35

Expected functional outcomes	Equipment	FIM/Assistance data	Exp	Med	IR
Respiratory		Low endurance and vital capacity secondary to paralysis of intercostals; may require assist to clear secretions			
Bowel	Some to total assist	Padded tub bench with commode cutout or padded shower/comode chair	1–2	1	1
	Other adaptive devices as indicated				
Bladder	Some to total assist with equipment; may be independent with leg bag emptying	Adaptive devices as indicated	1–2	1	1
Bed mobility	Some assist	Full electric hospital bed			
	Side rails				
	Full to king standard bed may be indicated				
Bed/wheelchair transfers	Level: some assist to independent	Transfer board	3	1	1–3
	Uneven: some to total assist	Mechanical lift			
Pressure relief/positioning	Independent with equipment and/or adapted techniques	Power recline wheelchair			
	Wheelchair pressure relief cushion				
	Postural support devices				
	Pressure-relief mattress or overlay may be indicated				
Eating	Independent with or without equipment; except cutting, which is total assist	Adaptive devices as indicated (e.g., U-cuff, tendenosis splint, adapted utensils, plate guard)	5–6	5	4–6

Expected functional outcomes	Equipment	FIM/Assistance data	Exp	Med	IR
Dressing	Independent upper extremity; some assist to total assist for lower extremities	Adaptive devices as indicated (e.g., button; hook; loops on zippers, pants; socks, Velcro on shoes)	1–3	2	1–5
Grooming	Some assist to independent with equipment	Adaptive devices as indicated (e.g., U-cuff, adapted handles)	3–6	4	2–6
Bathing	Upper body: independent	Padded tub transfer bench or shower/commode chair	1–3	1	1–3
	Lower body: some to total assist	Adaptive devices as needed			
	Handheld shower				
Wheelchair propulsion	Power: independent with standard arm drive on all surfaces	Manual: lightweight rigid or folding frame with modified rims	6	6	4–6
	Manual: independent indoors; some to total assist outdoors	Power: may require power recline or standard upright power wheelchair			
Standing/ambulation	Standing: total assist	Hydraulic standing frame			
	Ambulation: not indicated				
Communication	Independent with or without equipment	Adaptive devices as indicated (e.g., tendenosis splint; writing splint for keyboard use, button pushing, page turning, object manipulation)			
Transportation	Independent driving from wheelchair	Modified van with lift			
	Sensitized hand controls				
	Tie-downs				
Homemaking	Some assist with light meal preparation; total assist for all other homemaking	Adaptive devices as indicated			
Assist required		Personal care: 6 hours/day	10*	17*	8–24*
Homecare: 4 hours/day					

*Hours per day.

Level C7–C8

Functionally relevant muscles innervated: Latissimus dorsi; sternal pectoralis; triceps; pronator quadratus; extensor carpi ulnaris; flexor carpi radialis; flexor digitorum profundus and superficialis; extensor communis; pronator/flexor/extensor/abductor pollicis; lumbricals (partially innervated)
Movement possible: elbow extension; ulnar/wrist extension; wrist flexion; finger flexions and extensions; thumb flexion/extension/abduction
Patterns of weakness: paralysis of trunk and lower extremities; limited grasp release and dexterity secondary to partial intrinsic muscles of the hand
FIM/Assistance data: Exp = Expected FIM score; **Med** = NSCISC median; **IR** = NSCISC interquartile range
NSCISC sample size: FIM = 43 / Assist = 35

Expected functional outcomes	Equipment	FIM/Assistance data	Exp	Med	IR
Respiratory	Low endurance and vital capacity secondary to paralysis of intercostals; may require assist to clear secretions				
Bowel	Some to total assist	Padded tub bench with commode cutout or shower commode chair	1–4	1	1–4
	Adaptive devices as indicated				
Bladder	Independent to some assist	Adaptive devices as indicated	2–6	3	1–6
Bed mobility	Independent to some assist	Full electric hospital bed or full to king standard bed			
Bed/wheelchair transfers	Level: independent	With or without transfer board	3–7	4	2–6
	Uneven: independent to some assist				
Pressure relief/positioning	Independent	Wheelchair pressure relief cushion			
	Postural support devices as indicated				
	Pressure-relief mattress/ or overlay may be indicated				
Eating	Independent	Adaptive devices as indicated	6–7	6	5–7
Dressing	Independent upper extremities; independent to some assist lower extremities	Adaptive devices as indicated	4–7	6	4–7
Grooming	Independent	Adaptive devices as indicated	6–7	6	4–7
Bathing	Upper body: independent	Padded transfer tub bench or shower/commode chair	3–6	4	2–6

Expected functional outcomes	Equipment	FIM/Assistance data	Exp	Med	IR
	Lower extremity: some assist to independent	Handheld shower			
	Adaptive devices as needed				
Wheelchair propulsion	Manual: independent all indoor surfaces and level outdoor terrain; some assist with uneven terrain	Manual: rigid or folding lightweight or folding wheelchair with modified rims	6	6	6
Standing/ambulation	Standing: independent to some assist	Hydraulic or standard standing frame			
	Ambulation: not indicated				
Communication	Independent	Adaptive devices as indicated			
Transportation	Independent car if independent with transfer and wheelchair loading/unloading; independent driving modified van from captain's seat	Modified Vehicle			
	Transfer board				
Homemaking	Independent light meal preparation and homemaking; some to total assist for complex meal preparation and heavy housecleaning	Adaptive devices as indicated			
Assist required		Personal care 6 hours/day	8*	12*	2–24*
Homecare: 2 hours/day					

*Hours per day.

Protocol for deltoid to triceps surgery

Indications and essential prerequisites	
4+ deltoid and no elbow contracture	
Strongly motivated	
Ability to participate in 12 week program	
Contraindications	
Severly spastic biceps	
Elbow flexion contracture greater than 30°	
Poor motivation, support	
Patient evaluation	
Muscle evaluation to establish candidacy: 4+ deltoid desired	
If deltoid strength below 4+	Programmed course for deltoid strengthening
If deltoid strength is 4+	Measure for dynamic elbow orthosis
Contact orthotist	
Preoperative	
Orthosis measurement taken	
Wheelchair controls on proper side	
Patient and car-giver education completed	
Surgical procedure	
Posterior 1/2 deltoid detached, extended with graft, attached to triceps tendon	
May include release of elbow contracture, distal tendon transfer	
Post-surgery course	
Day 1:	Patient in cylinder cast with elbow fully extended

	In bed shoulder abducted to 30° and arm elevated on pillows. Protect the shoulder and arm against sudden or uncontrolled movements. Do not pull on the arm (±) Cast or splint for wrist support if indicated
Day 2:	Begin hand exercises – active and passive Goals: maintain supple joints and good wrist motor strength
Day 2–3:	Out of bed in power wheelchair Use overhead sling placing shoulder in 30° abduction or more. (May exercise deltoid actively by supporting weight of the arm and the cast in the sling.) *No extra resistive exercises, no isometrics*
Day 28–35:	Out of cylinder cast, and sutures removed Remove overhead sling – shoulder is free to move
Post cast removal (PCR)	
Day 1:	In elbow orthosis with elbow locked in full extension; this normally allows 30° flexion. Examine arm in orthosis, if more flexion, orthosis or straps need to be modified Wear orthosis only during waking hours. At night wear a soft splint with elbow fully extended. Carefully monitor skin integrity for possible pressure points caused by the elbow orthosis or soft elbow splint. Educate patient on how to verbally instruct others on how to properly don/doff the orthosis and soft elbow splint, and skin inspection. Therapist can begin scar massage and begin patient on horizontal adduction exercises.

Day 28 (eighth week postoperatively)
Begin passive resistive exercises (PRE) to deltoid with elbow fully extended
When elbow flexed to 90° in orthosis (between sixth and seventh week PCR or 10–11 weeks postoperatively) orthosis may be discontinued. When orthosis is removed, begin PRE to the elbow. Patient can begin full ROM of elbow in gravity-eliminated position with resistance. Therapist can evaluate patient. Propelling manual wheelchair and transfer training, once patient reaches 90° of elbow flexion and is out of orthosis. Patient is to return orthosis to orthotist for future needs.

Discharge instructions:

1. How to advance orthosis

2. Night splinting regime – wear for 6 months

3. Program of resistive exercises for:

   a. shoulder

   b. elbow – when allowed

4. Precautions for caregiver and patient – printed instruction sheet

Outcome:

Ability to stabilize elbow in space, reach overhead objects, propel wheelchair

Protocol for Moberg (tenodesis) key-pinch procedure

Indications and essential prerequisites
C5–C6 tetraplegic (typically IC Group 2–3)
Grade 3+ extensor carpi radialis longus (ECRL) or provisions for increasing wrist extension, e.g., Grade 4 brachioradialis (BR)
Approximately 1-year post injury
Motivation to participate in 8-week program
Good hand posture with free passive range of motion (PROM)
Contraindications:
Spasticity of fingers (moderate to severe)
Limited range of motion (ROM) of fingers [meta-carpophalangeal (MP), proximal interphalangeal (PIP) flexion of index finger essential]
Poor motivation
Patient evaluation:
Adequate ECRL/B, BR strength
Mobile wrist, check gravity assisted flexion
Can pronate forearm
Thumb MP ROM
Preoperative
Orthosis measurement taken
Wheelchair controls on proper side
Patient and caregiver education completed
Surgical procedure:
Passiver transfer. Flexor pollicis longus (FPL) anchored to the volar surface of the radius. Optional procedures may include:
tendodese index finger,

pin and/or fuse thumb IP joints, or
Split 'New Zealand FPL–EPL tenodesis',
Tenodese EPL and EPB over thumb metacarpal if MP joint flexes > 45°
Transfer BR to ECRB if necessary.

Post-surgery course	
Week 1 through 4:	
Goals:	Educate patient in anatomy and protective measures of hand (i.e., transfers for 10 weeks postoperatively with thumb tucked into the palm, avoid stretching thumb on wheelchair rim while pushing, avoid extending thumb with wrist extended)
Activities:	Arm in cast with thumb and wrist flexed
Cautions:	Elevate arm in overhead sling or on pillows to control edema
	No resistive motions with elbow in flexion if BR has been transferred
	No pulling up from supine to sit, using flexed elbow on operated extremity as leverage point
	No hooking of operated arm around the push handle of wheelchair
Cast removal at 4 weeks	
Week 4 through 6	
Goals	Active ROM (AROM) only to regain wrist extension
	Dorsal splint to prevent accidental wrist or thumb extension
Activities:	Tuck thumb between middle and index fingers to prevent resistive pinch during AROM to wrist

	Fingers should be encouraged to follow the tenodesis pattern
	Begin scar massage
	Hand therapy treatment sessions, 20 minutes per twice a day
Cautions:	No passive stretch as this may loosen the transferred tendon
	Wear splint when not in therapy
Week 6 through 8:	
Goals:	ROM at wrist should be approaching normal limits
Activities:	Begin picking up small, light objects
	Review 'finger rolling' technique of curling the index for maximum lateral pinch ability
	May commence PROM to wrist to full range should full range not be realized
	Progress to using fork, utensils, and pushing lightweight wheelchair toward the end of this period
Cautions:	Avoid strong static pinch
	Wear splint during heavy activity (i.e. pushing wheelchair)
Week 8 through 10:	
Goals:	Full activity
Activities:	Wear dorsal splint during strenuous activities, especially transfers
	Begin upper extremity dressing using strong pinch
Cautions:	Wear night splints indefinitely to promote good hand posture
Outcome:	
Approximately 2–10 lb (0.9–4.5 kg) of lateral pinch that is enough to perform most activities of daily living without use of adaptive devices	
May occasionally need tightening of the FPL tendon	

VI

Protocol for two-stage restoration of active grasp and release of thumb and fingers

Phase 1 (opening phase)
Indications and essential prerequisites:
C6–C7 quadriplegic (International Classification Groups 4 or 5)
Minimum of four Grade 4 muscle groups in the forearm free from moderate to severe spasticity and contractures
Good hand posture
2 point discrimination on thumb and index <1.0 cm
Approximately 1 year post injury
Strong motivation to complete 6 month course and comply with protocol
Support system at home to assist with care for 6 month period
Contraindications:
Spasticity of fingers (moderate to severe)
Limited range of motion (ROM) of fingers [meta-carpophalangeal (MP), proximal interphalangeal (PIP) of index finger essential]
Poor motivation
Patient evaluation:
Adequate extensor carpi radialis longus and brevis (ECRB and ECRL), brachioradialis (BR), pronator teres (PT), and flexor carpi radialis (FCR) strength
Mobile wrist, fingers
Thumb MP ROM

Preoperative	
Orthosis measurement taken	
Wheelchair controls on proper side	
Patient and caregiver education completed	
Surgery:	
Passive opening: Tenodesis of extensor pollicis longus (EPL), abductor pollicis longus (APL), and EDC to radius; or	
Active transfer: BR to EPL, ABPL, and EDC	
May fuse carpometacarpal (CMC) joint in palmar abduction	
Post-surgery course:	
Week 1 through 4:	
Goals:	Educate patient in physiology of tendon transfer: practice activating muscles on opposite arm
Activities:	Power wheelchair; arm elevated in cast for 1 week and *pro re nata* thereafter for edema (check for proper blood circulation to hands)
Cautions:	Avoid elbow flexion against resistance if BR transferred
Week 4 through 6 (cast removal)	
Goals:	Regain wrist flexion partially
	Determine timing of flexor phase
Activities:	Begin only active ROM (AROM) to wrist flexor

	Edema control as needed
	May push manual wheelchair with splint on
	Wear splint when not actively ranging
	Passive ROM (PROM) to PIP and digital IP (DIP) joints with MPs slightly flexed and wrist extended
	Therapist begins scar massage
Cautions:	Protect thumb CMC joint if this has been fused
	Ventral splint fabricated to prevent excessive wrist and thumb flexion
	Do not hyperextend the MP joints
Week 6 through 8:	
Goals:	Regain full wrist flexion
Activities:	Begin PROM to wrist flexors
	Begin re-education process of the BR through various facilitations; may need to stabilize the arm and have patient pull hand toward shoulder initially (the BR is a 'slow learner')
	If triceps are weak, rehabilitation may take longer
Cautions:	Avoid sudden movements into wrist flexion

Phase 2 (closing phase)

Indications:
7–10 weeks or longer posture extensor phase of hand surgery
Full wrist flexion (passive = active)
Two or three Grade 4 muscles for transfer
Surgical procedure:
When finger extension is via brachioradialis transfer and CMC joint has been fused in 1st procedure then:
ECRL transferred to flexor digitorum profundus (FDP)
PT may be transferred to FPL via a free tendon graft (i.e., palmaris longus or plantaris tendon)

	Zancolli lasso (FDS anchored to A1 pulley), or House intrinsic tenodesis (free tendon graft extends PIP as MP extends, blocking MP hyterextension)
	Split FPL (New Zealand) procedure
	When extension is via tenodesis of the extensors into the radius and CMC joint is mobile, then:
	ECRL to FDP
	PT to FPL (tendon graft if necessary)
	BR to insertion of FPOB via rerouted ring finger FDS graft
	Zancolli lasso (FDS anchored to A1 pulley), or House intrinsic tenodesis (free tendon graft extends PIP as MP extends, blocking MP hyperextension)
	Split FPL (New Zealand) procedure
Post-surgery course:	
Week 1 through 4:	
Goals:	Patient education in anatomy and physiology
Activities:	Hand in cast; elevate arm for 1 week and *pro re nata* edema control thereafter
	Monitor blood supply to fingers
	Power wheelchair for mobility
	Practice triggering wrist extensors or unaffected arm
Week 4 through 6 (cast removal):	
Goals:	Regain partial wrist extension
	Weak active exercise against no resistance
Activities:	Only AROM to wrist; protect thumb between index and middle fingers during wrist extension to prevent resistive exercise
	Wear splint whenever not actively ranging
	Therapist begins scar massage
Cautions:	No resistive exercise to fingers or thumb
	Dorsal splint to prevent wrist and thumb extension
	No elbow flexion against resistance because of transfer of BR
Week 6 through 8:	
Goals:	Weak active exercise against little or no resistance

	Regain almost full wrist extension
	Teach thumb protection techniques (avoiding extension)
Activities:	Gentle PROM to wrist extensors
	Retrain ECRL and resume retraining BR
	Begin picking up small, light objects
	Continue protecting thumb between middle and index fingers during wrist extension
	Wear splint when not exercising
	May push lightweight wheelchair with splint
	PREs to wrist extensors
Cautions:	No hyperextension of the thumb or fingers
	No static pinch
Week 8 through 10:	
Goals:	Strong active exercises against resistance
Activities:	Begin using resistive and static pinch/grasp
	Will need short-resting hand splint to be worn nights indefinitely to preserve good hand posture
Cautions:	Wear splint during strenuous activities (e.g. transfers, dressing) for protection
Week 10 through 12:	
Goals:	Full activity
Activities:	Observe transfers, advance bed mobility, and propelling manual wheelchair to verify precautions
	Continue with night splints
Cautions:	Reinforce thumb protection techniques to prevent stretching of lateral pinch

*Normally, only one hand is operated on at a time to allow some independent functioning to take place

VII

Functional Independence Measure and American Spinal Injury Association impairment scale

Functional Independence Measure (FIM)

7 Complete Independence (Timely, Safely) 6 Modified Independence (Device)	No Helper
L **Modified Dependence** **E** 5 Supervision **V** 4 Minimal Assist (Subject = 75%+) **E** 3 Moderate Assist (Subject = 50%+) **L** **Complete Dependence** **S** 2 Maximal Assist (Subject = 25%+) 1 Total Assist (Subject = 0%+)	Helper

	ADMIT	DISCH
Self Care		
A. Eating	□	□
B. Grooming	□	□
C. Bathing	□	□
D. Dressing-Upper Body	□	□
E. Dressing-Lower Body	□	□
F. Toileting	□	□
Sphincter Control		
G. Bladder Management	□	□
H. Bowel Management	□	□
Mobility Transfer:		
I. Bed, Chair, Wheelchair	□	□
J. Toilet	□	□
K. Tub, Shower	□	□
Locomotion		
L. Walk/wheelChair	W□ C□	W□ C□
M. Stairs	□	□
Communication		
N. Comprehension	A□ V□	A□ V□
O. Expression	V□ N□	V□ N□
Social Cognition		
P. Social Interaction	□	□
Q. Problem Solving	□	□
R. Memory	□	□
Total FIM	□	□

NOTE: Leave no blanks; enter 1 if patient not testable due to risk.

American Spinal Injury Association (ASIA) impairment scale

A = **Complete:** No motor or sensory function is preserved in the sacral segments S4–S5.

B = **Incomplete:** Sensory but not motor function is preserved below the neurological level and extends through the sacral segments S4–S5.

C = **Incomplete:** Motor function is preserved below the neurological level, and the majority of key muscles below the neurological level have a muscle grade less than 3.

D = **Incomplete:** Motor function is preserved below the neurological level, and the majority of key muscles below the neurological level have a muscle grade greater than or equal to 3.

E = **Normal:** Motor and sensory function is normal.

Clinical syndromes

Central Cord
Brown–Sequard
Anterior Cord
Conus Medullaris
Cauda Equina

VIII

Spinal cord injury functional questionnaire* instructions

Please take a few moments to fill out the attached activities of daily living (ADL) Functional Questionnaire. This portion of the questionnaire includes areas of activities of daily living that are most commonly encountered.

This questionnaire is a 'subjective' measurement of what level of ADL Function you perceive yourself to be at in relation to performance of the task listed.
Each activity will have five choices in answering the question. Please use the following when answering the questions:

MUCH BETTER:	The level of independent hand function has IMPROVED SIGNIFICANTLY in the quality of performance because of *speed, dexterity*, and *efficiency*
BETTER:	The level of independent hand function has IMPROVED in the ability to use the hand more *efficiently*
NO CHANGE:	The level of independent hand function has STAYED THE SAME
WORSE:	The level of independent hand function has WORSENED since the surgery
MUCH WORSE:	The level of independent hand function has WORSENED SIGNIFICANTLY in the quality of performance because of *speed, dexterity*, and *efficiency*

Spinal cord injury functional questionnaire

(Instructions on page three)

Please read through ADL (Advanced Daily Living skills) category and mark an 'X' in the box that best answers the question.

	(2) Much better	(1) Better	(0) No change	(–1) Worse	(–2) Much worse
I. Hygiene and grooming					
Washing					
Shaving					
Brushing hair					
Brushing teeth					
Clipping nails					
Faucets					
Shower					

* From James House M.D. with permission

	(2) Much better	(1) Better	(0) No change	(−1) Worse	(−2) Much worse
II. Eating					
Cutting meat					
Opening containers					
Pouring liquids					
Using utensils					
III. Dressing					
Upper extremity					
Lower extremity					
Fastening					
IV. Communication					
Using telephone					
Writing					
Typing					
V. Homemaking					
Preparing meals					
Making bed					
Wash/rinse dishes					
VI. Transfers					
Car					
Bed					
Shower/tub					
Toilet					
Couch					
VII. Wheelchair					
Mobility/propulsion					
VIII. Miscellaneous					
Handling small objects					
Opening doors					
Opening mail					
IX. Vocational					
Job opportunities					
X. Avocational					
Recreational activities					
Total score					

Index